ADVANCES IN
MEDICAL ONCOLOGY, RESEARCH
AND EDUCATION

Volume II

CANCER   CONTROL

ADVANCES IN MEDICAL ONCOLOGY, RESEARCH AND EDUCATION

Proceedings of the 12th International Cancer Congress,
Buenos Aires, 1978

General Editors: A. CANONICO, O. ESTEVEZ, R. CHACON and S. BARG, Buenos Aires

Volumes and Editors:

 I - CARCINOGENESIS. *Editor:* G. P. Margison

 II - CANCER CONTROL. *Editors:* A. Smith and C. Alvarez

 III - EPIDEMIOLOGY. *Editor:* Jillian M. Birch

 IV - BIOLOGICAL BASIS FOR CANCER DIAGNOSIS. *Editor:* Margaret Fox

 V - BASIS FOR CANCER THERAPY 1. *Editor:* B. W. Fox

 VI - BASIS FOR CANCER THERAPY 2. *Editor:* M. Moore

 VII - LEUKEMIA AND NON-HODGKIN LYMPHOMA. *Editor:* D. G. Crowther

VIII - GYNECOLOGICAL CANCER. *Editor:* N. Thatcher

 IX - DIGESTIVE CANCER. *Editor:* N. Thatcher

 X - CLINICAL CANCER - PRINCIPAL SITES 1. *Editor:* S. Kumar

 XI - CLINICAL CANCER - PRINCIPAL SITES 2. *Editor:* P. M. Wilkinson

XII - ABSTRACTS

(Each volume is available separately.)

Pergamon Journals of Related Interest

ADVANCES IN ENZYME REGULATION
COMPUTERIZED TOMOGRAPHY
EUROPEAN JOURNAL OF CANCER
INTERNATIONAL JOURNAL OF RADIATION ONCOLOGY, BIOLOGY, PHYSICS
LEUKEMIA RESEARCH

ADVANCES IN MEDICAL ONCOLOGY, RESEARCH AND EDUCATION

Proceedings of the 12th International Cancer Congress,
Buenos Aires, 1978

Volume II
CANCER CONTROL

Editors:

A. SMITH
Department of Epidemiology and Social Research
Christie Hospital and Holt Radium Institute, Manchester

and

C. A. ALVAREZ
Department of Clinical Oncology
School of Medicine of "del Salvador" University, Buenos Aires

PERGAMON PRESS

OXFORD · NEW YORK · TORONTO · SYDNEY · PARIS · FRANKFURT

U.K.	Pergamon Press Ltd., Headington Hill Hall, Oxford OX3 0BW, England
U.S.A.	Pergamon Press Inc., Maxwell House, Fairview Park, Elmsford, New York 10523, U.S.A.
CANADA	Pergamon of Canada, Suite 104, 150 Consumers Road, Willowdale, Ontario M2J 1P9, Canada
AUSTRALIA	Pergamon Press (Aust.) Pty. Ltd., P.O. Box 544, Potts Point, N.S.W. 2011, Australia
FRANCE	Pergamon Press SARL, 24 rue des Ecoles, 75240 Paris, Cedex 05, France
FEDERAL REPUBLIC OF GERMANY	Pergamon Press GmbH, 6242 Kronberg-Taunus, Pferdstrasse 1, Federal Republic of Germany

First edition 1979

British Library Cataloguing in Publication Data

International Cancer Congress, 12th, Buenos Aires, 1978
Advances in medical oncology, research and education.
Vol. 2: Cancer control
1. Cancer - Congresses
I. Title   II. Smith, A   III. Alvarez, C A
616.9'94   RC261.A1   79-40704
ISBN 0 08 024385 1
ISBN 0-08-023777-0 Set of 12 vols.

In order to make this volume available as economically and as rapidly as possible the authors' typescripts have been reproduced in their original forms. This method unfortunately has its typographical limitations but it is hoped that they in no way distract the reader.

Printed and bound in Great Britain at
William Clowes & Sons Limited, Beccles and London

Contents

DIAGNOSIS

PSYCHOLOGICAL IMPACT OF CANCER

DATA PROCESSING IN CANCER

Foreword

This book contains papers from the main meetings of the Scientific Programme presented during the 12th International Cancer Congress, which took place in Buenos Aires, Argentina, from 5 to 11 October 1978, and was sponsored by the International Union against Cancer (UICC).

This organisation, with headquarters in Geneva, gathers together from more than a hundred countries 250 medical associations which fight against Cancer and organizes every four years an International Congress which gives maximum coverage to oncological activity throughout the world.

The 11th Congress was held in Florence in 1974, where the General Assembly unanimously decided that Argentina would be the site of the 12th Congress. Argentina was chosen not only because of the beauty of its landscapes and the cordiality of its inhabitants, but also because of the high scientific level of its researchers and practitioners in the field of oncology.

From this Assembly a distinguished International Committee was appointed which undertook the preparation and execution of the Scientific Programme of the Congress.

The Programme was designed to be profitable for those professionals who wished to have a general view of the problem of Cancer, as well as those who were specifically orientated to an oncological subspeciality. It was also conceived as trying to cover the different subjects related to this discipline, emphasizing those with an actual and future gravitation on cancerology.

The scientific activity began every morning with a Special Lecture (5 in all), summarizing some of the subjects of prevailing interest in Oncology, such as Environmental Cancer, Immunology, Sub-clinical Cancer, Modern Cancer Therapy Concepts and Viral Oncogenesis. Within the 26 Symposia, new acquisitions in the technological area were incorporated; such acquisitions had not been exposed in previous Congresses.

15 Multidisciplinary Panels were held studying the more frequent sites in Cancer, with an approach to the problem that included biological and clinical aspects, and concentrating on the following areas: aetiology, epidemiology, pathology, prevention, early detection, education, treatment and results. Preferred Papers were presented as Workshops instead of the classical reading, as in this way they could be discussed fully by the participants. 66 Workshops were held, this being the first time that free communications were presented in this way in a UICC Congress.

The Programme also included 22 "Meet the Experts", 7 Informal Meetings and more
than a hundred films.

METHODOLOGY

The methodology used for the development of the Meeting and to make the scientific
works profitable, had some original features that we would like to mention.

The methodology used in Lectures, Panels and Symposia was the usual one utilized
in previous Congresses and functions satisfactorily. Lectures lasted one hour each.
Panels were seven hours long divided into two sessions, one in the morning and one
in the afternoon. They had a Chairman and two Vice-chairmen (one for each session).
Symposia were three hours long. They had a Chairman, a Vice-chairman and a Secretary.

Of the 8164 registered members, many sent proferred papers of which over 2000 were
presented. They were grouped in numbers of 20 or 25, according to the subject, and
discussed in Workshops. The International Scientific Committee studied the abstracts
of all the papers, and those which were finally approved were sent to the Chairman
of the corresponding Workshop who, during the Workshop gave an introduction and
commented on the more outstanding works. This was the first time such a method had
been used in an UICC Cancer Congress.

"Meet the Experts" were two hours long, and facilitated the approach of young professionals to the most outstanding specialists. The congress was also the ideal place
for an exchange of information between the specialists of different countries during
the Informal Meetings. Also more than a hundred scientific films were shown.

The size of the task carried out in organising this Congress is reflected in some
statistical data: More than 18,000 letters were sent to participants throughout the
world; more than 2000 abstracts were published in the Proceedings of the Congress;
more than 800 scientists were active participants of the various meetings.

There were 2246 papers presented at the Congress by 4620 authors from 80 countries.

The Programme lasted a total of 450 hours, and was divided into 170 scientific
meetings where nearly all the subjects related to Oncology were discussed.

All the material gathered for the publication of these Proceedings has been taken
from the original papers submitted by each author. The material has been arranged
in 12 volumes, in various homogenous sections, which facilitates the reading of the
most interesting individual chapters. Volume XII deals only with the abstracts of
proffered papers submitted for Workshops and Special Meetings. The titles of each
volume offer a clear view of the extended and multidisciplinary contents of this
collection which we are sure will be frequently consulted in the scientific libraries.

We are grateful to the individual authors for their valuable collaboration as they
have enabled the publication of these Proceedings, and we are sure Pergamon Press
was a perfect choice as the Publisher due to its responsibility and efficiency.

          Argentina   Dr Abel Canónico
          March 1979   Dr Roberto Estevez
                                             Dr Reinaldo Chacon
                                             Dr Solomon Barg

                                             General Editors

Introduction

The concept of disease control embraces the co-ordinated and purposive mobilisation of a community's resources with a view to reducing the total unfavourable impact of a disease on that community. It involves the setting of realisable objectives relating to preventive, curative and alleviative measures: it involves the systematic implementation of plans designed to achieve those objectives; and it involves the necessity for continuous monitoring of progress as a mechanism for the maintenance of the momentum and direction of the control programme.

Control of cancer involves educational, political and administrative measures as well as preventive, curative and palliative techniques.

A. SMITH
March 1979

Cancer Education

Cancer Education in the United States Since 1948

Margaret H. Edwards

National Cancer Institute, Bethesda, Maryland 20014

ABSTRACT

The National Cancer Institute initiated a support program for cancer education in 1948. Its goals were to coordinate cancer teaching in medical and dental schools and to improve its quality. Changes in this program over a 30-year period as well as its present status are described.

Medical education has undergone many changes during the same period such as an increase in elective time. Similarly, knowledge concerning cancer has expanded, and more must be taught so that physicians are able to provide optimum care to their patients. Chemotherapy is an example of such new knowledge.

Significant improvements in medical and dental education have been noted in institutions which are the recipients of the National Cancer Institute's support grants. These include a wide variety of educational offerings and opportunities for periods of intensive study. There is still a need, however, for more emphasis on certain neglected areas of cancer teaching, such as radiation therapy and the psychosocial aspects of cancer.

Graduate education in the clinical specialties varies in cancer content, and examination of these programs is underway to learn the optimum amount of cancer experiences desirable in each specialty training program. Training in the clinical subspecialties pertaining to cancer has grown rapidly but some types of oncologists, notably radiation therapists, are still in short supply. A new specialty in dental oncology is emerging.

Continuing education of medical and dental practitioners is not carried out systematically in the United States, but a wide variety of courses and other offerings are available. The medical specialties all require periodic re-examinations for maintenance of certification.

Cancer education has evolved as medical knowledge has advanced, and therefore future changes and improvements may be anticipated.

KEY WORDS

Cancer   Education   Clinical   Medical   Dental

3

INTRODUCTION

Education regarding cancer has been provided to physicians and dentists in the
United States by governmental and voluntary agencies since 1938, as well as by
private sources.

The National Cancer Institute, a governmental agency, has supported clinical
training since its founding in 1938 (1,2), when clinical traineeships as well as
research fellowships were initiated. The clinical traineeships were transferred
to the Division of Chronic Disease Control in the Bureau of Health Services in
1948, where they remained active until that Division was phased out in 1968. In
1948, the National Cancer Institute, at the direction of the National Advisory
Cancer Council, initiated a program to promote coordination of cancer education
for undergraduate students within schools of medicine and dentistry, known as the
Undergraduate Cancer Training grants (3). These grants supported institutional
activities such as tumor boards, seminars, conferences, guest speakers, and
stipends for students working on cancer projects during vacation periods. A
national Cancer Achievement Test was developed and administered in all institutions having these grants; by 1950 these included virtually all of the nation's
medical, osteopathic, and dental schools. Grants to medical schools were limited
to $25,000 per institution, and those to dental schools to $5,000 per institution.

In 1963, the National Advisory Cancer Council, after a review and evaluation of
the Undergraduate Training Grant Program and consultation with cancer educators,
decided to phase out this program and replace it with one which would 1) be
competitive, 2) expand the scope of activities to include graduate and continuing
education, and 3) place no ceiling on the funding of individual grants. In 1966,
73 Clinical Cancer Training grants were awarded, and by 1972, 104 institutions were
funded for a total of $7,257,000.

Graduate post-resident trainees were supported on these grants from the outset in
a variety of clinical specialties. In 1966, the only officially recognized oncologic specialty was radiation therapy, but the largest proportions of graduate
trainees on Clinical Cancer Training grants were in medical oncology, followed by
surgical oncology, pediatric oncology, radiation therapy, gynecologic oncology,
and pathology. Since that time, national subspecialty boards have been established for medical oncology, pediatric hematology-oncology, and gynecologic
oncology. The majority of the trainees on Clinical Cancer Training grants,
however, have always been undergraduate medical and dental students working during
vacation periods on cancer projects (65 to 75 percent). The annual numbers of
graduate trainees have ranged from 55 to 205.

In 1974, the Clinical Cancer Education grants were established to replace the
Clinical Cancer Training grants. These grants have similar objectives and guidelines (4) for both undergraduate, graduate, and continuing education as the
earlier grants, but do not carry stipends for trainees. However, individuals can
be funded for periods of graduate post-resident instruction coupled with teaching
responsibilities for periods up to one year; such individuals are classified as
"clinical associates," and no more than $12,000 of the salary for each individual
may be charged to the grant. Undergraduate medical and dental students may still
be supported during vacation periods to work on cancer projects. As in the past,
the numbers of undergraduate students receiving support exceed those of the graduate students.

The amount of support for this program in the past ten years has ranged from
$5.0 million to $9.5 million, and the number of institutions supported annually
has ranged from 51 to 113. Presently, 53 of our country's 114 medical schools,

20 of its 59 dental schools, and 13 larger teaching hospitals receive support from the National Cancer Institute in grants totaling $9.5 million. Two hundred ninety undergraduate and 221 graduate students received support this year for engaging in special periods of study related to cancer. A total of 5,847 such individuals have received such support since the program was initiated in 1948.

For almost 40 years the American Cancer Society has provided support for a variety of professional educational activities. The Society has, since 1948, awarded more than 4500 one-year Clinical Fellowships to institutions with the appropriate quali- fications, to provide advanced training relative to cancer in seven medical and four dental specialties. These include internal medicine, gynecologic oncology, pathology, pediatrics, diagnostic radiology, radiation therapy, nuclear medicine, surgery, oral pathology, oral surgery, orthodontics, and prosthodontics. Junior Faculty Clinical Fellowships are also offered by the Society in Diagnostic Radi- ology, Radiation Therapy, Pathology, Surgery, Internal Medicine, Pediatric Onco- logy, Gynecologic Oncology, and four dental specialties. This year, 140 of these are Junior Faculty Fellowships. In addition, occasional grants for fellowships are made to institutions by local Divisions of the Society. Currently $2.49 million is budgeted by the Society to support 435 fellows in both clinical fellow- ship programs. Of these, 142 are in medicine, 82 in surgery, 77 in radiology, 41 in pediatrics, and 28 in gynecologic oncology. Reviews (5) of the program have shown that it is producing a rich harvest of highly talented and well-trained cancer teachers and investigators.

The Leukemia Society (6) also provides fellowships to 117 individuals annually at a cost of $1,750,000. A few of these are physicians engaged in clinical research relative to leukemia. The Damon Runyon - Walter Winchell Cancer Fund likewise supports postdoctoral research fellowships, approximately 125 annually, of which a small number are awarded to M.D.'s (7).

Hospitals and medical centers use funds from other sources to support interns, residents, and advanced trainees. The Council of Teaching Hospitals of the Asso- ciation of American Medical Colleges (8) reports that in 1976, 169 non-federal and 20 federal hospitals supported Clinical Fellows, the support for which was derived from patient revenue (44 percent), National Institutes of Health (23 percent), Veterans Administration and other Federal sources (14 percent), private foundations (ten percent), state and local governments (six percent), medical school sources (one percent) and other sources (two percent). Sixty-one percent of the funds for Clinical Fellows was expended by hospitals in 11 northeastern states. The proportion of these fellows in cancer-related training programs is undetermined.

CANCER EDUCATION

Medical education has undergone many changes in the United States since 1948. The increase in research conducted in medical and dental schools, a "systems" approach to teaching in the basic and clinical sciences, reduction in the time devoted to laboratory work, the use of computers and sophisticated audiovisual aids, increasing input on curricular structure from students, a shift in the proportion of required courses with the rise of student electives, and growing emphasis on the production of family physicians (general practitioners) are examples of such changes.

Similarly, our knowledge concerning cancer has increased dramatically since 1948, and has changed the instruction provided to all students of the health profes- sions. Improvements in radiation therapy, developments in the use of chemotherapy, advances in immunotherapy, in support capabilities during the course of any therapeutic modality, uses of multimodal therapy, and advances in diagnostic capabilities have altered the content of cancer instruction.

Significant improvements in medical and dental education relating to cancer, which have been noted in the United States in recent years and which are carried out in many of the institutions supported by National Cancer Institute education grants include:

> a required core of cancer content in the curriculum
>   for all students
> comprehensive cancer syllabi as required reading for
>   all students
> self-instructional teaching aids regarding cancer
> curricular reviews and analyses regarding cancer
> development of educational objectives regarding cancer
> systematic evaluation of cancer teaching activities
> a variety of cancer electives
> rotations on cancer units or in cancer hospitals
> summer (free-period) cancer projects
> use of other health professionals in educational roles:
> > cancer nurse specialist
> > pharmacist
> > medical librarian
> > medical social worker.

There is still a need, however, for more emphasis in the curricula of medical and dental schools on the following areas:

> the epidemiology of cancer
> cancer prevention
> early diagnosis and screening for cancer
> carcinogenesis (especially environmental)
> psychosocial aspects of cancer
> role of radiation therapy
> nutritional aspects of cancer
> systematic evaluation of therapeutic modalities
>   (cooperative studies)
> uses of a tumor registry
> evaluation of student responses to educational methods.

Graduate education in the medical and dental specialties is variable in its cancer content among the many hospitals in the United States which provide such residency programs. There is a need to determine guidelines for the optimum amount of cancer experiences to be furnished during residency training, and the skills to be developed. A beginning has been made to do this for the specialty of gastroenterology; other specialty groups need to provide similar guidelines.

Graduate education in the cancer subspecialties of medical oncology, gynecologic oncology, pediatric hematology-oncology, and radiation therapy is provided by many institutions, but specific standards and guidelines for such programs have been developed only for radiation therapy. A series of workshops has been held with the medical, surgical, and pediatric oncologists to develop such standards. The grants for clinical education from the National Cancer Institute presently support graduate students in these subspecialties related to cancer.

A new type of oncologist is emerging, namely, the dental oncologist, who is a dentist with specialty training usually in oral pathology or oral surgery who assists surgeons, radiation therapists, and others in the treatment of patients with cancer, particularly of the head, neck, and oral cavity. Such persons perform much-needed functions in large medical centers or cancer hospitals.

Continuing education for practicing physicians and specialists in the United States is not systematically carried out. No controls are maintained on the quality or amount of postgraduate education in which physicians participate. However, 23 state licensing agencies require that physicians report the number of hours of continuing education courses taken annually preceding relicensure, and 16 states have adopted procedures leading to continuing education relicensure requirements. All 22 medical specialties have established a policy to require recertification; six are actively implementing this policy. The American Medical Association, to which a majority of physicians in the United States belong, regularly publishes lists of approved continuing education courses in its journal, and issues recognition awards to physicians who have completed 150 hours of accredited courses over a three-year period. One-fifth of the physicians in the United States have received such awards.

Continuing education regarding cancer is provided by many professional organizations, the American Cancer Society, and by medical schools and teaching hospitals. Examples of these supported by the National Cancer Institute which are ongoing include:

> conferences, courses, symposia
> self-instructional materials
> hospital visits by consultants
> telephone consultation networks
> preceptorships at medical centers
> visits by health assistants to physicians' and dentists'
>   offices with educational materials.

SUMMARY

An overview of cancer education provided in the United States by governmental and other sources since 1948 has been presented. The impact of changes in medical and dental educational methodology and of advances in cancer knowledge during this period has been noted. Existing weaknesses in cancer education at the undergraduate level have been enumerated. Significant aspects of cancer education at the undergraduate, graduate, and postgraduate levels are described.

References

1. Edwards, M.H. (1975). National Cancer Institute Training Programs.
    Journal of the National Cancer Institute, 55, 1023-1026.

2. Edwards, M.H. (1975). Training Programs in the National Cancer Institute.
    Cancer Research Journal, 35, 2891-2894.

3. Edwards, M.H. (1967). Report on Cancer Teaching Programs 1947-1967.
    National Cancer Institute. Prepared for the National Advisory Cancer
    Council.

4. Interim Guidelines for Clinical Cancer Education Grants. National
    Cancer Institute. July 15, 1974.

5. A Study of American Cancer Society Fellows' Current Involvement with Cancer-
    Related Activities. Prepared for the American Cancer Society, November 1974,
    by Lieberman Research, Inc., N.Y.C.

6. Leukemia Society of America, Inc., N.Y.C. Florence Phillips, Public Education
    and Information. Personal Communication.

7. Damon Runyon - Walter Winchell Cancer Fund, N.Y.C. Alice Morrison, Research
    Programs. Personal Communication.

8. COTH Survey of House Staff Policy and Related Issues, 1976. Association of
    American Medical Colleges, Washington, D. C.

The Professional Education Program of the American Cancer Society

Sidney L. Arje

*Vice President for Professional Education, American Cancer Society, Inc.
New York, N.Y.*

ABSTRACT

Professional education by the American Cancer Society stresses early diagnosis and prompt and adequate treatment. It provides information on cancer to motivate the medical and allied health professions to practice the latest techniques in detection and diagnosis. The program is aimed at the primary physician defined as the physician who sees the patient first. The methods used include publications, audiovisual materials and conferences. Clinical fellowships are supported to increase the number of physicians with expertise in the management of cancer. To insure the inclusion of cancer in the education of medical students, the American Cancer Society supports Professors of Clinical Oncology in Medical Schools. The American Cancer Society also assists other professional organizations in carrying out their educational programs. The effectiveness of professional education activities of the American Cancer Society results from the organization of the Society into its National Headquarters, 58 Divisions and 3,000 Units. This allows for broad coverage at national, regional and local levels and provides professional education where the target audience lives and works.

TEXT

Because of the constantly growing body of medical knowledge necessary to provide optimum medical care, the medical and allied health professions have an increaseing need for continuing education in all fields of medicine. This is nowhere more apparent than in the field of cancer. The American Cancer Society is the only organization with a sustained interest and a proven capacity for professional education in cancer on a broad scale throughout the United States.

In addition to providing factual information and the means for education to physicians, dentists, nurses and to members of the allied health professions, the program of the American Cancer Society must persuade and stimulate them to carry out new or special procedures in the detection, diagnosis, treatment and rehabilitation of cancer and to recognize the importance of their individual roles in determining the extent to which cancer is controlled.

It is important to emphasize that much of the effort of the American Cancer Society in its professional education program is concerned with the cultivation of attitudes. Cultivating a hopeful attitude, a belief in the curability of cancer and in the im-

9

portance of early detection and prompt and adequate treatment for this purpose is
basic to the program.

The aim of the professional education program of the American Cancer Society, therefore, is to make sure that the members of the medical and allied health professions
in every community are convinced of the importance of and are carrying out the best
cancer detection and management techniques.

Since the burden of prevention and early detection of cancer rests primarily on the
doctor who first sees the patient, the professional education program of the
American Cancer Society is particularly directed to the primary care physician, as
well as to dentists, nurses and other allied health professional personnel both
directly and through their colleagues in the local community.

In establishing priorities for the educational programs of the American Cancer
Society, emphasis has been properly placed on those forms of cancer which have a
high incidence and lend themselves to control by prevention or early diagnosis.
Both public and professional educational programs concentrate on six sites -- lung
cancer, breast cancer, colon and rectal cancer, uterine cancer and skin cancer.
Lung cancer and skin cancer can be effectively attacked by preventive measures and
the others through detection, early diagnosis and prompt and adequate treatment.

Programs are designed to supplement the roles of the medical, dental and nursing
schools and the professional societies. Medical schools and medical societies are
more therapy-oriented in their educational efforts and stress the management of
cancer after it has been diagnosed. They give insufficient attention to prevention or screening and this gap provides the American Cancer Society with a unique
educational role in concentrating on prevention and detection and early diagnosis.

The tools of the professional education program of the American Cancer Society
encompass all the educational techniques in common use. As most surveys show that
health professionals still rely on the printed word as their chief source of education, the American Cancer Society makes major use of this medium. It publishes
"CA-A Cancer Journal for Clinicians" six times a year and distributes it free in
the United States and at cost outside the U.S. The circulation of "CA" is over
400,000 and has the widest distribution of any medical journal in the world.

Another professional journal of the American Cancer Society is CANCER, a monthly
technical journal for those members of the medical and scientific professions with
special interests or responsibilities in the cancer field. This journal is sold
through the publisher but the financial support of the American Cancer Society
makes it available at a price which greatly increases its circulation-currently
over 17,000.

In addition to these two journals the American Cancer Society publishes the
Proceedings of its National Conferences which are held twice a year and provide a
continuous update on cancer management, both by site and discipline. In the past
five years, for example, there have been conferences on detection and diagnosis of
cancer, treatment and rehabilitation of cancer, radiation oncology, virology and
immunology in human cancer, gynecologic cancer, urologic cancer and a series on
specific sites, such as breast, colon and rectum, leukemia & lymphomas, etc. The
Proceedings of these conferences when published provide the latest information
covered by experts in each field and fill the gap between the publishing of the
textbooks on the same subjects.

Augmenting this library of professional education publications are two for which
the American Cancer Society provides financial support to their development. In
return, the Society is granted the privilege of publishing them. These are the

series "Current Concepts in Cancer" and "Clinical Oncology for Medical Students and Physicians -- A Multidisciplinary Approach" 50,000 copies of a fifth edition of "Clinical Oncology" have been published this year and a Spanish translation has been supported by the American Cancer Society and is now available.

To meet specific needs the American Cancer Society provides many shorter publications dealing with all aspects of cancer management in the form of reprints, original articles, monographs, etc. There are about 200 such publications available for physicians, dentists, nurses and allied health personnel.

While the printed word is a major means of communication in professional education, audiovisual materials are also provided by the American Cancer Society. A film library is maintained and updated constantly. About 40 films are available in 8mm and 16mm and in film and video cassettes. They address the detection and diagnosis of various sites of cancer and cover the nursing management of selected sites. Audiotapes of the Highlights of National American Cancer Society Conferences are available and audiotapes on specific subjects are produced and distributed.

Many other means of communication are used. The national conferences have been mentioned but these are duplicated on a smaller scale at regional and local levels. Travelling teams of cancer specialists provided by the American Cancer Society discuss aspects of cancer management requested by community physicians. Continuing medical education related to cancer is supported in community hospitals through hospital cancer coordinators, support for tumor boards and the provision of educational materials.

Supplementing these direct efforts in professional education, the American Cancer Society maintains a clinical fellowship program. Regular clinical fellowships are awarded annually to institutions to improve the management of the patient with cancer by supporting clinical oncology training for young physicians and dentists. Institutions must be able to provide 12 consecutive months of oncology training in a program leading to board certification in selected disciplines. Junior Faculty Clinical Fellowships are awarded annually to fellows to provide a three-year individualized program for outstanding young clinicians to follow academic careers upon completion of their specialty training. Assisting such promising individuals in academic assignments during the critical years when their career decisions are being made is intended to increase the number of teachers and clinical researchers in cancer. In awarding these fellowships the American Cancer Society places primary emphasis on the qualifications of the prospective fellow and his potentialities as a future leader in the cancer field as well as on the capacity and ability of the institution to provide him with training. The American Cancer Society also provides the Audrey Meyer Mars International Fellowship in Clinical Oncology which is awarded annually to a qualified physician from a selected country outside the United States for one year of advanced training in clinical cancer management at a training center in the United States.

To bring about more effective management of cancer patients by improving cancer teaching in medical schools and other appropriate institutions at undergraduate, graduate and continuing education levels and to extend the benefits of such teaching to both students and practitioners of the medical, dental, nursing and allied health professions, the American Cancer Society maintains a program of Professorships of Clinical Oncology. Grants for Professors of Clinical Oncology are awarded to medical schools in the U.S. who appoint a full professor authorized to carry out activities to achieve the stated goal of the program. There are presently 17 such American Cancer Society Professors of Clinical Oncology.

Besides these educational programs which are identified with the American Cancer Society, there are others which are identified with other organizations and

institutions but which are supported by the American Cancer Society. A major example is the Society's financial support of the American College of Surgeons'
Hospital Cancer Program which is aimed at upgrading the care of cancer patients in
hospitals. Financial support is provided to the American Joint Committee for
Cancer Staging and End Results Reporting to assist it in developing standards for
staging cancer and standardizing terminology. These are but a few examples of
financial support provided for a variety of projects that further the objectives
of the professional education program of the American Cancer Society.

For the nursing profession, the American Cancer Society provides stipends for
instructors in nursing schools to permit them to attend refresher courses in
cancer centers offering such courses during their summer vacations. Such practical
experience is designed to improve their teaching of cancer nursing.

Having briefly described the goals, the audience and the methods used in the professional education program of the American Cancer Society, the operation of the
program can now be examined.

To understand how the program operates it is necessary to appreciate the organization of the American Cancer Society. There are 58 Divisions of the Society
which roughly correspond to the states of the United States. These Divisions are
made up of about 3,000 Units which roughly correspond to counties in the states.
The Divisions of the Society are joined together to form a National organization
in which they are proportionately represented and to which they contribute financial support to maintain a National program. With funds provided for professional
education, the National program develops and produces the tools of professional
education such as the journal CA, the films, the publications and conferences;
and supports the clinical fellowship program and the others described above. The
Divisions with their funds distribute CA, support the ACS Professorships of
Clinical Oncology, and through their Units distribute the publications, use the
films and carry out other professional education activities.

It can be seen then that the professional education program of the American Cancer
Society operates at three levels -- National, Regional (Division) and Local (Unit)--
and therin lies its strength for it can be implemented where the medical and allied
health professionals live. It insures a distribution outlet for educational
materials that are useless if they do not reach those they are intended for. And,
if the program operates properly at the National and Division levels, it should
provide Units with a variety of educational materials and methods for their use
which can be adapted to their local needs. Without question, professional
education is most effective when it is carried out where the medical, dental,
nursing and allied health professionals live and work.

Development and Use of Cancer Education Materials

**W. Lawrence, Jr., T. Hazra, J. Steinfeld, P. Munson,
J. Wilson and L. Leary**

*School of Medicine and MCV/VCU Cancer Center, Medical College of Virginia,
Richmond, Virginia, U.S.A.*

ABSTRACT

A collection of instructional objectives in oncology has been developed in response
to a perceived need for identification of the body of knowledge in oncology that is
required by the graduating medical student. These objectives are now being utilized
in some parts of the medical school curriculum at the Medical College of Virginia
and various resource materials based on these objectives have been developed for
student self-study. The two major ongoing thrusts of the oncology education program
at MCV are (1) a curriculum analysis program to determine the degree to which the
objectives developed are actually included in the present medical curriculum and,
(2) continued efforts to increase usage of the objectives and the resource materials
in the medical curriculum.

Keywords: CANCER EDUCATION   CURRICULUM ANALYSIS   ONCOLOGY OBJECTIVES
RESOURCE LIBRARY

Is undergraduate medical training in oncology adequate? Those of us who have a
specific interest in oncology have always maintained that it is not, but we have only
documented deficiences anecdotally, such as the limited number of specific oncology
courses in our curriculum, and the lack of emphasis on cancer in our national certi-
fying and licensing examinations. It is our belief that the eventual attainment of
adequate cancer education in schools of medicine will depend on oncologists joining
forces with other medical specialists to identify and develop a balanced and realistic set of specific expectations – a body of required knowledge – so that the "un-
differentiated" medical student is prepared to begin postgraduate training in any
clinical field at the time of his or her graduation. Once these expectations in oncology are defined to most everyone's satisfaction, the methods of attaining them in
our educational process also require our attention. The purpose of this presentation is to outline the approach at our institution to both aspects of this process.

Whether cancer education is approached using specific courses in oncology, or by
introducing the necessary concepts and information in the various portions of the
medical curriculum in a broader fashion, is of no great importance. The crux of
the matter is to define the objectives to be achieved and then to develop methods
for insuring this. In our own school of medicine, the curriculum in the first two
years is oriented towards "subject matter" with separate curriculum committees for
the cardiovascular system, the gastrointestinal system, the endocrine system, the
reticuloendothelial system, and other subject categories. In order to effectively

insert an adequate number of oncologic concepts in each of these areas, a representative who has an interest in oncology education usually participates on each of
the planning committees and, hopefully, insures the introduction of appropriate oncology education for the area concerned. To achieve this goal we must have objectives to be attained and instructional methods and materials for accomplishing this.
There are similar needs for students and faculty participating in the clinical portion of the curriculum in the third and fourth years.

Development of a Handbook of Objectives in Oncology

Approximately five years ago a group of interested faculty members representing five
separate medical institutions with differing curricula joined forces with the expressed purpose of developing a list of instructional objectives intended to answer
the question, "What does the graduating medical school student need to know about
cancer?". This group of participants[1] from the Medical College of Virginia, Wayne
State University, Medical College of Georgia, University of Virginia and the Southern Illinois University developed a handbook of objectives for twenty-three broad
categories in oncology education through a series of meetings conducted with the
assistance of the Virginia Division of the American Cancer Society. Each of the
participating faculty members drew upon their own experience and the educational
materials that had been developed in their specific institutions. The resulting
handbook represented a compromise between the many and varying ideas presented. It
represented what the committee felt to be appropriate goals to be reached by the
time the student had completed his undergraduate medical education. Some of the
many objectives that were eventually included may be too advanced for this level
of the educational process and many important objectives may have been omitted.
This first draft was then reviewed by clinicians and basic scientists from several
other medical schools in a health sciences consortium and the handbook was further
revised on the basis of the feedback received.

The final result, completed in 1976, was considered a working document that would
require further revisions in the future as new information is developed in the field
of oncology and as field experience with these objectives is gained. To facilitate
student usage of the objectives that were developed, a concise list of appropriate
responses or "answers" to each objective was developed and these were included in
the handbook.

A table of contents of the categories of oncology objectives included in this handbook appears below:

    I. Cancer Cell Biology
        A. Cancer Cell Metabolism
        B. Cell Cycle in Normal and Cancer Cells
        C. Tumor Growth Characteristics
        D. Cancer "Spread"

[1]Walter Lawrence, Jr., M.D.   Lawrence Baker, D.O.
 William L. Banks, Jr., Ph.D.   Ronald Izbicki, D.O.
 E. Richard King, M.D.   (Wayne State University; Detroit, Mich.)
 Harold M. Maurer, M.D.   Armand Karow, Ph.D.
 Albert E. Munson, Ph.D.   (Medical College of Georgia; Atlanta, Ga.)
 Paul J. Munson, Ed.D.   B. W. Ruffner, Jr., M.D.
 Paul Richter, M.D.   (Univ. of Virginia; Charlottesville, Va.)
 Robert B. Scott, M.D.   Charles Whitfield, M.D.
 Wade K. Smith, M.D.   (Southern Illinois University; Spring-
 (all of the Medical College of Virginia; field, Illinois)
 Richmond, Virginia)

    II. Carcinogenesis
        A. Chemical Carcinogens
        B. Viral Carcinogens
        C. Radiation
   III. Pathology - Practical Aspects
    IV. Diagnostic Procedures in Reference to Cancer
     V. Cancer Screening
    VI. Principles of Early Cancer Management
   VII. Principles of Cancer Chemotherapy
        A. General
        B. Alkylating Agents
        C. Antimetabolites
        D. Miscellaneous Agents
  VIII. Principles of Radiation Therapy
    IX. Principles of Immunology
        A. Immunobiology
        B. Immunogenetics
        C. Tumor Immunology
     X. Head and Neck Cancer
        A. Upper Respiratory and Alimentary Tract Cancer
        B. Neoplasms of the Salivary Glands and Thyroid Gland
    XI. Carcinoma of the Lung
   XII. Cancer of the Gastrointestinal Tract
        A. Carcinoma of the Esophagus
        B. Gastric Cancer
        C. Pancreato-biliary Cancer
        D. Neoplasms of the Liver and Small Intestine
        E. Cancer of the Colon and Rectum
  XIII. Breast Cancer
        A. Primary Cancer
        B. Recurrent or Metastatic Cancer
   XIV. Genito-Urinary Tract Cancer
    XV. Gynecologic Cancer
   XVI. Neoplasms of the Skin and Soft Parts
  XVII. The Leukemias
 XVIII. The Lymphomas
   XIX. Solid Tumors in Children
    XX. Paraneoplastic Syndromes
   XXI. The Patient with an Unknown Primary Cancer
  XXII. Supportive and Palliative Management of Cancer Patients
 XXIII. Psycho-Social Aspects of Cancer

The detailed objectives for the individual sections listed above will be available
for review at the seminar session. A sample of the format is shown in Table I.

Methods for Analyzing Cancer Education at the Medical College of Virginia

Since medical education is an ongoing process, the utilization of these instructional objectives required some analysis of our existing educational process before
implementing new teaching programs and methods for fulfilling objectives that we
feel are not now properly addressed. This important step differs in each institution just as their curricula differ. At the Medical College of Virginia (MCV) we
are in the process of exhaustively analyzing our current curriculum with the assistance of a curriculum analyst to determine which objectives are now included in
the curriculum, and the efficiency of the method employed for achieving each specific goal.

A review of the literature reveals that approaches to curriculum analysis have been

TABLE I   Example of Objective Listing

XV Gynecologic Oncology

Cancer of the female genital tract is frequent, responsive to therapy, and can frequently be detected at an early stage. To channel his patient for appropriate treatment, the student/physician should be able to:

1. Given a 65 year old female with a vulvar abnormality:
   a. Describe the procedure for establishing a diagnosis.
   b. Describe each of the following: leukoplakia, carcinoma, "in situ", and invasive carcinoma.
   c. Describe the lymphatic drainage of the vulva.
   d. Name the primary treatment method if a malignant tissue diagnosis is established.
2. Given a patient with an abnormality on the uterine cervix, diagnose and formulate a plan of management. Specifically, the student/physician should be able to:
   a. List two (2) signs of carcinoma of the cervix.
   b. List two (2) epidemiologic characteristics of carcinoma of the cervix.
   c. Describe two (2) methods for establishing a diagnosis in the patient with an ulceration of the cervix.
   d. Differentiate the terms carcinoma in situ, microinvasive carcinoma, and invasive carcinoma.
   e. Describe in outline form one (1) staging system for carcinoma of the cervix and list the appropriate procedures in the work-up of the patient for "staging".
   f. Describe two (2) methods of treatment of carcinoma of the cervix, and a specific reason for choosing each.
3. Describe the common sites of metastatic spread from carcinoma of the cervix and primary cause of death of an untreated or unsuccessfully treated patient with this disease.
4. In a patient with carcinoma of the endometrium,
   a. Describe the typical age group, symptoms, endocrine features, and physical findings.
   b. List the techniques required to establish this diagnosis.
   c. Describe the approach to clinical staging and treatment and give one (1) major reason for treatment failure.
   d. Describe the pattern of metastatic spread that may occur.
5. In a patient with carcinoma of the ovary, establish the diagnosis, stage the patient, and formulate a plan of management. Specifically, the student/physician should be able to:
   a. List three (3) symptoms and/or signs of ovarian cancer.
   b. List three (3) common types of ovarian cancer.
   c. Briefly describe a method of staging ovarian cancer and list the techniques for accomplishing this.
   d. Indicate reasons for choosing surgery, radiation therapy and/or chemotherapy for patients with ovarian cancer and the class of drugs most efficacious for this disease.
6. List three (3) common benign non-functional and two (2) functional ovarian neoplasms and list one (1) specific characteristic of each.
7. State which site of the common invasive gynecological cancer is (a) the most common, and (b) the leading cause of death.

almost exclusively limited to analyzing test results and student course evaluations. In this regard, curriculum analysis has been historically based on an "output" model, or the knowledge and attitudes students exit with. For the purpose of our analysis of cancer education, this model is insufficient because it does not

include content analysis as an important factor in determining the merit and competence of the curriculum. Our approach is best represented as an "input-output"
model. This model couples a comprehensive analysis of content (input) with the
development of a cancer knowledge test (output) based on the Handbook of Objectives
in Oncology.

Content analysis of the curriculum is being conducted thru two methods. The first
involves a thorough analysis of student notes and syllabus materials as they relate
to the objectives in the handbook. That is, all of the written materials, especially those in the first two years, are being compared with the oncology objectives in
order to discover where in the curriculum oncologic information is being presented
to medical students. In this way we are investigating curriculum input and its
relation to the 23 topics and the 360 objectives in the handbook. Also within the
input portion of the model, faculty and student perceptions of oncology education
are being sought through survey methods. The faculty survey seeks the perceptions
of which objectives are being taught to medical students and in which courses they
 are exposed to these materials. The student survey is identical to the faculty
survey but its intent is to discover, from the student's point of view, the extent
to which the handbook objectives are being covered in the curriculum. Both surveys
use a qualitative scale which allows the respondents to judge coverage in terms of
how well the curriculum includes the objectives in the handbook. The input portion
of the model is, then, a combined effort involving direct analysis of the written
portions of the curriculum and analysis of student and faculty perceptions of how
well the curriculum reflects the objectives in the handbook.

The output portion of the model is being developed through the construction of a
comprehensive Cancer Knowledge Test. The test will consist of items generated directly from the oncology objectives and will actually be a series of topic specific exams which coincide with the 23 cancer topics in the handbook. This test will
be administered, using a matrix sampling technique, to medical students at all
undergraduate levels of their education. In this way, we should obtain a baseline
oncology education level for entering medical students and then observe the degree
of oncology knowledge gained during all four years of undergraduate education at
MCV. Also, a set of exams will be developed which will be used in conjunction with
supplementary resource materials in order to provide self-assessment capabilities
to the student using these materials.

The input-output model for cancer education analysis at MCV is, then, a new approach
to curriculum analysis. It is a model which can be used to evaluate (1) the adequacy of the curriculum in terms of specific objectives, and (2) the level of oncologic knowledge students obtain through each year of medical school. In addition,
a natural "spinoff" of the model is an array of self assessment tools for students
to further enhance their medical education in the area of cancer.

Specific Methods for Use of the Objectives in the Medical School Curriculum

The three major approaches employed for utilization of the Handbook of Objectives
in Oncology are: (1) distribution of the objectives for a specific segment in
advance of a seminar or lecture or other educational experience so that the student
can identify the concepts, information or skills that are considered basic elements
of oncology knowledge; (2) a body of educational resource materials has been identified, developed, and collated, and this is currently housed in one place in a
media resource library that is available to students for their own self-study activities; and (3) specific self-instructional materials have been developed for a
few selected areas in the oncology curriculum that will allow learning to take
place more efficiently by means of specifically constructed instructional packages,
slides, and similar materials.

1. Distribution of objectives with brief appropriate responses. Although this
approach can be utilized at all levels of the curriculum, it is most appropriate
for the less structured aspects of the medical school curriculum occurring during
the clinical years. Students having weekly seminars in the clinical disciplines
are given an opportunity to review the objectives, study appropriate resource
materials, and develop questions regarding areas that need elucidation by the faculty member at the time of the later seminar session. The collection of resource
materials addressed to each section of the handbook is also available to the students for further reading at their own time and rate. Not all faculty members in
the clinical disciplines have employed this approach, but the involvement of clinical faculty in this planning process has led to an increasing interest in this
method of utilizing these materials. It has been particularly useful in the cancer sessions presented by the Department of Surgery in the third year of our curriculum.

2. The use of the resource materials for supplementary study related to objectives
listed in the handbook. Faculty members participating in a portion of the curriculum that relates to sections of the Handbook of Objectives in Oncology have participated in the development of a resource book for each of the sections represented.
A sample listing is shown in Table II. Although these resource books are housed
in the media library along with appropriate texts for student access, additional
copies of these materials are planned for specific satellite teaching areas throughout the medical complex. This need for wider distribution of resource materials
applies particularly to students who are assigned to the teaching wards where special student study areas have been developed. These resource materials will be
progressively included in these study areas, where applicable, as enthusiasm is
developed by the clinical faculty in utilization of this approach.

3. The development of specific self-instructional materials for achieving selected
objectives. At the outset of this project, it was the goal of the interinstitu-
tional committee writing the objectives to develop specific self-instructional
packages for all groups of objectives identified. As the project progressed, it
became apparent that formal self-instructional packages were very time consuming
to produce and were not always applicable to the objectives listed. Specific
reading assignments, slide sets, or teaching films were often just as successful,
and often more readily available, than up-to-date well-constructed self-instructional packages. Some faculty members involved in a specific portion of the curriculum found these alternate approaches more feasible than the self-study packages,
while others found the S.I.P. the ideal method for assisting the student in his
own learning process. The list of some of the self-instructional units developed
to fulfill the oncology objectives at this institution are listed in Table III.
All of these materials are available in our media library and are distributed to
student groups at the appropriate time in the curriculum when this method is to
be employed. These range from instructional packages related to biochemical concepts in oncology to the clinical approach to a patient with possible breast disease. The latter package has been particularly useful in assisting students
during the clinical rotation in surgery as it consolidates the needed concepts and
information for this phase of the student's education. Similar packages and slide
sets have been developed whenever this approach seems the most appropriate.

Future of the Project

With a constantly changing body of information in oncology, and comparable changes
in the overall medical school curriculum, it is apparent that this effort is a
never ending project. At present, our own efforts in cancer education still fall
short of our stated goals, but progress is being made along the lines described.
There are obviously other innovative approaches to cancer education which could be
employed including a more vigorous effort in the development of self-instructional

TABLE II   Activity Sheet for Relating Instructional Objectives to Educational
           Resource Materials (Example)

Unit   XV-Gynecologic Oncology

Objectives   Educational Resource Materials

    1   Ackerman, L.V. and Del Regato: Chapter 14, Vulva. Pages 820-
                           829 in: Cancer-Female Genital Organs, 4th ed., C.V. Mosby
                           Co., 1970.

                           Krupp, P., et al: Current status of the treatment of epider-
                           moid cancer of the vulva. Cancer Supplement 38:587-595, 1976.

    2   Silverberg, E.: Gynecologic cancer: Statistical and epide-
                           miological information. American Cancer Society Professional
                           Educational Publications No. 3308, 1976.

                           Nelson, J.H., Averett, H.E. and Richart, E.M.: Dysplasia and
                           early cervical cancer. American Cancer Society Professional
                           Educational Publications No. 3387, 1975.

                           Moss, W.T., Brand, W.N. and Battifora: Chapter 17. Pages
                           408-453 in: The Cervix in Radiation Oncology, C.V. Mosby Co.,
                           1973.

                           Rubin, P.: Cancer of the Cervix-Stage I. JAMA 193:596-600,
                           1965.

                           Rubin, P.: Cancer of the Cervix-Stage II. JAMA 193:822-826,
                           1965.

                           Rubin, P.: Cancer of the Cervix-Stage III. JAMA 193:1101-
                           1107, 1965.

                           Rubin, P.: Cancer of the Cervix-Stage IV and Recurrent Car-
                           cinoma. JAMA 194:273-278, 1965.

    3   Peeples, W.J., et al: The ocurrence of metastasis outside
                           the abdomen and retroperitoneal space in invasive carcinoma
                           of the cervix. Gyn. Oncol. 4:307-310, 1976.

                                                                        ETC.

packages, the use of programmed learning texts, or the use of complex computer
techniques with sophisticated feedback methods for assisting the student in his
learning process. Nevertheless, the development of a specific set of objectives
in oncology is still the basis of most of the efforts to be employed. It is also
important to recognize the fact that continual revision of both the materials and
methods employed is required if the graduating medical student is to be well prepared, in terms of oncology, for his responsibility to his patients of the future.

TABLE III   Examples of Self-Instructional Materials Available

General Pathology of Neoplasia - Part I; definition, structure and characteristics
(self-instructional package)
General Pathology of Neoplasia - Part II; classification, pathologic diagnosis and
pathologic basis of clinical effects (self-instructional package)

TABLE III Examples of Self-Instructional Materials Available (continued)

Neoplasia - Carcinogenesis and General Characteristics of Neoplasms (short-framed programmed text)
Surgical Pathology of Various Organs (there are a large number of microfiche that cover neoplasms of specific organs as well as other disease processes)
Oral Cancer Detection (videotape)
Neoplasm of the Thyroid Gland (self-instructional package)
Gastrointestinal Cancer - Part I; Neoplasms of the Upper Digestive Tract (slide series with syllabus)
Gastrointestinal Cancer - Part II; Neoplasms of the Stomach (slide series with syllabus)
Gastrointestinal Cancer - Part III; Neoplasms of the Pancreato-biliary System and Liver (slide series with syllabus)
Gastrointestinal Cancer - Part IV; Neoplasms of the Small Bowel (slide series with syllabus)
Gastrointestinal Cancer - Part V; Neoplasms of the Colorectum (slide series with syllabus)
Polyps of the Colon (self-instructional package)
Ulcer vs. Carcinoma of the Stomach (self-instructional package)
Bone Tumors - Part I (microfiche)
Bone Tumors - Part II (microfiche)
An Introduction to Tumors of the Skin (slide series with syllabus)
Pathology of Intracranial Tumors (self-instructional package)
Breast Masses - Differential Diagnosis (self-instructional package)
Carcinoma of the Vulva (self-instructional package)
Radiologic Diagnosis of Carcinoma of the Lung (self-instructional package)
Staging of Hodgkin's Disease (self-instructional package)
Nucleotide Nomenclature (self-instructional package)
Steroid Nomenclature (self-instructional package)

UICC's Role in Cancer Education of Medical Students

Bruno Salvadori

*Istituto Nazionale per lo Studio e la Cura dei Tumori,
Milan, Italy*

The amount of knowledge acquired on the pathology and natural history of malignant tumors, the development of new techniques for the detection on cancer, the progress in the field of diagnostic procedures and of therapeutic means, the philosophy of interdisciplinary treatments, the methodology of clinical trials are convincing proofs of the fact that oncology is to be considered as a well defined discipline. As a matter of fact, all over the world, there is an increasing interest for this branch of medicine: on the other hand, in spite of this, it must be admitted that in most countries, apart from praisable exceptions, methods and programs employed for training personnel at all levels are, to use the words of Umberto Veronesi, "rudimentary, inadequate or non-existant". As a consequence professional education is a live and urgent problem: responsability for the fight against cancer are general practitioners, hospital doctors and specialists working in cancer centers, whose main tasks are respectively diagnosis, treatment and clinical research.

Perhaps the greatest responsability for the success of treatment lies with the general practitiones who, scattered throughout the community, must be able to spot the symptoms suggestive of cancer among the mass of diseases they are confronted with, must know what means are available for treating each case and make an approximate prognosis. A general practitioner can only cope with this task if he has been given a solid grounding in oncology in his undergraduate days. Regarding this point, in the majority of countries there is a widespread feeling of dissatisfaction with the whole approach to the teaching of oncology to medical students.

The chief shortcomings are: duplication in the teaching of some aspects of the subject, complete omission of others, unsystematic coverage, diversity and often conflict of opinions expressed by different teachers, lack of correlation between interdepartmental courses, theo-

B. Salvadori

retical bias, with a minimum of clinical and practical training.
Tests carried out in different countries have shown that a large number of medical students have a sketchy knowledge of oncology and that
their ideas on the prognosis of the various types of tumors are rudimentary, to a large extent incorrect and overpessimistic.

U.I.C.C. has devoted particular interest to Professional Education
since 1954, when a special Committee ad hoc was created at the 6th
Cancer Congress in Sao Paulo: to the purpose, Drs. Canonico, Maren-
go, Grant and Veronesi, who acted as Chairmen of these Committees o-
ver sixteen years, deserve a word of thanks for the rewarding job
they did. The action of U.I.C.C. in this field continues with the
present Education Program in the framework of which a special Project,
chaired by Dr. Sherman, is devoted to undergraduate education in oncology.

As regards undergraduate cancer teaching the greatest obstacle we
must face is the structure of teaching, which is based either on the
type of treatment (medicine, surgery, radiotherapy) or on organ pathology (gynecology, padiatry, ear, nose and throat, urology, and so on).
This structure is well suited to diseases that are treated mainly by
a single type of therapy or that are specific to one organ. On the
contrary, a disease that can affect all organs and can be treated
with several therapeutic means does not fit easily into this scheme.
The problem has thus remained unsolved for many years and is still a-
waiting for a rational and satisfactory solution. As things are, oncology is taught patchily in many disciplines with the inevitable gaps,
overlapping and conflict of opinion.

From a historical point of view, oncology attracted a certain interest by universities in the forties. It was in the United States in November 1944 that a special committee, the Government Consultive Committee, after an investigation of several years, reported that among
graduates in medicine there was a "deplorable ignorance" of cancer,
that they were not prepared to confront the problems of diagnosis and
therapy of tumors. Another committee, presided by Frank Adair, was
created to prepare within two years a new program for oncology education to be introduced into the American universities. From a reviw of
the curriculum of the various medical faculties, it seemed more reasonable, at least at that moment, to apply a so called horizontal rather than vertical teaching program in oncology. The teaching of the
horizontal type consisted in the coordination of the various principles of oncology taught within the various disciplines, placing them
in a logical order to avoid or reduce to a minimum the number of du-
plications or omissions. In order to effectively apply this horizontal coordination, it was evident that it would be necessary to appoint
someone to be responsible in each medical faculty, and this was done:
each U.S. university has a "cancer coordinator" who had ample power
and the task of following from the first to the last year the teaching of oncology to the medical students. The cancer coordinators imme-

diately formed an association, the Association of Cancer Coordinators, that then became the American Association for Cancer Education, and at their annual meetings they decided the policies and the techniques to be employed.

This program, started by the United States Government, lasted for 20 years, it costed the federal government about 40 million dollars and improved substantially the preexistent situation. Every year the level of oncology education in graduate students was verified with appropriate multiple choice tests, assisting in a progressive and consistent improvement.

Federal support was discontinued in 1966 in order to initiate a new program of postgraduate training in oncology, but most of the cancer coordinators remained at their posts. In every case the new philosophy of an integrated and multidisciplinary oncology education was by this time an important part of the American university.

The example set by the United States was followed by many other countries. Moreover, many universities went on from there, creating permanent committees to assure the continuity of oncology education among the various disciplines, and introducing special courses in oncology of 30 to 40 hours, taught in the various departments.

However, in the last 10 years more people came to the opinion that at least part of the oncologic knowledge could become a separate discipline in itself and therefore taught independently. It is that which is commonly defined as "vertical" oncologic education that presupposes the institution of an oncology chair. There were thus created in many countries chairs of oncology (about 100 in the world), even though they may have diversified objectives.

What can they teach in a department of oncology? First of all, they can teach that part of oncology not include in the other disciplines. There is a part which includes the fundamental principles of oncology that is not, as a rule, handled in the specialized departments; thus, such basic ideas can be gathered together in a separate course.

Included in the programs of the oncology chair are the epidemiology of tumors, the most important causative factors, the early diagnostic means, mass screening methodology, the most relevant diagnostic instruments, the clinical classification of tumors according to the TNM system, the principles of therapeutic programs, the significance of periodic control of cured patients, the techniques of rehabilitation, and the prognosis and the psychological problems concerning the patient with neoplasias. All these separate problems, which can be combined to form a single special course, are essential for an adequate cancer education of the student and are not treated in a complete and comprehensive manner in other medical courses.

In the second place, the chair of clinical oncology must prepare the
student for the interdisciplinary approach to oncology, by means of
an articulate and polyspecialized instruction with the participation
of professors of various extractions outside of the regular staff,
with seminars and multidisciplinary panels, creating exemplary situations which instill the principles of collaboration between the various
therapeutic branches.

There is a last task that the director of the chair of oncology can
assume: that of coordinating the instruction of oncology for the entire period of the university study. Thisformula, that an oncologist,
on one hand, imparts an education on the principles of clinical oncology and, on the other, coordinates according to a logical and coherent succession the oncologic instruction given by other members of
the faculty, has had considerable success in the last few years. Vertical teaching has the advantage of supplying the student with a coherent and complete picture of cancer as an entity and not merely as
a topic that arises in other b ranches of medicine. The vertical plan
apparently fits best into the last years of the curriculum. Here the
student has a basic science background, some clinical experience and
a greater familiarity with medicine in general, all essential for understanding the complexities of cancer. Apart from that, the student
in his last years is able to draw together the fragments of cancer
knowledge acquired during the earlier years of medical school.

What are then the chairs of clinical oncology existing in the world
today? In 1958 there were 13 oncology chairs throughout the world; in
1968 there were 43; and today there are almost 100. But more important and encouraging than that is that an inquiry conducted by the
Union Against Cancer found that by 1968 there were already 182 universities ready to institute a department of oncology.

Among the projects of the Educational Program, the undergraduate education is the one to which the U.I.C.C. devotes the largest interest.
Over the past years the Union has undertaken a number of projects according to a series of logical steps. The first step was to carry out
a survey of Medical Schools round the world to find out the present
situation of oncology teaching and the outlook in the various countries. The survey furnished revealing results, presented by dr. Veronesi on several occasion, which were helpful to the people working
out the program of activity. Secondly, it was decided that clinical
oncology could become established more extensively if the content
were outlined in a book which has been called "Manual of Clinical Oncology". The manual, which was published in 1972, was very successful,
20,000 copies being printed and disseminated throughout the world,
with translation into four national languages. A special Committee
prepared a new edition, enlarged and updated, which has been issued
on the occasion of this Cancer Congress in Buenos Aires.

Lastly, it was decided to organize regional meetings in order to stu-

dy on the spot ways and means of improving the   teaching of oncology,
and this program of meetings is now under way. The Education Committee has had occasion to note how greatly the teaching of medicine differs from one country to another, according to the   university structure and to social, cultural and economic conditions. It therefore
seemed pointless to produce a document containing general recommendations on how to strengthen the teaching of oncology for application in
the various countries. It was felt that the problem should be tackled
on a sectorial basis, that is country by country, or rather by groups
of countries with similar university structures and similar socio-economic conditions. To do this we planned the Regional Conferences on
Cancer Teaching, the first of which was held in Krakow in 1972. It
was attended by representatives of Medical Schools and Ministries of
Health in the countries of Eastern Europe (USSR, Poland, Rumania, Hun-
gary, Czechoslovakia, Yougoslavia and German Democratic Republic) together with experts in oncology of the Committee on Professional Education of UICC. After three days of proficuous discussion which made
it possible to gather important information and to compare different
experiences, the participants agreed on the following main points:
1) cancer is, all over the world, a social problem, due to the increasing incidence of the disease;
2) medical doctors must then be provided today with a larger amount
   of knowledge on cancer that in the past;
3) the curriculum of medical students should be modified in order to
   include in it a more efficient oncologic teaching;
4) it is possible to identify the general guidelines for this purpose;
   a number of basic information and principles concerning or as the
   content of chairs of oncology. The other aspects of cancer, which
   are usually part of different specialized disciplines, should be
   taught inside a coordinated program;
5) it was stressed out that the practical application of these guidelines must be adopted according to the organization of medical education and cancer controll existing in each country;
6) it was considered advisable that in the cities where a Cancer Institute or a Cancer Hospital exist, these institutions cooperate in
   the University programs, specially to improve students' bed-side
   teaching, through the so called "patient oriented learning";
7) a suggestion was made to promote the creation of a special Committee at national level or inside each Medical School; it should be
   either responsability to draw the program for oncological teaching
   to be included in the curriculum;
8) The "Manual of Clinical Oncology" edited by UICC should represent
   a common text to be used internationally. The results of the Conference in that part of Europe were spectacular: most of the Medical Schools have already set up special cancer programs for students or are in the way to do so and we are therefore very encouraged.

The second Conference was held in Sao Paulo, Brazil, in 1976; it was
attended by representitives from Argentina, Brazil, Chile, Colombia,

Equadro, Paraguay, Peru and Uruguay. Dr. U. Veronesi and Dr. C. Sherman of the UICC Education Programme, Dr. J. Litvak of the Pan American Health Organization (PAHO), Dr. A. Linsell of the International Agency for Research on Cancer, and Dr. G. Auvert of the Pan American Federation of Associations of Medical Schools (FEPAFEM). At the end of two days of work, after a number of surveys and eight workshops, it was stated that "cancer education in Latin American Medical Schools is at present inadequate since it is uncoordinated, disorganized and too limited in scope". Of particular interest was the contribute of the students themselves who took part in the discussion.

Finally, we have to remind the workshop organized by the UICC Education Programme at the 3rd Asian Cancer Conference, held in Manila in 1977; in this workshop the results of three different surveys conducted to determine the present status of cancer education in Asian medical schools, the students' viewpoint of their cancer education, and the role of the cancer cocieties in various Asian countries in cancer education of medical students. The final recommendations that emerged from these meetings are similar to those expressed in Krakow.

In conclusion, objectives to be reached by UICC's action, by using the tools I have shortly illustrated can be summarized as follows:
1) inform the student of the fundamental characteristics of cancer development and dissemination, including the tumor-host relationships;
2) develop in the student capability in the detection and early diagnosis of cancer;
3) keep the student informed of the development of new diagnostic means and techniques for the diagnosis of cancer;
4) inform the student of the necessity and possibilities of planning an appropriate therapeutic program;
5) train the student in the cancer patient care even when a definite cure is impossible;
6) make the student aware of the continued responsability of the physician for the cancer patient, not only as regards the medical requirements but also the emotional, economic and social aspects;
7) furnish the student with a clear concept of clinical trials and of their design and conduction.

Cancer Education in United States Medical and Dental Schools: The AACE-NCI Survey

Richard F. Bakemeier,* John Deegan, Jr.,* and Gordon S. Black**
for the American Association for Cancer Education

*University of Rochester School of Medicine and Dentistry
**University of Rochester College of Arts and Science, Rochester,
New York, U.S.A.

ABSTRACT

Since July, 1975, a survey of programs of cancer education in medical, osteopathic, and dental schools in the United States has been conducted by the American Associa- tion for Cancer Education under the sponsorship of the National Cancer Institute. Data has been obtained from 110/114 medical schools, 8/9 osteopathic schools and 55/58 dental schools; also from 1,311 faculty, and 3,856 students. In addition, 55 institutional visits were made.

Determinants of desirable educational program charcteristics were sought through several approaches, including multiple regression analysis. In addition to the attributes of successful and innovative programs, of which there are many, certain deficiencies were detected. These included instruction in cancer patient rehabili- tation, in psychosocial aspects of cancer, in radiation therapy principles, and exposure to certain relatively common malignancies. The career options of senior medical students were assessed in relation to potential manpower needs in various oncologic fields.

INTRODUCTION

It is the purpose of this paper to discuss briefly the survey of student cancer edu- cation in United States medical and dental schools which has been supported by the National Cancer Institute and has been conducted by members of the American Asso- ciation for Cancer Education, an organization of about 700 academic clinical oncol- ogists and basic scientists.

In the allotted space will be discussed the survey design and present in a descrip- tive manner some of the data available at this time concerning preclinical and clin- ical student cancer education. Certain areas will be pointed out which require strengthening if student cancer education is to be made more effective.

The Cancer Education Survey had its origin in early 1975, stimulated by the interest of Dr. Margaret Edwards of the United States' National Cancer Institute. It has been funded through a contract from the Institute's Division of Cancer Control and Rehabilitation, directed by Dr. Diane Fink.* Table 1 outlines the Survey design.

* Contract No. - CN - 55191

27

TABLE 1   AACE-NCI Cancer Education Survey

1. EDUCATIONAL RESOURCES QUESTIONNAIRES
         administration, facilities, programs
         110/114 medical schools; 55/58 dental schools

2. FACULTY QUESTIONNAIRES
         teaching, research, clinical activities
         1311/2516 medical faculty (52% response)

3. STUDENT QUESTIONNAIRES
         random sample; 25% of 2nd and 4th year
         3618/6046 medical students (60% response)

4. INSTITUTIONAL VISITS
         44 medical schools; 3 osteopathic schools;
         8 dental schools

The mechanism of data collection centered on three types of questionnaires and a series of institutional visits. First, the educational resources questionnaire was completed by a faculty member, designated by the dean of each school as being thoroughly familiar with the institution's cancer education program. This questionnaire acquired information concerning the administrative structure, financial support, facilities (such as hospitals and clinics), and the general nature of programs of cancer education for students, fellows, practicing physicians, nurses and paramedical personnel. Of the 114 medical schools, 110 agreed to participate in the survey.

The faculty questionnaires were sent to all faculty members named as having important roles in the programs of that school. Data collected included details of the faculty members' teaching, research, and clinical activities. Of those contacted, 52% responded.

Thirdly, a student questionnaire was sent to a random sample of the second year and fourth year classes through the dean's offices. At least 25% of the class members, selected at random, were asked to complete the questionnaires. Of this random sample, 60% responded.

Finally a series of 55 institutional visits were carried out including 44 medical schools comprising a representative sample of large and small schools, public and private schools, schools with a long tradition of major emphasis on student cancer education, and schools attempting to develop new or expanded programs.

A sampling of some of the data currently available and pertinent to this educational symposium will now be presented.

Based on the experience of many cancer educators in the American Association for Cancer Education, and on observations made during the course of institutional visits, a list of cancer education program characteristics was created which included those considered most desirable in conveying modern information about cancer biology, diagnosis, and treatment to students.

These characteristics can in general be divided into two groups: a) In Table 2 are listed characteristics of institutional environments such as the availability of cancer patients for student education programs, the variety of services provided for patients, and the presence of other cancer education programs in an institution

such as those for residents, fellows, practicing physicians, nurses and social
workers.

TABLE 2   Cancer Education Program Characteristics
(Dependent Variables: "Outcomes")

a.   Environmental

1.   Availability of cancer patients
2.   Variety of patient care services
3.   Multiple levels of non-student education
residents, fellows, practicing physicians,
nurses, social workers

and b) In Table 3 characteristics of student cancer education program content, such
as the variety of educational opportunities (e.g. student cancer fellowships, lecture series, and treatment planning conferences); the multidisciplinary nature of
the program; outpatient exposure to permit students to observe patients responding
to therapy and doing well; education in the psychosocial aspects of cancer; and
student education activities conducted by oncologic subspecialties such as medical,
pediatric, or radiation oncology.

TABLE 3   Cancer Education Program Characteristics
(Dependent Variables: "Outcomes")

b.   Content

1.   Variety of student cancer educational
opportunities
2.   Multidisciplinary cancer education
3.   Cancer outpatient exposure
4.   Psychosocial aspects of cancer
5.   Oncologic subspecialty education activities

These program characteristics were measured and a numerical score assigned for each
participating institution on the basis of answers provided to relevant items in the
educational resources questionnaire.   A tabulation of these answers resulted in a
numerical score being recorded for each characteristic.   The scores quantitatively
represented the degree to which an institution possessed each of the characteristics.
The institutional scores for each characteristic were then treated in the data analysis as dependent variables, or "outcomes," which were conceptualized as resulting
from the effects of certain other measured institutional characteristics termed
independent variables, or "causes."

To establish those institutional characteristics which might contribute to these
desirable education program characteristics, a list of potential determinants or
causes was created for use in subsequent analyses.   These potential determinants,
which are also referable to as independent variables, included the following, listed
in Table 4.   The general medical curriculum design; the number of medical students
enrolled; whether a school was private or a state supported institution; the length
of support from National Cancer Institute Education Grants; the presence of a representative of the cancer education program on the Curriculum Committee; the presence
of an interdepartmental Cancer Education Committee; and the presence of certain
administrative structures, such as an NCI Cancer Center; a Department of Oncology;
and various oncologic subspecialty divisions.

TABLE 4   Institutional Characteristics
(Independent Variables: "Determinants")

Curriculum design
    Traditional (departmental; 2+2 yrs)
    Non-traditional (innovative types)
Number of students
Private or public institution
NCI education grants
Ca. Ed. Representative on Curriculum Comm.
Administrative structures
    Cancer Centers; Depts. of Oncology; Divisions

A description of the details of analyses conducted to investigate the interrelationships between each dependent variable and the previously enumerated set of independent variables is beyond the scope of this paper. But in brief, the analytic technique employed, called multiple regression analysis, permitted a determination of
those independent variables which, when all are considered simultaneously, were
most closely associated with each of the dependent variables; that is, with each of
the cancer education program characteristics measured.

Table 5 presents a general summary of the results obtained from this portion of the
Survey, listing the institutional attributes considered as potential determinants
which were found to be most closely associated with the presence of desirable
characteristics in an institution's student cancer education programs. These
important institutional attributes include: the presence of an NCI education grant;
the functioning of a multidisciplinary cancer education committee; the appointment
of a cancer education program representative to the institution's curriculum committee; the presence of medical, pediatric, and radiation oncology divisions; the
presence of a Department of Oncology; and the presence of an NCI Cancer Center.

TABLE 5   Institutional Attributes Associated with
Desirable Cancer Education Characteristics

NCI Education Grant
Cancer Education Committee
Cancer Ed. Representative on Curriculum Comm.
Medical Oncology Division/Unit
NCI Cancer Center
Department of Oncology
Pediatric Oncology Division/Unit
Radiation Oncology Dept./Division

It is difficult, and perhaps misleading, in this type of analysis to attempt to
assign cause and effect relationships to these characteristics. But observations
obtained from institutional visits have indicated that these various determinants
may indeed assist an institution in strengthening its student cancer education
programs.

Let us now turn to data from student questionnaires and look for nationwide
strengths or weaknesses in student education.

Beginning with the preclinical sciences, there is evidence from the Survey that the
majority of American medical students are provided with some foundation in tumor
biology with the major exposure being in pathology courses. Institutional visits
indicated that the presence of organized multidisciplinary integrated tumor biology
courses, usually with some degree of clinical correlation, resulted in considerable
interest among preclinical students, and that this could often lead to more active

student participation in later clinical cancer education programs.

Table 6 lists the percentages of the 1757 senior medical students responding to the Survey who indicated they had received over six hours of instruction concerning a given type of cancer. Each reader will have to decide for himself whether or not a larger number of students should have received at least this arbitrarily selected amount of instruction. To help in this, the annual incidence of these tumors is included in the righthand column. It appears that students have a fairly good exposure to such common malignancies as gynecologic, lung, breast, and gastrointestinal cancers. In view of the lower incidence of leukemias and lymphomas, students receive a relatively greater exposure to these diseases.

TABLE 6   Per Cent of 1757 Senior Students Receiving
Over 6 Hours of Instruction Concerning:

		USNC/Yr*
Gynecologic cancers	78%	98,000
Lung cancer	74%	68,200
Breast cancer	69%	89,700
Gastrointestinal cancers	69%	171,400
Leukemias	64%	21,300
Lymphomas	62%	21,900

*United States New Cases per Year (1977)

On the other side of the coin are obvious deficiencies in the overall student cancer education programs. The data in Table 7 indicates that rather large percentages of students nearing the completion of their undergraduate medical education recall having examined or followed no patients with malignant melanoma (42%); pancreatic carcinoma (32%); ovarian carcinoma (29%); head and neck carcinoma (27%); and prostatic carcinoma (21%). Again the annual incidence of these malignancies in the United States is included to provide a perspective of the relative importance of these tumors.

TABLE 7   Per Cent of 1757 Senior Students
Having Seen no Patients with:

		USNC/Yr*
Malignant melanoma	42%	9,500
Pancreatic carcinoma	32%	21,800
Ovarian carcinoma	29%	17,000
Head and neck carcinoma	27%	23,900
Prostatic carcinoma	21%	57,000

*United States New Cases per Year (1977)

An approach to correcting this deficiency is the increased utilization of community hospitals and outpatient departments in student teaching. Many patients with common malignancies, particularly patients who are doing well, may not be referred to academic centers where most student teaching is conducted. Therefore, adequately supervised instruction in community hospitals may provide students with more realistic experience concerning common malignancies. Access to ambulatory patients, even in the academic centers, can also provide students with a better understanding of the natural history of these malignancies and help them to develop more positive attitudes toward the care of cancer patients.

Finally, several important topics appear to be receiving insufficient attention in many medical schools. Table 8 shows percentages of students, in their final year of medical school, who reported having received less than one hour of instruction concerning cancer patient rehabilitation (73%); psychosocial aspects of cancer (43%); radiation therapy principles (37%); and cancer chemotherapy principles (13%).

TABLE 8   Per Cent of 1757 Senior Students Receiving
Less Than One Hour of Instruction Concerning:

Cancer patient rehabilitation	73%
Psychosocial aspects of cancer	43%
Radiation therapy principles	37%
Cancer chemotherapy principles	13%

Radiation therapy appears to present significant unique educational problems which merit special attention. Today, there is a greater need for radiation oncologists in the United States than is currently being met by qualified applicants to train-ing programs. It was apparent from students' responses to the questionnaire, and during institutional visits, that exposure to radiation oncology has been minimal or absent for most medical students. Radiation oncologists in many schools do not participate in basic science courses, in physical diagnosis courses, or in clinical clerkships. Partly because of this lack of contact with radiation oncologists, few students choose electives in this subject. In addition, the structure of the cur-riculum may provide no real opportunity for students to become familiar enough with radiation oncology to consider it as a viable career option.

In the Survey, students were asked about their current preferences regarding future career development. Table 9 indicates the percentages of senior students indicating a given field as his or her first choice. Also listed are the numbers of physicians who would enter a given field, assuming all 15,000 medical graduates actually pur-sued a career that corresponded to their current first choice. Most students, as in other surveys, indicate internal medicine, family practice, surgery, pediatrics, and obstetrics/gynecology as major fields of interest. It is perhaps not surprising that oncologic subspecialties rank far behind these categories. Medical Oncology was the first choice of 1.6% of senior medical students or about 240 per year. The corresponding figure for radiation oncology was 1.1% or 165 per year; and for pedia-tric oncology was 0.6% or 90 new oncologists per year. Obviously other individuals may decide later to enter an oncologic field, and some of the oncologically-oriented students will change from their current first choices. It seems likely that the estimated need of approximately 300 new medical oncologists annually between now and 1985 will be difficult to achieve, and radiation oncology also appears likely to face a continuing shortage of applicants, particularly if student exposure to the field is not increased.

TABLE 9   Senior Student Career Choices

Specialty	First Choice (%)	MD's/Yr*
Internal Medicine	24.6	3690
FAmily Practice	18.6	2790
Surgery	14.5	2175
Pediatrics	11.1	1665
Obstetrics/Gynecology	7.2	1080
Medical Oncology	1.6	240
Radiation Oncology	1.1	165
Pediatric Oncology	0.6	90

n = 1757 4th year students
*Assuming 15,000 new MD's per year.

Time does not permit discussion of additional educational program deficiencies uncovered by the Survey, or their possible solutions. It should be pointed out, however, that only 54% of senior students had personally performed a proctosigmoid-oscopy. Only 75% of senior students had observed a mastectomy, and only 42% of the

students reported having seen a breast cancer patient undergoing estrogen therapy
for metastatic disease. These appear to be rather significant, but correctable,
educational deficiencies.

A variety of cancer educational techniques appear to be appropriate for improving
the current state of student cancer education. These include more effective use
of multidisciplinary preclinical teaching; more emphasis on cancer diagnosis and
therapy during standard medical and surgical clerkships; more availability of student cancer fellowships, especially during vacation periods; more attractive clinical electives with emphasis on interdisciplinary cooperation; better utilization
of ambulatory cancer patients for student teaching; increased exposure of students
to common malignancies in community hospitals; and more emphasis on the psychosocial
and rehabilitative aspects of cancer.

These and other educational approaches will be discussed in a set of guidelines
for student cancer education which should emerge from the data of the AACE-NCI
Cancer Education Survey during 1979.

Oncology Teaching—Latin American Survey***

R. A. Estévez* and C. A. Alvarez**

*Director, Professor of Clinical Oncology
**Associate Director, Professor of Clinical Oncology
***Chair of Clinical Oncology, School of Medicine, "del Salvador"
University, Av. Luis Ma. Campos 726, 7° piso, 1426 Buenos Aires, Argentina

INTRODUCTION

During the course of an International Congress of Oncology, which took place in Buenos Aires in July 1975, a preliminary survey on Oncology Teaching in Latin America was carried out among the participants (1) (8). Said survey, organized by a Clinical Oncology Chair at the "Hospital Militar Central de Buenos Aires" (Buenos Aires Central Military Hospital) had the collaboration of the "Oficina Sanitaria Panamericana" (Panamerican Health Department)(OPS/OMS), and its main purpose was to contribute to the knowledge of the present condition of said specialty education in Latin America, and, taking as a basis the information collected from the attending American oncologists, to stimulate a discussion and interchange of experiences for the best development of this specialty, according to the condition and necessities of each country.

The interest showed by the participants and the conclusions arised from said survey, gave a clear proof of the true concern on that subject and pointed out the responsibility it should be dealth with (2). Taking into consideration the above mentioned, at that time we thought that this kind of consultations could and should be enlargened and improved (3) (4) (5). We thought an adequate way would be to carry out similar investigations, but this time, among Medical Schools in Latin America (6) (7).

What we are now trying to achieve - by means of the complementation of both studies, is the full representation of Latin American medical doctors' opinion with respect to Oncology teaching in this region. This is the aim of this work, which includes the results arising from the analysis of the answers of several Medical Schools Directors, Oncologists, Medical Teachers and Specialists concerned with Oncology in all Latin America.

This study, coordinated and carried out by the Clinical Oncology Chair of the School of Medicine of the "del Salvador" University at the "Hospital Militar Central de Buenos Aires" and which had the collaboration of the VI Department of the "Oficina Sanitaria Panamericana" (OPS/OMS) and the sponsor of the Committee of Professional Education of the U.I.C.C., tries to be another contribution towards the obtention of resources for the struggle against Cancer in our region.

MATERIALS

In both surveys, a total amount of 380 forms specially made and consisting of 8 pages with 28 questions divided into several subjects, were distributed. These included indications to answer the questions, and sections for the identification of the surveyed personnel. At Medical Schools, the opinion of the teaching classes was requested in order to answer some questions, and on the contrary, other questions had to be answered by the ones in charge of Oncology teaching in each educational center. A sheet containing the indications to answer the questions was included, as well as another sheet for the identification of the surveyed professional. The great majority of questions was made following the multiple choice and complementation system, however, some of them requested a true opinion on certain specified subjects.

METHODOLOGY

A total amount of 200 forms was distributed among oncologists of several Latin American countries during the first survey which took place during a Congress of Oncology held in Buenos Aires in July 1975. There were no inconveniences to collect the answers, as the participants handed them in at the end of the Congress.

Afterwards, forms were sent by mail to 180 Medical Schools in Latin America. The collection of data coming from the Schools was continuously hindered by mailing defficiencies, which in some cases, compelled us to make a second and sometimes even a third delivery of forms during the course of a year. The first delivery to all Schools was made in November 1975.

In order to enable a more easy study of the data and to obtain results having a real significance, the replies were divided into seven subjects, to wit:
  I) Academical Background.
  II) Teaching Activity of Surveyed Persons.
  III) Prevailing Specialty among them.
  IV) Oncology Teaching to Pre-graduates.
  V) Oncology Teaching to Post-graduates.
  VI) Oncology as a Medical Specialty.
  VII) General Position of Oncology Teaching.

Finally, for the detailed and comparative analysis of each question, three parameters were used:

a) To point out the generic meaning of the answer, irrespective of the country or region it came from.
b) To point out the differences among answers coming from participants of large cities (large Schools) and those coming from smaller rural centers. The difference was recorded, only when significant.
c) To point out the difference existing among countries.

RESULTS

I) Academical Background

The need to know the importance and characteristics of the Schools of Medicine involved, originated questions on the number of graduates per year and on the number of subjects in the curriculum thereof.

From the 121 surveyed persons, 50 gave a background, and the rest gave no answer.

Regarding the number of graduates per year, the figures range between 2.000 physicians per year - corresponding to the "Universidad Autónoma de Mexico" (Mexico Independent University) - and 44 graduates per year at the "Universidad de Caxias do Sul" (Caxias do Sul University), Brazil. There is a majority of schools having 44 to 100 graduates per year (22 of 50 Schools).

The number of subjects in the curriculum ranges between 21 and 90, with an average of 44.10. We conclude stating that 79% of the consulted Schools have a number of subjects fluctuating between 30 and 58.

II) Teaching Activity of Surveyed Persons
The following table includes the results obtained:

The columns Professor through Others (first) fall under **TEACHING CATEGORY**; the columns Oncology through Others (second) fall under **SUBJECTS THEY TEACH**.

COUNTRY	Number of Surveys	Teaching Staff (No.)	Professor	Full Professor	Assistant Lecturer	Assistant Professor	Others	Oncology	Surgery	Radiotherapy	Internal Medicine	Pathology	Gynaecology	Others	Deans
Argentina	55	20	3	2	4	2	10	7	3		2		4	4	
Bolivia	1	1	1					1							
Brazil	34	28	12	7	3		6	3	6	1	4	5	1	6	2
Colombia	6	4	3		1							1	1	1	
Chili	5	5	3				2	3							2
Guatemala	1	1		1											
Mexico	4	3	1				2					1		1	1
Panama	1	1		1										1	1
Paraguay	2	1			1				1						
Peru	2	1	1						1						
Salvador	2	2		2					1		1				
Uruguay	6	5	2		1		2	3	2	1				1	
Venezuela	2	2	2					2							
TOTALS	121	75'	28	13	10	2	22	19	13	2	7	7	6	13	6

Members of Teaching Staff: 75 which means: 61.66% of surveyed persons.

III) Oncology Teachers

19 surveyed persons called oncology teachers:

COUNTRY	Number of Oncology Teachers	TEACHING CATEGORY				
		Professor	Assistant Lecturer	Assistant Professor	Auxiliary Professor	Other Teaching Categories
Argentina	7	1				6
Brazil	3	1	1		1	
Venezuela	2	1		1		
Uruguay	3	1				2
Chili	3	3				
Bolivia	1	1				
TOTAL	19	8	1	1	1	8

IV) Oncology Teaching to Pre-graduates

From the answers collected, we may summarize the following: Oncology teaching to medical pre-graduates is made by means of the curriculum of several subjects: 102 surveyed persons answered in this way.

The subjects more frequently mentioned as a means of Oncology teaching were: Pathological Anatomy, Internal Medicine and Surgery.

On the existence of a Chair to teach Oncology to pre-graduates, 16 participants answered affirmatively, 4 negatively and the rest did not answer.

Four participants chose an alternative means: the creation of Coordinating Committees or Units of Oncology Teaching. Said Committees or Units would be formed by professors of other subjects and their function would be to direct this subject's teaching.

With reference to the years of the curriculum in which Oncology is taught, the following data were collected: 6th. year: 76 answers; 5th. year: 63 answers; 4th. year: 41 answers; 3rd. year: 25 answers. We must explain that in many cases, more than a year is recorded, for example: 4th., 5th. and 6th. year, etc.

The advised average of hours for the teaching of Oncology during all the medical career was 138.

The present teaching of Oncology as an independent subject is almost not mentioned, however the attitude of the teaching staff towards this matter is considered favourable in 73.5% of the cases, and that of the students is highly favourable (86.3%).

Regarding the importance Cancer Epidemiology Teaching to pre-graduates deserves, from a total of 50 answers, 26% answered: VERY IMPORTANT; 30%: QUITE IMPORTANT; 34%: NOT VERY IMPORTANT and 5%: NOT IMPORTANT AT ALL.

During the survey, we tried to learn which were the books on Oncology Teaching more used by students. To that end, we begged them to mention the three most common books. 27 surveyed persons answered (especially those who had mentioned the existence of independent Chairs). The three books mentioned more times were:

      1) CANCER - Ackerman and Del Regato.

      2) CLINCAL ONCOLOGY MANUAL (U.I.C.C.)

      3) CANCER MEDICINE - Holland and Frei.

When Oncology appeared as an independent subject within the curriculum, it was placed in the 6th. year of the career, having an average of 60.83 hours of teaching.

As to the teaching methodology, 2/3 of those who answered, stated that practical activities cover from 60 to 80% of the teaching task. Said activities were specified as follows: hospitalized patients care, attendance to Tumors Committee and Seminars of the specialty, attendance to the Laboratory and other Hospital Services related to Oncology.

One of the differences to be noticed in relation with the importance of Universities, is that of the existence of Oncology Chairs as an independent subject; generally, this existence was true in those large Schools belonging to important cities; on the contrary, seldom were there Oncology Chairs in minor Schools.

Oncology Teaching to pre-graduates is generally considered poor: 83.8% of the answers. 91.17 agreed that the creation of Chairs for pre-graduates would enable a better oncology teaching. From all those who thought in this way, 90.32% conclude that said Chairs should be integral, trying to comprise the whole subject and not only branches of Oncology.

V) Oncology Teaching to Post-graduates

When we asked the surveyed persons whether there were Oncology Chairs or Departments for post-graduates at their Schools, we obtained 92 replies: 50 were affirmative and 42, negative.

From a total number of 27 replies referred to the methodology employed to teach Oncology to post-graduates, 14 participants said that this was developed by means of improvement or up-dating Courses; 10 replies mentioned 2 years' Training Courses for Clinical Oncology Specialists and finally 3 mentioned Internships at Cancer Institutes.

59.4% replies indicated that Oncology Teaching by means of Chairs or Departments for post-graduates dependent on the Schools is satisfactory. An average of 2,073.3 hours for Specialists' Courses for graduates, organized by Oncology Chairs was indicated.

National Oncology Institutes, Cancer Hospitals, Oncology Services of General Hospitals and specialized Medical Associations were mentioned as the entities in charge of oncology teaching to post-graduates.

As to the question on the importance assigned to the teaching of Cancer Epidemiology in the continuous education of a general physician, 41.5% answered affirmatively, and the remaining 48.5%, negatively.

VI) Oncology as a Medical Specialty

With respect to this matter, we asked whether there was a title of Oncologist in each country. From 80 replies, 55 answered YES and 25, NO.

Regarding the way to obtain the title of Oncologist, we collected the following information from 54 replies:

1) A 3 years' internship at a Cancer Hospital: 30 replies.
2) Official Courses for post-graduates with a maximum duration of 2 years in Oncology Chairs: 16 replies.
3) 3 to 5 years continuous attendance to an Oncology Unit and presentation of curriculum before an official agency: 8 replies.

As to this matter, the answers indicate that in some countries, e.g. Argentina, Brazil and Venezuela, there is a title of "Oncology Specialist". In Argentina, two ways of obtaining the title were mentioned: five years' attendance to a known Oncology Unit; a 2 years' (full time) specialization Course at Oncology Chairs. In Brazil, the ways are: a 3 years' internship at a Cancer Hospital; and in the case of radiotherapists, after this internship, they must undergo an examination before the Radiologists Association. The agencies which grant the title of specialist in Argentina are: the "Secretaría de Estado de Salud Pública" (Public Health State Department) and the "Colegio de Médicos" (Physicians Association); in Brazil: the Brazilian Cancer Society, the Brazilian Medical Association and the Radiology Society (Radiotherapists).

There is almost a general agreement on the fact that Oncology should be a medical specialty. As for the system considered more adequate for the obtention of the title of "Oncology Specialist", the following may be stated: 2 years or more (full time) improvement courses for post-graduates should be carried out in specialized Chairs or Institutes, as it happens with other specialties; afterwards, an adequate practice of the specialty shall be carried out in suitable places during a period of 3 years or more. Another prevailing opinion is that of undergoing a three years' internship at a Cancer Hospital and afterwards passing a confirming evaluation test. Finally, the possibility of self-training and (non-supervised or non-organized) attendance to Units related to the specialty, is mentioned, though the progressive inefficiency of this practice is acknowledged.

VII) General Position of Oncology Teaching

The present state of this subject's teaching in Latin America was categorically considered unsatisfactory; 83.5% of the opinions indicated thus. The post-graduate level was considered the poorest as regards the knowledge of this subject; the post-graduate level defficiency was specially marked in the training of specialists, except in Argentina and Brazil where it is considered satisfactory

There follows a complete table referred to the above mentioned matter.

Question: Condition of Oncology Teaching in the Country.

Replies:

Ideal   : 1
Satisfactory : 16
Unsatisfactory: 89   Pre-graduate level: 70
                            Post-graduate level: 108
                                        Continuous Education: 35
                                        Specialists Training: 43
                                        Technicians Training: 30
No answer: 15

ONCOLOGY CHAIRS IN LATIN AMERICA

COUNTRY	CHAIRS	Title of On- cologist	Tumors Re- gistries
Argentina	2 in Buenos Aires: "Instituto de Oncología" and "Hospital Militar Central"	YES	YES
Bolivia	No Chairs - There is a National Cancer Institute	YES	YES
Brazil	6 Chairs: "Servicio Nacional del Cáncer", "Clínica del Cáncer de Recife", "Universidad de Sorocaba", Belén (Para), "Universidad de Sao Paulo"	YES	YES
Colombia	1 Chair at the School of Medicine of the "Universidad Javeriana de Bogotá"	NO	YES
Chili	2 Chairs: "Universidad de Chile", "Universidad Cató- lica"	NO	YES
Guatemala	No Oncology Chairs	NO	NO
Mexico	6 Chairs: "Clínica del Cáncer", "Hospital Civil de Guadalajara", "Hospital Español de Mexico", Hospi- tal Militar Central de Mexico".	YES	YES
Panama	No Oncology Chairs	NO	YES
Paraguay	No Oncology Chairs. There is a National Cancer Ins- titute	NO	YES
Peru	No Oncology Chairs. There is a National Institute of Neoplastic Diseases	YES	YES
Salvador	No Oncology Chairs	NO	YES
Uruguay	1 Oncology and Radiotherapy Chair in Montevideo	NO	NO
Venezuela	No Oncology Chairs. Oncology Teaching at the "Uni- versidad de los Andes", in Merida.	YES	YES

NO AVAILABLE DATA: Costa Rica, Cuba, Ecuador, Guayanas, Haiti, Honduras, Puerto Rico, Rep. Dominicana.

Almost unanimously, (91.17%) the conclusion was that the creation of Chairs or Departments for Pre- and Post-graduates would improve this subject's teaching. It was also considered (in 90.32%) of the cases, that the Chairs to be created should be of "Oncology", covering the subject in all its aspects and turning down the possibility of creating Chairs of oncological sub-specialties, e.g.: Oncological Radiotherapy, Oncological Surgery, etc.

Some of the surveyed persons suggested the creation of Committees or Units coordinating the teaching of Oncology to pre- and post-graduates within University Schools.

As an important complement of Oncology Education, we asked on the existence of National or Regional Registries of Cancer:

> 76 answered YES
> 15 answered NO
> 30 did not answer

CONCLUSIONS

From the total number of analyzed answers, we conclude that:

1) The present level of Oncology Teaching to pre-graduates and post-graduates, is considered unsatisfactory. The creation of Oncology Chairs or Departments within Medical Schools with the purpose of improving the overall teaching of this subject is considered useful almost unanimously.

2) The teaching of Oncology to medical students was and is carried out through different subjects of this career and not as an independent subject. Nowadays, there is a favourable trend among students and teachers towards the creation of Oncology as an independent subject, but there are still some difficulties caused by the poor academical coordination to that end and by the small number of Oncology Professors.

3) The teaching of Oncology to post-graduates is carried out by means of Oncology Chairs or Departments which generally function within National Cancer Institutes or Cancer Hospitals. Specialized units at General Hospitals and Medical Societies also play an important role in this respect.

4) Oncology teaching to post-graduates could be grouped in two main areas. A) Immediate post-graduate level (dedicated to those physicians who wish to specialize in some particular field of Oncology). Within this level, we can mention: a) Oncology Internships at Cancer Hospitals. b) A minimum two years (full time) specialization courses in Oncology Chairs or Institutes. B) Continuous Education: (dedicated to physicians in general). It comprises short term improvement courses - 30 to 50 hours - dictated by Hospital Services and Medical Societies.

5) The title of "Oncology Specialist" exists only in some countries. The Health Department and Specialized Medical Societies are the ones in charge of granting this title.

6) It is almost a general opinion that Oncology should be considered as a medical specialty.

7) The title of "Oncology Specialist" was generally obtained by the mere attendance during some years to a service of this specialty and by the subsequent ratification by official entities or Medical Societies. Nowadays the main systems suggested in order to obtain said title are the following: A) 3 years' Oncology internship at Cancer Hospitals (with a subsequent capacity test before specialized Medical Societies). B) 2 years' (full time) specialization courses in Oncology Chairs or Institutes.

8) From the Schools involved, there is a majority of schools with 44 to 100 graduates per

year. The number of subjects in the curriculum ranges from 21 to 90, with an average of 44.10.

9) From the 121 surveyed persons, 75 were university teachers. Among these, the majority were Oncology, Surgery or Internal Medicine teachers.

10) The existence of Cancer Registries is well known (at hospital's level and at the Regional and National level), however, the teaching of Cancer Epidemiology in the continuous education of the general physician is not given much relevance.

BIBLIOGRAPHY

1) C.A. Alvarez: Estudio sobre la Enseñanza de la Oncología, Actas del II Congreso Argentino de Oncología Clínica. Julio 1975 - Buenos Aires

2) C.A. Alvarez: La Enseñanza de la Oncología en América Latina. Revista Latinoamericana de Quimioterapia Antineoplásica. Vol. VII, Año 1976

3) W.I. Mc Keachie: Research on teaching at the college and university level. Handbook of Research on Teachings. (N.L. Goge, editor). Rand Mc Nalby, Chicago, 1963.

4) F.N. Kerlinger: Foundations of Behavioural Research. Educational and Psychological Inquiry. Holt, Rinehart and Winston, Inc. New York, 1964.

5) G. Miller, M.D.: Teaching and Learning in Medical School. Editor: Commonwealth Fund. Book, Harvard University Press, 1965.

6) Ensino da Cancerologia. Relatorio sobre os Congressos Integrados de Cancerologia - Sao Paulo, Brasil. Setembro 1969.

7) La Educación Médica en América Latina. Publicación Científica Nro. 255. Oficina Sanitaria Panamericana (OPS/OMS), 1972.

8) Surveys, Polls, and Samples - New York: Harper and Row, 1950, Chap. 1

The Students' Viewpoint of their Cancer Education (A Survey carried out among Latin American Students who have finished their Medical Studies)

M. Gaitán Yanguas* and H. Kasdorf**

*Instituto Nacional de Cancerología, Bogotá, Colombia
**Dep. Oncología, Fac. de Medicina, Montevideo, Uruguay

ABSTRACT

Students are best qualified to asess the efficiency of cancer teaching programs. A questionnaire was sent to 186 interns in 41 medical schools of 20 Latin American countries. Students rate of response was 68% from 78% of the schools in 60% of the countries. Only 15% have an organized course of Oncology which is mainly theoretical.Of the remaining schools about 20% give students an integrated knowledge in Cancerology. Teaching is provided mainly in surgical and medical clinics. Radio and chemotherapy is poorly taught. About half of the students have the chance of being in contact with or looking after cancer patients. A minority performs small diagnostic procedures (simple/punch biopsy, PAP, etc.) sees or takes part in treatment (radium insertion, external radiation).Only 24% are enlightened about the psychological aspects; 20% of the schools have symposia, seminars, conferences, congresses, but attendance is compulsory only in two. Available cancer textbooks are rated as acceptable in 48%. Knowledge in cancer acquired at end of medical training is qualified as mediocre 28%, defficient 33%. To improve teaching, students suggested creating a Chair of Oncology or compulsory attendance to a Cancer Centre. Survey, though incomplete, reflects defficient cancer education in medical schools in Latin America and the urgent need to improve.

KEYWORDS

Teaching, Cancer education, Medical education, Undergraduate teaching.

RESULTS AND DISCUSSION

When considering the various aspects of the teaching of Oncology in medical schools it is the students themselves who are best qualified to assess how good and efficient these programs are. This is so, since only they can appreciate how much useful theoretical knowledge they have received and the kind of opportunities they were given in practical teaching.

A survey on this basis was conducted among students who had just completed their medical training. A questionnaire, specially designed for

this purpose was sent to 186 interns in 41 schools of Medicine in 20
countries of Latin America (table 1). The students rate of response
was 68% from 78% of the schools in 60% of the countries.

TABLE 1 - Students Survey and Rate of Response

	Countries	Schools	Hospitals	Students
Questionnaires	20	41	36	186
Answers	12	32	25	127
% of Replies	60	78	69	68

The analysis of the answers to each of the questions shows the following results.

1 - Is there an Oncology Course in your Medical School?

Only 10 replies were positive: 8% (table 2). These 10 students came
from 5 schools; that is to say that only 15% of the schools have an organized course of Oncology. A really very low figure. Moreover very
few hours are devoted to the teaching of Oncology which is mainly theoretical, including hardly any practical training.

TABLE 2 - Is there an Oncology Course in your School?

5 of a total of 32 schools (15%) have a course of Oncology

The course is compulsory in all 5 schools

Duration of the course is under 3 months

Number of hours dedicated to the course are:
>   In 1 school - 200 hours
>   In 2 schools - 96 to 100 hours
>   In 1 school - 20 to 24 hours
>   In 1 school - 16 hours

The course is:
>   In 1 school - 100% theoretical, 0% practical
>   In 2 schools - 80% theoretical, 20% practical
>   In 2 schools - 20% theoretical, 80% practical

2 - How is the Teaching of Cancer carried out if the Schools do not have an Oncology Course?

Table 3 shows that only 8% of the schools have a coordinated teaching
in Oncology. The remaining 92% do not give their students an integrated knowledge, merely providing fragmentary information.

However, this integrated information can be acquired at specialized
Cancer Centres as it presumably happens in 13% of the schools. This
would raise the number of schools with an integrated teaching of Oncology to about 20%, which is still a very low figure.

3 - Time dedicated to Oncology in the various Chairs

The distribution of answers in Fig. 1 illustrates clearly that only -
the professors in the surgical clinics dedicate an acceptable amount

TABLE 3 - Does your University Hospital have a Tumour Clinic, a Tumour Committee, a Coordinator of Oncology or is the Hospital affiliated to a Cancer Centre?

YES: 99 students (78%) from 12 hospitals (48%)

NO: 28 students (22%) from 13 hospitals (52%)

Type of Teaching Unit:

Tumour Committee	38 students (38%)	from 5 hosp. (42%)
Tumour Clinic	48 students (48%)	from 6 hosp. (50%)
Coordinator of Oncology	46 students (46%)	from 4 hosp. (33%)
Affiliation to Cancer Centre	44 students (44%)	from 6 hosp. (50%)
	* ⠀⠀⠀⠀*	* ⠀⠀⠀⠀*

* The totals are more than 99 students, 12 hospitals and 100% because several answers include two or more modalities.

TIME DEDICATED TO ONCOLOGY IN THE VARIOUS CHAIRS

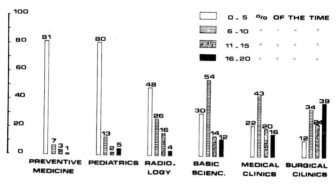

Fig. 1

of hours to the teaching of cancer, and that those of the medical sciences contribute to a lesser degree. But it is really amazing to see how poor the teaching of cancer in Preventive Medicine, Radiology and Pediatrics is.

4 - Teaching of Radiotherapy

Radiotherapy is one of the three orthodox and effective methods for - the treatment of cancer. In spite of that only 7 schools (22%) (table 4) give some kind of information to the students about this modality of treatment. In addition to that, in more than half of them, teaching is only theoretical, taking up less than 5% of the total studying time.

5 - Teaching in Cancer Chemotherapy

As shown in table 5, the teaching in cancer chemotherapy is almost as poor as that of radiotherapy. Only one third of the schools give "some" information about this treatment resource, which is one of the most promising weapons. Furthermore, in half of the schools, teaching is - only theoretical, with little time dedicated to it.

TABLE 4 - Teaching of Radiotherapy

Received some teaching in Radiotherapy:

YES: 51 students (40%) in 7 schools (22%)
NO: 76 students (60%) in 25 schools (78%)

Time dedicated to Radiotherapy in 7 schools:

1 - 5% of total time: 4 schools
6 - 10% of total time: 2 schools
11 - 15% of total time: 1 school

Teaching only theoretical: 4 schools

Teaching theoretico-practical: 3 schools

TABLE 5 - Teaching of Cancer Chemotherapy

Received some teaching in Tumour Chemotherapy:

YES: 82 students (64%) from 11 schools (34%)
NO: 45 students (36%) from 21 schools (66%)

Time dedicated to Chemotherapy in 11 schools:

1 - 5% of total time: 7 schools
6 - 10% of total time: 2 schools
11 - 15% of total time: 1 school
16 - 20% of total time: 1 school

Teaching only theoretical: 5 schools
Teaching theoretico-practical: 6 schools

6 - Does your University have a Tumour Clinic, Committee, Coordinator of Oncology or is the Hospital affiliated to a Cancer Centre?

From the 127 students, 28 (22%) answered NO (table 6). The remaining 99 who said YES came from 12 University Hospitals. It is really surprising that only less than half of the hospitals have some kind of Oncological Unit that would allow the students to become acquainted with the practical aspects of cancer management.

TABLE 6 - Kind of Teaching Units

78% of students from 12 hospitals (47%)

	% Stud.	% Hosp.
Tumour Committee	38	42
Tumour Clinic	48	50
Coordinator of Oncology	46	33
Affiliation to a Cancer Centre	44	50
	*	*

* Total more than 100% since schools include 2 or more types

7 - Contact with Cancer Patients

When questioned about the opportunities they had of being in contact with or taking care of patients having one of the 25 main sites of cancer, 20 students did not reply (probably because they did not have

the opportunity of seeing patients or because they did not remember
the exact figures).

In 28 of the remaining 107 answers the information is not useful for a-
nalysis, because they do not supply detailed figures, since they give
only a minimum, a maximum or an average of the total number of patients
seen. Therefore, only 79 replies were meaningful (Fig. 2). It is evident that there are big differences in geographical pathology amongst
the countries surveyed, still, there is not a single site of cancer
which has been seen by all the students. The most frequent sites in the
survey are stomach, leukemia, colorectum and cervix; but even in these cases at least four to eight students did not have the opportunity
to see patients with these localizations. And there are some sites,
such as bladder, penis, kidney, soft tissues that were seen by less
than half of the students.

fig 2

79 STUDENTS HAD THE OPPORTUNITY OF BEING
IN CONTACT WITH THE FOLLOWING NUMBER OF
PATIENTS OF CANCER

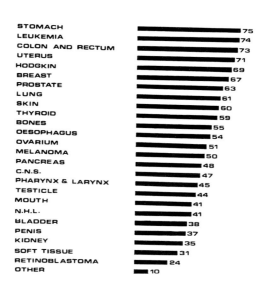

STOMACH	75
LEUKEMIA	74
COLON AND RECTUM	73
UTERUS	71
HODGKIN	69
BREAST	67
PROSTATE	63
LUNG	61
SKIN	60
THYROID	59
BONES	55
OESOPHAGUS	54
OVARIUM	51
MELANOMA	50
PANCREAS	48
C.N.S.	47
PHARYNX & LARYNX	45
TESTICLE	44
MOUTH	41
N.H.L.	41
BLADDER	38
PENIS	37
KIDNEY	35
SOFT TISSUE	31
RETINOBLASTOMA	24
OTHER	10

8 - Participation in Diagnosis

Students were then asked what opportunity they had to "observe", "take part" or "do themselves" any of the most common diagnostic procedures. As 25 of them did not give information on this point we have only
102 valid answers (Fig. 3).

Only two thirds, and in some cases only half of the students could observe these very important diagnostic procedures; and except for cervical citology, biopsies and indirect laringoscopy, less than 10% of
the students could perform them personally.

9 - Participation in Treatment

There were 25 answers without information about "observing", "taking
part" or "doing personally" some of the commonest therapeutic procedu-

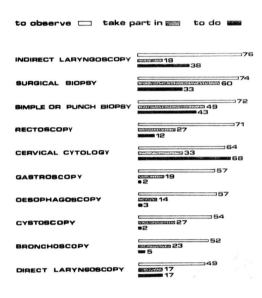

fig 3

102 students had the opportunity "to observe" or "take part in" or "do themselves"
the following diagnostic procedures

to observe ☐   take part in ▨   to do ▰

INDIRECT LARYNGOSCOPY	76 / 18 / 38
SURGICAL BIOPSY	74 / 60 / 33
SIMPLE OR PUNCH BIOPSY	72 / 49 / 43
RECTOSCOPY	71 / 27 / 12
CERVICAL CYTOLOGY	64 / 33 / 68
GASTROSCOPY	57 / 19 / 2
OESOPHAGOSCOPY	57 / 14 / 3
CYSTOSCOPY	54 / 27 / 2
BRONCHOSCOPY	52 / 23 / 5
DIRECT LARYNGOSCOPY	49 / 17 / 17

fig 4

102 students had the opportunity "to observe" or "take part in" or "do themselves
the following therapeutic procedures

to observe ☐ take part in ▨ to do ▰

gastroctomy, any type	75 / 69 / 0
hysterectomy any tipe	74 / 1 / 79
thoracocentesis	67 / 55 / 51
thyroidectomy any type	62 / 55 / 1
laparocentesis	61 / 46 / 51

fig 4 cont.

conization of the cervix	58 / 49 / 2
ovariectomy	55 / 58 / 4
mastectomy any type	53 / 53 / 3
pneumonect, any type	36 / 16 / 0
amputation for cancer	27 / 22 / 2
radium insertion or simil.	22 / 17 / 2
laringectomy any type	17 / 12 / 0
external radiation treat.	17 / 4 / 2

res, as listed in Fig. 4.

There is a great difference between the opportunities a student has
to "observe" or 'collaborate with' surgical procedures and those he has
in what concerns radiotherapy. Only one in five students can see an insertion of radium or treatment session of X-Ray or Telecobalt.

On the other hand, some students say that they "did" major surgical procedures, as mastectomy, hysterectomy, and thyroidectomy. It is obvious that this implies a lack of responsability of the professors.

10 - Teaching on Psychological Aspects

Only 24% (30 students) admitted to having received some teaching on this very important part of the management of the patient with cancer.

11 - Continued Education

Another of the questions sought to establish whether at their school they had meetings on cancer such as symposia, conferences, etc.; 99 answered YES (80%) and 27 said NO (20%). The participation in these - activities is compulsory in only two of the schools.

12 - Textbook of Oncology

Of the 119 answers received, 82 (69%) said that textbooks, sillabi , outlines, etc. for studying Oncology were available in their School - Library. The value of these books was classified as shown in table 7.

TABLE 7 - Cancer Books available at Schools are

(From 82 replies - 69%)

Excellent 12%
Satisfactory 34%
Acceptable 48%
Bad 4%
Very Specialized 2%

As a conclusion it must be pointed out that there is an urgent need of a textbook on cancer for medical students, written in spanish, keeping in mind the particular circumstances of Latin America's geographical pathology, the conditions of medical practice and hospital facilities for diagnosis and treatment.

13 - Acquired Knowledge of Cancer

This is one of the paramount aspects of this survey, since it represents the students assessment of how efficient they consider the teaching of cancer at their respective schools has been. The answers were as shown in table 8. No comments are needed on this point, because it is very significant in itself.

TABLE 8 - Acquired Knowledge of Cancer was

Excellent 0%

Satisfactory 8%

Mediocre 28%

Defficient 33%

Very Poor 31%

14 - Recommendations

The students were asked to express their ideas about what they considered most convenient to improve the quality of the teaching of Oncogy at their medical school. Some of the replies offer two or more proposals (table 9). What most of them suggested was the creation of a Chair of Oncology or that students should attend a Cancer Centre. The fact that only a small number mentioned Tumour Clinics can be explained as it was shown above, by the existence of these clinics in several hospitals.

TABLE 9 - Recommendation to improve Teaching of Cancer

(From 209 replies)

Create Chair of Oncology.......................51%

Through Cancer Centre..........................50%

Intensive Cancer Courses.......................26%

Oncologist coordinates Teaching in various
Chairs...24%

Cancer Committee or Cancer Clinic at University
Hospital.......................................11%
*

* Two or more replies are given

Physiological Effects of Mass Communication Media and Necessity for Changes in Education

Gustav Gebels

Psychologist, Bad Sooden-Allendorf, Federal Republic of Germany

ABSTRACT

Messages communicated by mass and education media are described and criticised, the psychological after-effects being adverse too frequently. Attempts made to motivate the public to avoid cancer fail. Wrong, and in many cases dangerous, approaches are discussed, indicating the necessity of an holistic psychotherapeutic approach before, during and after treatment. As yet too many neglect the significance of complete Rehabilitation! New medical and psychotherapeutic approaches have a hard time to be fully accepted by the medical schools! At the same time, false ideas spread quickly; too little is being done to correct every-body's wrong ideas about cancer.

INTRODUCTION

The "bad" is always given too much attention in communication; whether actual or not is entirely a different matter, and must be sufficiently emphasised, continuously, for society to become aware of the negative and harmful effects which all forms of mass-media can have on the subject "cancer". It takes time for the medical world to learn to accept new, positive approaches. More so the public. In many countries mass-media have tried to help, yet failed.

Questions to be asked are: Why is so much negative communication –issues of deep concern– not prevented? Has cancer finally been recognised as a real problem by society, or is it unnecessarily being turned into a social problem with the help of mass-media? Don't newspapers, radio-news, TV and other forms do anything else but create cancer-phobia, resulting in not being examined? Posters of Cancer-Societies, Newspaper-articles, Advertisements, etc. were shown, pointing out the wrong approaches. Examples are poster-headlines, such as: "Every third person will contract cancer! Every fifth person will die of cancer! Cancer is curable only if recognised on time!", or: "Every form of cancer can be beaten......The chance to win against cancer: Annual precautionary examination!", or even a third example: "Breast cancer can be healed only if recognised on time and treated correctly!" Here again certain questions arise. How soon is "on time"? How high is the chance to win against (what type of) cancer? How is it treated correctly? Can such posters not cause anything else but panic? Paroles such as these are completely wrong; health-propaganda should let facts speak for themselves, avoiding wrong guarantees. Too much fear-evoking news is reported day-by-day: e.g., quoting two German weekly-magazines: "Mastectomy was frightening, but what followed was nearly worse...", or

"Medical examinations for prostate-cancer are highly dangerous!!". The best-selling
daily newspaper in the Federal Republic of Germany continuously quotes "news" about
cancer, such as "CANCER! Three pupils found dead-- Have 11 others been infected?"
A leading Australian newspaper quotes a well-known Professor as having claimed:
"The cancer-patient's fate is sealed...".

During an International Conference on "Public Education about Cancer" in Monaco,
1974, it was noted that "the printed and spoken words are the poorest ways of
imparting information...". This statement must be contradicted, since, except for
scientific and actual news (e.g.: "..smoking is a hazard and can cause cancer,
therefore beware!"), mass-media have exactly opposite effects, being the best means
to sow panic. Printed words invite only minimum criticism by readers; radio and
films make out of millions a complete mass of silent, helpless listeners.Even after
succesful operations, the belief brought about through mass-media ("cancer is death,
therefore I must die...") can remain too strong. Growing subdued unwillingly, fear
of cancer resulting in painful death may be the beginning. Cancer, resulting in
painful death, may ultimately be the end.....

Wrong Medical Approaches
It is time for all to realise that medical technology is merely a means to an end;
it is not allowed to become an end in itself. Patients should be approached as
fellow-beings; recognition of psychic problems is necessary-- they cannot simply
be patched-up physically. As an example::a person had biannual breast-examination
for many years with negative results. Three months after her husband's death, bi-
lateral mastectomy had to be performed. As an "after-effect", a strong tremor in
both hands and arms resulted, with an unability to write legibly, or simply draw
straight lines even eight months after completion of treatment. Medical care included two strong antidedepressiva, thrice daily. No improvement showed until Psychotherapy with an holistic approach took over, although medical diagnosis blamed
scar-contractions. Combinations of Indirective therapy, Couè'sPositive Approach
and Autosuggestion, Music-psychotherapy,Gymnastica and other eurythmic exercises
all showed positive results; the antidepressiva could be reduced considerably with
success. This should point out the great need for more "synthetical" Psychotherapy,
avoiding one-sidedness. Much can be done to heal what is left to heal, but the will
to live on cannot be restored solely through pharmaceutica or other unilateral
approaches.

Rehabilitation
Rehabilitation has been recognised as an important step to achieve full acceptance
in society, yet the extreme importance of psychological rehabilitation with post-
operative cancer-cases is still largely neglected. The "European Forum on Sex-
Counselling for the physically Handicapped", held in Brussels, 1977, by leaders in
such fields, treated topics such as "Disabled Persons--Relationships and Sexuality",
"Attitudes with regard to Sexuality of the Disabled", "Pitfalls and problems of
Sex Counselling" and others. Yet not one of these mentioned cancer-cases and problems which could arise with these. In other words: people who have had cancer and
are on their way to recovery (if not fully recovered) are not regarded as such.
Results of cancer-operations are not seen as possible handicaps; Laryngectomy,
mastectomy, etc. are too frequently not regarded as disabilities. Instead, those
concerned,directly and/or indirectly, are frustrated by too many factors, including constant medical after-treatment, as well as frightening news from daily
literature..... Distress is influenced by mental processes; therefore mental readjustment is of utmost importance for individuals, groups, as well as the public
as a whole.

New Ideas
Compared to money and work put into research on cancer, too little is being done
to find out how to avoid it completely. Further, unorthodox methods are not easily

accepted by the medical schools (e.g., Dr. J. Issels and Dr.E.van Aacken, Federal
Republic of Germany, both supporters of an holistic, immunological approach;
Dr. A. Meares, Australia, on Meditation instead of Operation; Professor B.L. Reid,
Australia, on Microwaves to cure cancer....).

At a Cancer Congress in Bonn, 1977, Professor U. Veronesi noted that for over 50
years there existed a controversy on the correct treatment of melanoma--- either by
means of surgery or radiotherapy. During these years not one research project was
undertaken which could have led to accept either one or the other form of therapy.
Further: after a critical analysis of approx. 800 planned and to some extent
already published research reports, only a maximum of 40 reached the required
standards. From the total annual carcinoma cases of represented countries at the
said congress, exact controlled studies were only carried out with a maximum of 1%
of cases.. Veronesi thus concluded that numerous successful treatments are not even
known of by the majority -not to mention the word "understood"-, and therefore too
often not accepted by the medical establishments. The present president of the UICC,
Professor P.F. Denoix, commented at the said congress that many Oncologists have
completely neglected the area "Prevention of Carcinoma" for the sake of "Treatments",
"Cures", etc.

Too few countries have as yet concentrated on "prevention" or "avoiding cancer by
means of living correctly", paying attention to keeping physical and psychic
harmony in complete balance. The cynic would maintain that Surgeons and Radiotherapists also need to make a living!!

CANCER-PREVENTION
In answering a question such as "What is the best way to prevent cancer", the reply should definitely include: By thwarting any damaging articles and other forms
of communication through continuously retorting these, using the same as well as
other media, but correctly, avoiding the building up of fear, frustration, panic,
by restoring the masses's assurance, teaching them a positive approach to life,
and attacking the sources whenever fear-arousing news appears. It is indeed a pity
that sufficient Journalists, Medical Practitioners, Psychologists, Social Workers
and others -including Post-Operatives- have as yet not been found to assist. Rather
headlines such as C A N C E R ! improve sales; if colleagues are financially or
politically in any way supported, many may even assist in writing such negative
reports. Too many M.D.s make a living "treating" post-operative "patients" instead
of giving them a chance to become cured completely.

Modern man is in all respects an unique being: What can't be bought or sold ex-
pensively carries little weight. Therefore proper ways of life -the cheapest method
to avoid diseases, including cancer, by building up physical and psychic resistance
- are not good enough! As a result, people carry on, wasting away in an ageing process through heir own fault....

In Ancient China the highest-paid medical-practitioner was he who had to treat the
fewest in his locality, this having been real proof of having taught them how to
live correctly. This agrees with the views of a past German Surgeon, Ernst von
Bergmann, who once remarked: "The best Doctors are those who treat a person in such
a way that in future he can afford the most famous and most expensive Medical
Specialist, since he does no longer require his help...."

CONCLUSION

In conclusion, the following picture (Fig. 1) should be noted, painted by a cancer-
struck person who had noticed the harmful effects which others had created by
continuously talking about their own personal cases, each wanting to have had the

most alarming, most dangerous disease, each telling others any- and everything
about cancer, using own imaginations and that of others to spread all forms of
rumour. Imagination can magnify fear, rumours can make anything suspicious. Rumours
and imaginations can be strengthened from tongue to tongue, causing panic. Not
telling each other about cancer is regarded as equivalent to "not knowing the whole
truth. And this spreading of information by and amongst laymen, especially, can
cause grave harm and shoul be attacked by the Professional World. If nothing is
done, mass-media can easily lead to false ideas. If the wrong things are done, the
human impact of cancer-news can have grave effects, especially where phobias have
thus been caused and the disease has then set in. The lack of recognition can be
severe; persons not being seen as   fully healed without the right to rehabilitate (
("cancer equals death, therefore there's no chance for him/me to recover....") require especially psychological/psychotherapeutic treatment. What is said in numerous cases need not affect the individual.   The fact that completely untrue data
can arouse fear, anxiety and even panic, and this may further lead to a worsening
of the disease is not considered- not even by the greater part of the medical
profession, as yet. All such factors necessitate educational changes. Educational
changes with Patients and the Public. Educational changes with Students and Professionals. Including Oncologists.

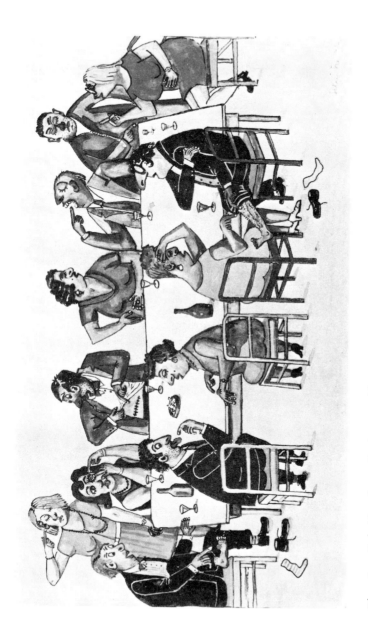

Fig. 1. Painting by a Post-operative cancer-case pointing out -according to her experience-
how all forms of "information" are spread by other patients,as rumours, imaginations,
possibly ending up as false information, evoking fear, anxiety and frustration and
preventing individuals from fully recovering through wrong beliefs.

Cancer Campaign

Reaching the Hard to Reach
(Chairman's Introduction)

R. L. Davison

*Executive Director, Manchester Regional Committee for Cancer Education,
Kinnaird Road, Manchester M20 9QL, England*

ABSTRACT

Cancer control implies the difficult task of changing the way people behave. If
people are "hard to reach" it is because there is a distance between ourselves as
communicators and those we wish to help. Distance can be physical, where large,
scattered populations are served by few trained workers, or in densely-populated
urban areas where the supply of workers is also inadequate.

Illiteracy also creates a communications distance; less obvious but no less real
is the problem of functional illiteracy where people can read, but do not. Psychological distance means that because of socially-transmitted fears of cancer, individuals avoid messages about cancer. And cultural distance raises further problems
when perceptions of health, the meaning of symptoms and definitions of illness may
differ widely between different sections of the same population and between professional workers and those they wish to help.

To reach people we must understand them. If a communication fails it is usually
the fault of the communicator, not the recipient.

CHAIRMAN'S INTRODUCTION

Effective cancer control, to prevent some forms of cancer and to maximise the potential for curing or controlling others, holds the promise of saving more lives
than does any one foreseeable discovery from fundamental research. Even though
this implies that most difficult of all tasks - that of changing the way people
behave - much has already been achieved, for many countries can point to improved
cure-rates through earlier diagnosis of cancer and to some success in programmes
of cancer prevention.

However, these successes have most often been achieved among sections of the population who are accessible to health education and whose members are able and willing to read or to listen to the message of cancer control. The problems of how to
reach the reachables have therefore largely been solved, and our main task here is
that of sustaining a steady educational effort. What is now of the utmost urgency
is that we should find ways of helping those who, for one reason or another, are
not reached or remain unaffected by such health education methods or messages as
many of us have relied on up to the present time. To narrow this gap and communi-

cate effectively is not easy, for, as Hyman and Sheatsley (1947) observed, "there is something about the uninformed that makes them harder to reach no matter what the level or the nature of the information". When the subject-matter is cancer, which even most of the "reachables" do not particularly want to hear about, our task is one of peculiar difficulty. But if our message of cancer control is to reach those who have not heard or do not understand it, then the initiative must come from us. We must build the bridges.

The description "hard to reach" implies that there is a distance, as yet not closed up, between ourselves as communicators and the specific target populations we wish to influence.

"Distance" in the sense we are discussing it today, can be of different kinds. It may be physical, where large territories inhabited by rural populations are served by very few trained health workers. But the difficulties of overcoming physical distance are not found only in large tracts of country. Many workers meet the same problems in our densely-populated cities and urban sprawls where trained work-ers are also in short supply, and the great problem is that of finding some means of access to those most in need of our message.

That the difficulties are rendered more acute when such populations contain a high proportion of illiteracy is obvious, for here some means must be found to spread the message by word of mouth. Perhaps less obvious is the problem of dealing with "functionally illiterate" communities. It is easy to assume that because universal schooling is provided in our country we can surmount our problems by providing app-ropriate literature, and that we can measure success by the volume of literature we distribute. But surprisingly high proportions of many communities are function-ally illiterate - they can read, but do not habitually gain information from the printed word. In such cases there may be a distance we ourselves are not even aware of.

But overcoming problems of geographical distance may not be enough. In every society there are individuals at a distance from our message because socially-transmitted misconceptions, fears, prejudices and superstitions make cancer a taboo subject, or at best do not encourage immediate action when symptoms appear. It is not difficult to understand an individual postponing a visit to the doctor if he believes cancer to be totally incurable and that the treatment he will receive cannot save him from an inevitably premature death. If he also experiences feelings of guilt and shame about cancer, (See, for instance, Peck 1972), then he will not only be even more reluctant to seek medical advice; he may also have been unwilling even to read or to listen to messages about cancer, however reassuring and encoura-ging their content.

Cultural distance is not only to be found in different perceptions of cancer. It is also present between different perceptions of the seriousness of symptoms and of the definition of illness. (See, for instance, Zola 1966). For example, a symptom that prompts a city worker who has a secure job to seek medical advice may well be dismissed as trivial by a nearby farmer whose livelihood depends on his own daily efforts. In the latter case messages that use the language and express the values of health personnel who are well educated and who are paid a salary for their work may well be virtually meaningless to him.

A knowledge of our specific target populations is therefore imperative if we wish to devise effective education for cancer control. No educator can do his job properly if he does not know something about those he wishes to teach. What do they know and believe about the subject? Is their existing information accurate? How do they feel about it? Are their attitudes such as to hinder or to help learn-ing? What are the pathways of everyday communications in their community? Too often in the past we have wrongly assumed that because we write and say certain things others will understand and act on our advice. But it has been well said that when a communication fails it is the fault of the communicator, not the recipient.

Our three main speakers today have each in their own way and in their own cultures recognised and tackled some of these problems in reaching the hard to reach. Some difficulties are common to all: others are peculiar to the widely different populations and cultures they serve. And though we recognise that what is appropriate in one country will not necessarily be effective in others, we know we shall gain from each presentation insights into reaching the hard to reach that we can take back and modify for use in our own programmes when this Conference is over.

REFERENCES

Hyman, H. and Sheatsley, P.B. (1947). "Some reasons why information campaigns fail". Public Opinion Quarterly II 412-413.

Peck, A. (1972). "Emotional reactions to having cancer". American Journal of Roentgenology 114 591-599.

Zola, Irving K. (1966). "Culture and symptoms - an analysis of patients presenting complaints". American Sociological Review. 31,65.

How to Reach the Hard to Reach

D. J. Jussawalla

Director and Chief Surgeon, Tata Memorial Centre, and
Hon. Founder-Secretary and Managing Trustee, Indian Cancer Society

For all practical purposes the subject is mainly concerned with mass communication efforts made in India to reach the vast pool of the rural population consisting of 80% of Indians who live in approximately 600,000 villages throughout the country, 70% of the people being engaged in agricultural pursuits.

To understand the magnitude of the problem and to clarify the issue, it will not be out of context to refer to the basic geographical and demographic data of the country, which is in fact a sub-continent, occupying 2.4% of the total land mass of the world, while striving to support over 15% of the population of our planet. 60% of the people are non-productive and only 12% of the working pool are covered by Central Health Insurance Schemes. To care for this colossal mass of humanity, only 30,000 physicians were engaged in medical practice at the beginning of this decade, giving an over-all ratio of approximately 1 doctor per 5000 persons, although in the large cities this proportion becomes a respectable 1 in 800.

A working force of 90,000 trained nurses is available (an increase from a mere 15,000 in 1950) and a total of 300,000 hospital beds are dispersed throughout the land. Medical colleges have been established at 110 centres (an increase from 61 in 1961).

On analysing 650,000 deaths that took place in the city of Bombay during the last decade, the incidence of cancer was found to have increased by a factor of 4, since 1950.

By 1961, cancer had come to occupy 6th rank as a cause of death. If, however, only the age-groups of 45 and above are analysed (the age after which cancer is most frequently encountered), the disease was found to be the third commonest cause of death, immediately following heart disease and tuberculosis.

The age pyramid illustrates the relatively young population:

$$0 - 4 \quad \text{years} \quad ... \quad 13.5\%$$
$$5 - 14 \quad " \quad ... \quad 24.8\%$$
$$15 - 54 \quad " \quad ... \quad 53.4\%$$
$$55 - 75 \quad " \quad ... \quad 8.3\%$$

The majority of the people live in approximately 575,000 villages, most of which have a population of between 500 and 5000.

Expectation of life at birth had by 1975 gone up to 52 years, and as the population as a whole gradually gets older, cancer will inevitably rear its head more frequently in the years to come. According to the population-based Bombay Cancer Registry, the crude incidence rate today is roughly 70 per 100,000, which on age correction according to the world population (UICC) rises to 135 per 100,000, clearly showing the effect increasing age of population can have on cancer incidence.

It is also evident that it is illogical in the circumstances faced by us today to try and undertake specific educational efforts in our villages for one disease entity alone, as the organisation called for will have to be so vast that only a general health-care and hygiene package deal becomes a practical proposition. Such, in fact, is the plan outlined by Government and the national voluntary anti-cancer agency, the Indian Cancer Society, for only undertaking general health educational activities (including those concerning cancer) in the villages throughout the country.

Rural India has been grouped for administrative purposes into 5000 blocks, and to facilitate the execution of public health measures each such unit is served by a primary health centre covering approximately 120,000 people and staffed by two qualified physicians, 4 trained nurses, 2 health visitors and 2 co-ordinators who, as a group, look after over a 100 villages in their area. Every such centre oversees 8 sub-centres, which in turn individually cater to about 12,000 villagers, with a health visitor and a nurse in attendance, and having additional help from the village head-man, who is traditionally the police officer, or the school teachers or other government employees.

The primary health centres refer their serious problems to a well-organised General Hospital, with diagnostic X-ray and clinical laboratory facilities, which functions at District level serving a number of administrative blocks where medical and surgical specialists are in attendance and the majority of cancers can be diagnosed and treated. Often, a major District Hospital of repute may drain a number of district areas. Each Indian State is divided into large Districts — again for administrative reasons — and the District Hospital serves as the medical headquarters of the area.

At the level of the individual larger village, the health care plan envisages the appointment of an individual trained as a health-care worker who may have the basic qualifications of a sanitary inspector, a health visitor or a pharmacist/compounder. He may be a resident of a neighbourhood village community and functions mainly as an adviser to the villagers on hygiene and preventive inoculations, and undertakes the implementation of these activities.

At the grass roots small village level, the village head-man or a respected elder or a midwife, after receiving the necessary basic training in hygiene and general health care, generally has the responsibility of looking after the simple every-day physical ills of the local villager. He/she is given training in the basic facts relating to preventive medicine, which includes maccinations and inoculations against infectious diseases and the essential tenets of hygiene and general health care.

One of the major problems facing the country today is illiteracy. If only the majority of the population could be taught to read and write, the communication problem would become much easier to resolve.

Under the present circumstances, however, the main problem is to establish an adequate mass communication network aimed at a target population which is poor, illiterate and continuously increasing in size at an alarming rate.

A recent survey of 400 villages undertaken by the Indian Agricultural Research

Institute reveals the fact that significant changes have occurred of late, in the attitude of the average Indian villager. He is nowadays more conducive to accepting new ideas and to following fresh progressive trends.

He also tends to be more practical than his forefathers and is willing to undertake new activities if he is personally convinced of their utility and benefit. This behaviour extends to all his actions on the farm, in his trade or in his home.

As the well-known sociologist Professor Richmond Hauser once commented, the Indian farmer is one of the most intelligent illiterates one could expect to find anywhere. To get through to this key individual, two avenues of approach are envisaged and both are being employed: the traditional and the technological.

Both have been tried out by sampling techniques and the best results would seem to be attainable by a judicious mixture of each.

A comprehensive controlled study was recently undertaken by the Indian Agricultural Research Institute and a fertiliser corporation, to assess the effectiveness of a variety of communication media in the rural set-up in India.

The conclusions reached are of great value to all those who plan to communicate with hard-to-reach target groups in developing countries. A short summary of the procedures undertaken and the design of the research project should prove illuminating. Eighteen villages were chosen for the study, together with four matched control areas. A number of parameters were chosen for study, such as:

a) the local caste structure, to examine different social strata and occupations;
b) the different sizes of land holdings, to examine the socio-economic situation;
c) the educational pattern existing in the area, to evaluate its impact on the
        population, and
d) the operative media utilised.

The gains in awareness, knowledge and symbolic adoption were then measured, after the involved respondents were fully exposed to the different media.

After collection, the data was coded to facilitate further analyses later at a suitable time, and a number of computer programs were developed to examine the data from different avenues. After conversion to standard scales, the extent in variation of the contribution made by the different media was examined in terms of awareness, knowledge, symbolic adoption and over-all effectiveness and an analysis of variance was also finally undertaken.

The following communication media were utilised in the study:

> Posters
> Wall paintings
> Pictorial exhibits
> Folders (pamphlets)
> Radio
> Film slides
> Film shows
> Group discussions
> Demonstrations
> Field trips.

The results were analysed from four angles:

1) Effectiveness of a single medium
2)   "   "   combination of two media
3)   "   "   combination of three media

4) Comparison with the non-exposed controlled group.

The field trip ranked first in creating awareness, whereas symbolic adoption of a new technology was best derived by field trips and demonstration techniques when paired together.

Demonstrations + slide shows ranked first in effectiveness jointly with field trips + slide shows.

In the three-media combination, radio + field trips + slide shows contributed the most in terms of overall effectiveness.

Cost analyses and cost-benefit ratios were also studied and a follow-up assessment was made, to examine the impact made on the villages from exposure to the various communication media at a subsequent visit, 8 to 10 months later.

The following conclusions were then drawn:

a) The majority of farmers exposed to the most effective media-mix were able to retain the new knowledge imparted to them.

b) Farmers exposed to the most effective media-mix were those who adopted the new teachings taught in the best possible manner.

c) Partial adopters were the ones who were exposed to media-mix of an effectiveness which was either or an average or low standard.

d) The majority of farmers had normally no access to any of the usual communication media and they had to rely for all information on their talks with friends and neighbours. As a result, all new knowledge was acquired by them through their exposure to the media-mix used in the study.

e) Farmers who did not adopt any new techniques pointed out constraints of inconveniences or insufficient credit to undertake the actions required.

f) The experiment could prove the fact that farmers were able to retain and apply the knowledge gained by them. Sufficient enthusiasm was also generated to motivate farmers to seek more information whenever needed by them.

This experimental study gives a direct pointer to the ways and means that could be used to REACH THE HARD TO REACH illiterate rural population in developing countries such as India, by utilising the traditional methods of communication so readily available today in most countries throughout the world.

Of the more sophisticated new communication technology, TV broadcasts via stationary orbit satellites are the most promising and have already been tested in India in order to reach the remote villages, where the vast majority of the population yet remains illiterate.

During 1975 and 1976, such special TV broadcast experiments called SITE (Satellite Instrumental Television Experiment) were conducted via an orbital satellite, through programmes directed to chosen villages in a number of Indian States, with the help of NASA in the USA and the Indian Space Research Organisation (ISRO), the All-India Radio and TV and a number of Central Government Ministries and State Governments. This was made possible through a commercial contract entered into between the U.S. and Indian Governments, whereby a satellite was placed in a pre-selected fixed orbit, from Cape Canaveral, above a chosen spot over Nigeria in Africa, in direct line with Nagpur, a city at the centre of India. Earth stations at Ahmedabad and Delhi were then asked to beam specially chosen educational programmes to this satellite, which beamed them back after adequate amplification. Such programmes were received in India in three ways:

a) by earth stations
b) by limited re-broadcast systems, and
c) by direct reception in selected village centres.

Although a number of snags soon became evident, on the whole corrective action
could easily be taken and the initial reaction in terms of software was most
encouraging. There was a lot of enthusiasm created among the villagers through
this experiment. After SITE was over in 1976 there was a great demand to continue
this service to the villages. Continuity is being provided by setting up new TV
stations and plans are also nearing completion to place domestic satellites over
India in 1979 to provide much wider coverage.

The main aim of this exercise initially was to provide information for four hours
per day on agriculture and health, in addition to entertainment in the local idiom.
Information on health problems was provided on general hygiene, on disease prevention and on family planning. In this general health package basic information on
cancer was also included.

It has now been agreed by Government and the Indian Cancer Society that information
on cancer shall form a part of the total health information package planned for all
the rural areas of the country. It was the unanimous opinion of all concerned
parties that to organise a separate cancer educational project would be too costly
and impractical in a developing country, which was poor, both in monetary and
trained manpower resources.

These efforts to establish communication possibilities were undertaken after
analysing the regional preference of the areas under assessment. The following
factors were found to be of great importance for successful implementation:

1) A knowledge of the profile of the target group (or what is better known as the
    consumer profile).

2) Creative and effective planning of the chosen message, so that the meaning can
    be clearly understood, believed and accepted by the target group.

3) The available variety of mass media in the target area and the possibility of a
    proper media-mix.

4) In the rural areas it is important to recollect that the end point target is
    the farmer and in the smaller towns, even if the average man is not directly
    engaged in farming, his indirect connection with the land and its productivity
    is considerable.

Reaching the Hard to Reach

Byron Lissaios

President of the Hellenic Cancer Society

SUMMARY

The following propositions have been the policy of the Hellenic Cancer Society
for the past years in our effort to reach the hard to reach.
a) To provoke the interest of the public by presenting the dark side
   of Cancer.
   Fear is probably the fastest way to achieve this goal.
b) To use public opinion to influence the media.
c) To educate public servants and politicians on the necessity of a
   national program on Cancer control.
d) To project the possibility of prevention and treatment of Cancer.
e) To maintain the Cancer campaign on a high scientific and social
   level.
f) To create at least a minimum of economic independence for
   competitive propaganda.
   These proposals have been the policy of the Hellenic Cancer
   Society for several years and have been met - in our opinion -
   with success.

The development of the subject requires the dissection of the
different targets .
Where are these people who for cultural or emotional attitudes
are allergic to confront the cancer problem ; Who present a personal
negative attitude and block any social effort of cancer fight ;
No one could accert - I presume -that this attitude is hereditary .
Then two possible possibilities: the environmental influence and personal susceptibilities,have to be considered.
Considering personal susceptibility,we understand that there are people who can not stand the sight of blood,a person in pain or even
hearing of a catastrophy .
Cancer for them is the taboo word,the one that must not be pronounced
or heard .Even if we accept that their comportement has to do with a
past experience over-emphasized by a weak constitution,these peaple

are of a minority,not to be taken on serious consideration in the mass
behavior we are interested in our discussion here .
Then it remains one and certain cause for the negative attitude of
people against cancer fight and this is the environmental influence.
We,the doctors and the difficulties of dealing withcancer patients
are the main cause of the negative comportment of the people .
Thiw attitude started some decades ago,when nothing was possible a-
gainst a disease of unknown origin,late diagnosis and high mortality.
As the incidence of the disease rise for different reasons,more peop
le comes in contact with cancer patients and this behavior is not going to stop unless we become able to humanize,socialize and make acceptable the face of the disease .The probleme is more difficult when
people with negative attitude against cancer have personal interest
or are on influencial positions and obstract any idea to ameliorate
the conditions of cancer control,proposing arguments that only ignorance or limited perception and knowledge could support them .
It seems then that the subject covers a non homogeneous group of people with the basic caracteristic feature their negative attitude to
any improvement in Cancer fight out of their narrow visual field .
This lack of uniformity of our target supports the idea that we have
to modulate a polymorphic plan into which each party must be considered according to its specific characteristics .
In our Society,Cancer is a new notion continually enriched by influential informations concerning its genesis and the different possibilities to confront it .Therefore it is not overestimated to consider
reaching the hard to reach as to sell something new to a difficult
client .Because reaching the hard supposes a continious fulfilement
of different necessities in the steps to follow,it must be accepted
as a good policy not to advertise something until it is at the shop`
s windows .
Each Cancer campain has as a final target the optimum cancer control
in a given geographical area .This optimum is usually measured by in-
ternationaly accepted criteria but in practice it is dependent upon
echonomical,technical and functional facilities which differ from
one country to another .
So - in our opinion - no cancer campaign has a promising future if it
is not promoted as a governement`s policy,no matter how enthousiasti-
cally it begins .Sooner or later it will have to face the obstacles
of some governemental policy on cancer if there is one .So-it seems
to me prepoderan that to over-run the first hard to reach is to make
cancer Campaign a governemental policy and to decide with the public
services the extend of its more appropriate level .It is here where
the first hard to reach reside .Persistance and patience are badly
needed in the effort to educate politicians and public servants .
The problem must be presented in a credible way utilizing evidence
either from similar experiences in other countries or from the economical,social and functional repercussions of cancer .
The comparison of the present condition with another more profitable
socially,economically and scientifically must be made to drive them
to the acceptance of the need for a national program on cancer control .
Although,personally,we don,t accept the necessity to policize medical or social matters,because in our opinion they contain biologically,I would say,the necessity of their confrontation I would not consider bad policy to make influential peope take political or social
credit and advantages from any important decision that could help the
realization of a national program on Cancer control .
Let me give you as an example the modus operandi for the tobacco/

cancer problem in a small tobacco producing country .
The one I have in mind takes a 5% of its annual national revenue from
tobacco .To persuade the political leadership to modernize its vues
in this social and health problem it was not sufficient to make them
aware of the deleterions effects of tobacco usage .
In our era consious acceptance of a social danger,either because it
is an accompaning phenomenum of more necessary measures,either for
profit or even pleasure is often socially and individually admitted .
But success - in the above example - resides in the way that the problem is presented .It is necessary to study and present the whole pro
blem from every possible side .National profit,working percentage of
the population from tobacco growing to cigarets selling,conditions
on cultivating,storing,packing,cigarets manifacturing and all these
in relation to export conditions in foreign countries,their habits,
their legislation and above all to confront the idea of public dis-
countent something that politicians cannot accept easily .All that
must be studied and presented by competent and desinterested people
because there is always danger to emerge with the other face of Janus
I used tobacco as an example of the necessary steps to take to persuade decisions making people on this particular subject .
In my opinion no cancer campaign has any possibility of success unless the state machinery is persuaded of the necessity of its existance,fears to be accused of insufficiency and finds political benefit .That means that people who undertake this responsibility must
not fear to usecontrolled persistant and patient pressure to promote
the necessities of cancer control .Attention must be paid to avoid
any personal projection for it is easy for any one to be accused for
personal benefit,social,political or even professional .
For that,persons who undertake the responsibility to educate the influential media must either posses the power to impose their ideas
or have scientific projection and social acceptance that will influence public opinion .Either way the oposition will be strong and will
depend on the strength,the influence and the morality of those with
different opinions .
High standing medical people is another group that could influence
adversely any coordinate efforts of cancer campaign.
They could do wrong by two ways:
a) Influence badly the common opinion
b) Give pretext to influential media to oppose any effort of organization in cancer control .
We think that the best way to fight all that is to challenge for comparison of their theories with facts and results that cancer campaign
must offer as a proof for the necessity of its existance .I say theories because bad critisism is always presented in abstract theoretical way and do not resist the comparison with any creative fact .
For this reason it is necessary to assure some social and economical
independance which will permit the realisation at least of a part of
what it is needed for an acceptable level of cancer control .Out-pa-
tient offices for detection,follow-up and out-patient treatments,nur-
sing at home,hospices for terminal cases,educational programs are
few examples to be exploited .
The projection of such facts is the more valuable way to oppose the
critisism of dubious value .
Donations,collects,any way of rasing funds,social events,social and
scientific manifestations are wellcomed and needed to procure the social standing of the campaign .
If and when the technical set up of a national program on cancer fight is ready that we can start to advertize to the public the benefits
of a cancer campaign .

Of a cancer campaign.
The possibility to reach this point by utilizing pressure of public
opinion -wich means that some program of public education must be run
in paralel with the education of influential milieu -is also to be
considered but without a national program every effort will atay in
a theoretical platform .
We come now to the moment when we must reach the people .
Anyone would like to deal with people with a consious participation
in prevention,detection and treatment of cancer but for different
reasons this is not the case .We must then move the interest of people on the cancer problem .
We have to mobilize the social interest of the common people and the
easier and faster way I know is fear .
Cancer and its complications must be presented in such a way that
could not leave indifferent the man in the street .
The frequency,the symptomatology,the evolution of the disease,its
complications,the condition of terminal cases and the different mechanism of death must be presented in some spectacular way .The dan-
gerto run of the track the public opinion has been proved unfounded
and on the other hand this effort has as an object to provoke the a-
dequat reaction for the acceptance of the following phases in public
education .
In our experience the phase of fear must not exceed the period of
two years but local conditions may influence its duration .
The next phase has as a target the education on the ways to prevent
and successfully treat cancer .This is the most difficult and sensitive phase because from its success depent the success of any future
effort .
Statistics,technical possibilities,spesialized centers,medical and
social personalities,cured patients are means to be utilized for the
success of this phase .
Information must be given in credible ways and presented to be easily consumed by the common people .
The idea that cancer is chronic disease from wich a lot of people-
under certain conditions-can be cured,a lot can live for years under
medical attention,provide moral and psychological help to recover the
loss of equilibrium the work "Cancer" provokes .
The possibility to confront the different complications of the disease and to help for the social rehabilitation of the patient are of
valuable mental and psychological strength for the patient and the
public .
I have tried in these few minutes,that have been allowed to me,to
touch the points of modulation of a general way by wich to reach the
hard to reach,rather to develop the different technicalities of such
an effort which naturally depend on a lot of local conditions .
In summary I would propose as an efficient way to reach the different
hard to reach the followings :
a) To provoke the interest of the public by presenting the dark sides
   of the cancer problem .Fear is probably the faster way to achieve
   this goal .
b) To use public opinion to press the decisions of influential media
c) To educate public servants and politicians on the necessity of a
   national program of cancer control .
d) To project the possibilities if prevention and treatement of cancer.
e) To maintain the cancer campaign on a high scientific and social
   level.
f) To create at least a minimum of economical independance for the

creation of provocative work for examplary and comparative exploitation .
      These proposals have been the policy of the Hellenic Cancer So-
ciety for several years and have been met -in our opinion - with
success .
                    Thank You.

Breast Cancer in Czechoslovakia

J. Švejda

*Research Institute for Clinical and Experimental Oncology, Brno,
Žlutý kopec 7, Czechoslovakia*

ABSTRACT

Breast cancer is the second commonest tumour in Czechoslovakia and its incidence
is increasing.   In 1965 the incidence was 32 per 100,000 but by 1975 it was
45 per 100,000. (Editorial note: These figures are low - perhaps they relate
to cases per total population.   It would be more usual to give the incidence for
women - which I should expect to be higher.)   In Czechoslovakia the cancer
control programme concentrates on prevention and early detection.   Despite some
evidence of success, it is still a serious problem that some women report their
symptoms late and prognosis is therefore poor.   Public education activity needs
to be developed - not only in Czechoslovakia but throughout the world.   The WHO
should encourage world-wide co-operation in this respect.

KEYWORDS

Experimental examination of the population, oncologicall program,
mammary committees, centres of clinical oncology, postgraduate anti-
cancer education.

INTRODUCTION

As in other countries also in Czechoslovakia the incidence of tumors
steady increases. In last time there are yearly in the czech part of
our republic 34 000 new registered malignancies and more than 26 000
persons die on tumors. The morbidity on neoplasmas increases yearly
about 2-2,5 %. There is also a steady increase in mortality, which
thanks the early diagnosis and improvements in the therapy is slower
than the increase in morbidity. The mean age of men who die on tumors is between 55 and 65 years, the mean age of women is between
45-55 years. These are 29 % from all death in men, and 42 % in wo-

men. The incidence of breast cancer is very serious and the cancer
is now the second most frequent tumor in women in our republic. Figure 1. shows the incidence of all new registered malignancies and
also the new registered breast cancers in the whole republic and
in its czech part in the interval of 10 years.

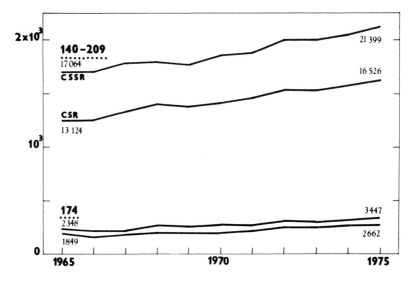

Fig. 1. Incidence of all new registered malignancies
        (140–209) and the new registered breast can-
        cers (174) in 10 years interval in CSSR and
        CSR.

The incidence of mammary cancer related on 100 000 inhabitants shows
the Fig. 2.

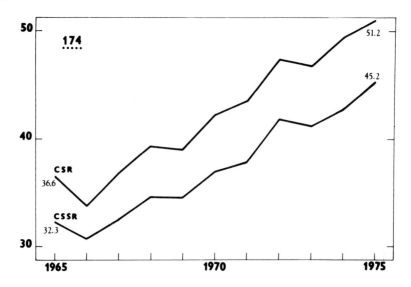

The age distribution of women malignancies and of breast cancer shows the Fig. 3.

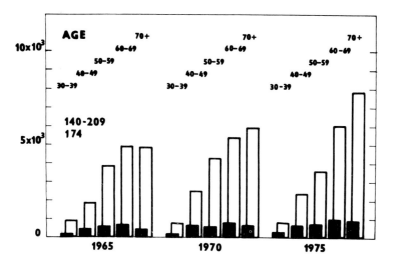

Fig. 3. Age distribution of all women malignancies (black columns) and breast cancer
(white columns) in 10 years interval.

The number of new registered cases of mammary cancer in the Oncological Institute in Brno during last forty years shows the Fig. 4.

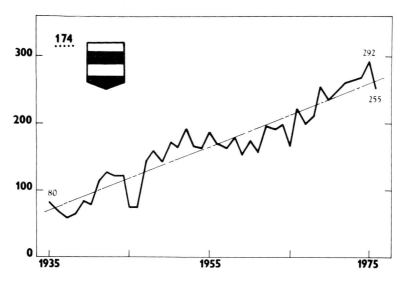

Fig. 4. New registered mammary cancers in the Oncological Institute in Brno in the interval
of 40 years.

DISCUSSION

The early diagnosis of the cancer remains therefore the principal
demand in the fight against this disease and the old problem how to
manage it gains more and more on importance. There are two possibilities: The examinations of the whole population, or the examination of the high risk groups. Two years ago the oncological program was established in our country with the aim to achieve a gradual dispensarisation of all population and to utilize the inter-
disciplinar teamwork of particular medical branches in oncology.
The main part of the program is the prevention through oncological
examinations to find out the precancerous lesions or the early stages of tumors.

The prevention is carried out in two directions:
a) The examinations of patients who are hospitalised for other
   diseases.
b) The experimental oncological examinations of selected groups of
   the population.
These examinations started two years ago in four districts of our
country and include women 30-64 years old and men between 40-64
years. In the year 1976 there were 46 327 persons examined (17 877
men and 28 450 women). New malignancies were registered in 110 cases (0,23 %), the precancerous lesions in 1840 cases (3,97 %). There were registered also some other diseases, e.g. hypertension,
diabetes and so on. Eighty one percent of persons were healthy. The
positive results may be seen not only in the discovery of new tumo-
rous lesions, but also in the deepening of the cooperation of medical staffs of various branches and in the introduction of some new
diagnostic methods or in their better exploitation. The action goes
until now without greater difficulties, but there is a question if
the technical equipment will be able to satisfy all these very
extensive tasks. As far as these examinations are for the present
in the experimental stage and the first evaluations were yet carried out, the only reasonable way remains therefore the examination
of high risk groups. The main problem is to find out the criteria
of the high risk. According to our opinion the van der Linde's
(1977) criteria would be the most suitable. The criteria include
the demographic and familiar factors, the factors connected with
pregnancy and suckling, the factors concerning the ovarian function
and predisposing breast lesions (fibrocystic disease with epithelial proliferation) and also the factors concerning the ionising
radiation. Independently on van der Linde (1977) we are using the
principal data of these criteria in our register. A very good work
in the early diagnosis of the breast cancer was done in our institute by the mammary committee which was established ten years ago.
It consists from a team of experts of various branches who once in
a week judge all suspect cases and establish the first diagnosis
which is verified by mammography, thermography by mens of liquid
crystals, by cytology and biopsy. The committee recomends also the
first steps in therapy, which is later approved or completed by the
whole medical staff of the institute when the case is discussed at
the general visite. The committee examines yearly about 700 patients sent to its consultary service by physicians or from some medical centers. In the year 1968, 201 new cases were registered, in
the year 1975 there were 292 cases. The committee has now 4 expec-
tant beds where suspected cases are under observation and 12 spe-

cial mammary beds destined for chemo and actinotherapy of patients
who are outside the area of our institute. From the therapeutical
point of view there were recently established chemotherapeutical
and immunotherapeutical procedures for stage I. a II. which will
enable a serious evaluation of the treatment. By stage III. the
therapeutical procedures are individual. To the mammary committee
belongs the so called advisory board for breast diseases which
functions twice in a week, controls the patients and returns relap-
ses to the mammary committee and to therapeutical departments. The
committees are now established nearly in all hospitals of our country. The action of the committees is connected with the action of
centres of clinical oncology established two years ago in all district hospitals. Members of the center are the experts of the hospital staff under the leadership of a district oncologist. The aim of
the center is not only the early diagnosis of all malignancies, but
also a suitable therapy. In this respect the centers ought to collaborate with our institute which publishes the methodological hints
as far as the diagnosis and therapy of particular tumors concerns.
In spite of all these arrangements it is necessary to remark on the
fact, that there are women who come to the treatment with an advanced cancer. The reasons are partly in women, partly in physicians.
The women do not pay enough attention to the lesion and do not con-
sult the physician at time. We pay therefore more and more attention to a reasonable anticancer education of the population and
stress the selfexamination of the breast as one of a very important
factors. As far as the physicians concerns it happens that the signs
of the disease are underestimated and the patient is sent to the
mammary committee or to the oncological center too late. The post-
graduate education is therefore by our Ministry of Health very
emphasized and is also one of important tasks of our institute which
in this respect collaborates with the Institute for Postgraduate
Study of Physicians in Prague.

CONCLUSION

The dangerous increase of breast cancer requires not only these regional arrangements, but needs a close international cooperation.
Here perhaps through WHO it will be necessary to establish a data
bank, general criteria of high risk groups, to find out the modes
how to bring women to regular examinations, to establish the principal methods for early diagnosis and to establish principal standard therapeutical processes. All these arrangements require the
cooperation with the departments of oncological epidemiology and
with the basic research. It is an enormous task, however it is necessary to start and so more, that a great work was yet everywhere
done. I believe that by connection of all these efforts and by a
real cooperation, good results may be achieved.

REFERENCES

Anderson, D. E. (1977). Genetics and the etiology of breast cancer.
   Breast, 3, 27-41.
Barth, V., R. Müller, H. K. Deininger, and P. Wöllgens (1974). Klinik, Mammographie, Cytologie, Stanzbiopsie und Plattenthermo-
   graphie in der erweiterten Mammadiagnostik. Dtsch. med. Wschr.,
   99, 175-180.
Levin, M. L., and D. B. Thomas (1977). The epidemiology of breast

J. Svejda

cancer. In A. C. W. Montague, Stonesifer, G. L., Lewison, E. F.
(Ed.), Breast Cancer, Vol. 12, A. R. Liss, Inc., New York. pp.
9-35.

Linde van der, F. (1977). Definition der Bevölkerungsgruppen mit
hohem Risiko beim Mammakarzinom. Schweiz. med. Wschr., 107,
962-968.

Moskowitz, M., S. Pemmarajn, P. Russel, L. Gardela, P. Gartside,
and S. DeGroot (1977). Observations on the natural history of
carcinoma of the breast, its precursors and mammographic coun-
terparts. Breast, 3, 14-19.

Prevention: Responsibilities and Methods

Nigel Gray

Director, Anti-Cancer Council of Victoria

The concept that people should take personal responsibility for their own cancer control - the early detection or prevention of their own cancers - is a very attractive one, but the process whereby they can be induced to take such responsibility is much more complex than it seems at first sight. The process involves well researched education programs, sometimes an extension into propaganda and, every so often, politics.

Whether or not we like the fact that the extension of education into propaganda was pioneered by Dr. Goebels, it is true that when you take a policy stance which attempts to induce the public to take personal responsibility for their own cancers, you are attempting to induce a behaviour change. This is not simply a process of education. In inducing behaviour change we are not merely giving people information and allowing them to modify their own behaviour as they think fit, we are attempting to persuade them to modify their behaviour as we think fit. We should not argue about definitions, but this is a very strong form of persuasion that we are using. We have got to be very sure of the scientific basis of the arguments on which the case rests before embarking on any sort of program which induces people to take responsibility for a process of early detection or prevention. Three programs warrant closer scrutiny. -

* Cervical cytology is properly based on science in this day and age, although, through the retrospectoscope, the evidence on which we introduced it was probably inadequate by today's standards.

* The program which aims at persuading people to undertake self-examination of the breast (BSE) has everything going for it because, first of all, it is a harmless process. Secondly, all the biological probabilities are in its favour. Thirdly, there is some scientific evidence which demonstrates the efficacy. However, when we approach the sort of cancer detection program which induces people to come in and accept even a tiny dose of x-ray, we have to be very sure of our scientific ground, since x-ray is a carcinogen of itself.

* Smoking control programs are, of course, amply justified both socially and scientifically and have been now for some decades.

1.   Cervical Cancer

The fact that people can be persuaded to accept responsibility for their
own cancer detection is best exemplified by the success of cervical
cytology which has been widely accepted by women in some countries (in
some contrast to BSE) - this, despite the fact that cervical screening
requires a visit to the doctor or clinic, invasion of privacy, sometimes
discomfort, and sometimes a fee, whereas BSE can be conveniently performed
on the bed or in the shower.

When the program began in Victoria only 15% of smears were initiated by
doctors, whereas now about 50% are.   This reflects establishment of the
procedure in medical practice and removes some of the need for a public
education program.

The success of cervical cytology can be seen from the following tables -

Penetration rates -

Table 1

Percentage of Population Screened Once

Aberdeen	90%	(1973)[1]
Jefferson County	90%	(1970)[2]
British Columbia	80%	(1974)[3]
Victoria (Australia)	62%	(1974)[4]

From a public health point of view these overall rates are impressive.

Table 2 shows the penetration rate by age for one or more smears in
the State of Victoria (Australia)

Table 2

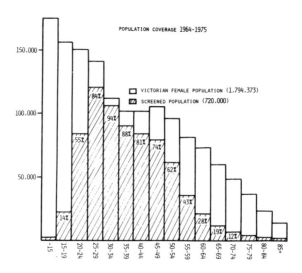

The percentage of the screened population (normal smears only) who had more than one smear is shown in Table 3

Table 3

Total women with 1 or more normal smears   676,611

1	smear	352,304	52%
2	smears	220,850	32%
3	"	67,000	9%
4	"	24,300	3.5%
5	"	8,510	1.2%
6	"	2,625	0.3%
7	"	725	0.1%
8	"	200	–
9	"	67	–
10	"	23	–
more than 10		7	–

To complete the picture, mortality in Victoria is shown in Table 4

Table 4

Mortality rates for Carcinoma of the Cervix in Victoria

5-year moving averages/100,00 total female population.

	20-49 years	50+ years
1965	5.17	21.10
1966	4.87	21.43
1967	4.72	30.94
1968	4.50	20.74
1969	4.41	20.81
1970	4.09	21.05
1971	3.69	20.16
1972	3.59	20.09
1973	3.01	20.87

While many would be disappointed by a repeat smear rate of slightly less than 50%, the natural history of the cancer involved is such that mortality can be reduced significantly despite sub-optimal penetration rates, and presumably almost abolished in that segment of the population which conforms to the recommended program of approximately biannual smears.

This program indicates clearly that people can be persuaded to take responsibility themselves and that the cooperation of the medical profession is an obvious co-factor.

Figures given, however, relate to affluent societies in which the incidence of cervical cancer is low to moderate. Some of the developing countries have a much higher incidence rate and would benefit substantially if the population would accept this type of program.

Clearly such a program could not be introduced to developing countries without being established as a pilot project, and an assessment needs to be made in advance of potential acceptance of the scheme.

2.   Breast Cancer

There are two important differences between the programs available for breast cancer and those for cervical cancer. The first is that there appear to be much more difficult psychological obstacles between cancer societies and their target population for breast cancer. Secondly, there are alternative methods of screening. Those exemplified by the HIP program are somewhat complex, require women to visit a central clinic and be subjected to x-ray to the breast. Despite this somewhat cumbersome program, 45% of those offered screening in the HIP Study participated in the full program. The major problem arising here is that the acceptance rates need to be higher for breast cancer since screening frequency is of critical importance and continuing practice of BSE is an important part of the program.

The alternative of a relatively cheap health education program involving BSE alone is attractive and one which, theoretically at least, could solve the screening frequency problem. Of course, the cancers detected by a BSE program would be a somewhat different group from those detected by an HIP program, but the predictable results[5] are good and delivery of the program ought to be within the resources of most cancer societies.

However, a health education program involving BSE is probably the ultimate in asking the population to take personal responsibility, and persuading them to do this is not as easy as it looks. In Victoria, approximately one-quarter of the female population appears to practise self-examination regularly. We have this information from a sample of 412 cancer patients and from a random survey. In an endeavour to boost this figure a rather complex psychosocial research program[6] was established with the intention of defining the obstacles which lay between us and the target audience.

The process of research, which has occupied several years, has given us some insight into the situation with women in my own State of Victoria. In asking ourselves why women do not behave as we felt they ought to, and why they did not accept the message we offered them so readily, we developed some special videotapes for use as test material. These tapes were made as experimental tools, they are not television advertisements, they are trigger tapes which were shown to small groups of women in order to extract their reactions to the situations portrayed. The tapes, therefore, do not offer solutions or conclusions. They left questions up in the air because we wanted to examine women's reactions; their reactions being obtained by a relatively complicated questionnaire. The analysis of the whole program can be boiled down into a single slide in which are the obstacles found which existed between us and our target population. There were seven of these obstacles :

    *   Uncertainty about ability to use the technique.

    *   Trivialisation of symptoms by doctor.

    *   Fatalism and pessimism as to benefits of treatment

    *   'It couldn't happen to me'

*   BSE screening arouses anxiety in some people.

*   Many women believe that any lump is a cancer.

*   Fear of male's reaction to treatment.

These seven obstacles are the target of a television program, including one advertisement aimed specifically at each one. They have been pre-tested but the program is now only beginning. It is impossible to even speculate upon the eventual level of regular BSE which may be achieved.

Only time will tell us how successful this program will be, but the basic message is quite simple. We are proceeding on the premise that women CAN be persuaded to take personal responsibility but they need to be encouraged in this by a carefully designed program which requires an analysis of cultural factors IN THE SOCIETY WHERE THE PROGRAM IS TO TAKE PLACE. I am doubtful whether the same obstacles as were found in the Victorian BSE program would necessarily be found in other countries, but imagine that others could well arise.

3.   Smoking Control

To come to the third area, which is the most obvious one and the one on which we have all worked hardest. This is prevention of smoking. We run into a very different psychological, sociological and political milieu. We are not offering a message to an acquiescent public without any obstacles and we have an additional and powerful obstruction in this situation; that is the tobacco industry.

We are trying to shrink the tobacco market and the tobacco industry is trying to do the opposite.

How do we persuade people to take personal responsibility for cancer prevention in this situation? It is easy enough to address a rational message to an adult and to ask an adult to give up smoking and thus take personal responsibility. Here are some Australian figures on how successful this process has been

SMOKING HABITS BY AGE AND SEX IN PEOPLE
OVER 16 YEARS. (PERCENTAGES)*

		TOTAL	AGE										
			16-19	20-24	25-29	30-34	35-39	40-44	45-49	50-54	55-59	60-69	70+
SMOKE CIGARETTES	MALE	41%	36	49	44	46	44	39	43	43	35	32	28
	FEMALE	29%	29	38	37	30	29	27	33	37	25	16	10
SMOKE CIGARS AND/OR PIPES	MALE	4%	1	3	5	6	4	6	4	3	5	4	3
	FEMALE	-	-	-	-	-	-	-	-	-	-	-	-
EX-SMOKER	MALE	22%	11	12	14	15	19	21	24	28	32	37	44
	FEMALE	10%	9	9	8	10	16	9	9	7	11	11	9
NEVER SMOKED REGULARLY	MALE	33%	52	35	37	32	33	33	29	25	27	26	24
	FEMALE	60%	60	52	55	59	54	63	58	55	63	72	79

* AUSTRALIA-WIDE SURVEY OF 3316 MALES AND 3037 FEMALES, JUNE-JULY, 1974.

Associated with this establishment of assistance in persuading people to take their own responsibility, we have had to do a lot of other things. In particular, we have had to try to remove the propaganda weapon of the enemy as this is a potent obstacle to our schools program. Whoever wins the battle for the minds of our children affects the smoking habits of the next generation of adults. If we wish them to be responsible we have to teach them early. If we fail, the tobacco industry wins.

There is a third area where we can help people take responsibility. We can ask them to smoke low-tar cigarettes. This is only possible if low-tar cigarettes exist. In general, they only exist where public and political pressure has been applied to the tobacco industry. Table 5 illustrates this. -

Table 5

Tar Content of Cigarettes

Country	Tar Range
Australia	5 - 22 mg
Philippines	26 - 44 mg
United Kingdom	4 - 34 mg
United States	1 - 21 mg

I think it is reasonable to say that the adult public have taken a lot of notice of us and have lowered smoking rates substantially over the years. This process has happened in most of the countries where there has been a widespread public education program. However, this sort of adult education program depends on the communications network which exists in sophisticated society but doesn't exist, for example, in an island community like the Philippines. So it is not going to be as easy in the Philippines to run a public education program as it is in America where we have the use of the media, a controversy which in many respects works in our favour, and we have an educated public able to appreciate our arguments.

The second area involved in getting people to take personal responsibility for their smoking habits is a much more difficult one because smoking habits are _established_ in childhood and adolescence. We are, therefore, trying to get people to take responsibility for their own cancer prevention at an age when, in the eyes of the law, they are not responsible enought to vote, to work, to leave school, to fight in the army or do a lot of other things such as drink alcohol. So we are faced with a substantial dilemma. Most of us have resolved this dilemma quite simply and satisfactorily by running school programs and our difficulties have been in designing practical and effective school programs.

Many cancer societies feel that a conflict exists between an anti-smoking program and one which encourages the use of low-tar cigarettes among the addicted. In practice, public health programs need to be tailored to their environment but low-tar cigarettes cannot be ignored as a public health weapon.

So, to sum up, this particular form of establishment of responsibility in the population requires us, first of all, to fight the politicians and the tobacco industry. Secondly, we have to design what is virtually an information cum propaganda program which _works_ among young people

who, at that stage, are too young to take the responsible decisions
that we are wanting to thrust upon them. Thirdly, we have to
organise and get together all the anti-smoking pressures we can think of
which will help us to lower smoking rates among the young. In other
words, we are fighting a war in this situation and we are using every
reasonable weapon we have. The rights of the non-smoker, for example,
has not a great deal to do with the health of the non-smoker. It is,
in fact, a sociological downward pressure on the smoker and on the
smoking rates of the community and the reason we use that weapon is simply
that we are fighting a war, that we are convinced our motives are
correct and our objectives are correct.

To summarise the whole situation, I would say that it is not enough to
expect people to be rational in their responses. You can't expect people
to take personal responsibility for their actions unless you inform them
of the rational basis underlying that program, unless you use a well-
researched information program which will make sure that your message
is translated correctly and not messed about with on the way. You have then
got to take certain areas and go beyond the area of education into the
field of propaganda which involves moral decisions and, finally, in the
case of tobacco, you have to fight a sociological war to get rid of the
opposition because one thing is absolutely certain - that is, no schools
program is going to succeed in the face of sophisticated opposition of
the advertising industry and the media.

Hence, the conclusions:

1.   Cancer mortality can be reduced if people will take personal
     responsibility for their own welfare.

2.   People may be _induced_ to take personal responsibility.

3.   The induction process may require substantial psychosocial research.

4.   Good programs need to be delivered.

5.   Opposition from tobacco promotion needs to be removed.

References:
1.   Macgregor, J.E. "Problems and results of comprehensive screening for
     cervical cancer." Joing European Assembly, Cyt.& Cancer Prev.
     Austria. July, 1973.

2.   Christopherson,W.M. et al. "Cervix cancer death rates and mass
     cytologic screening." Cancer 26: 4, 808-811, October, 1970.

3.   UICC Tech. Rep. Series, Vol16. Geneva, 1974

4.   Victorian Cytology (Gynaecological) Service, Annual Report 1974.

5.   Duncan, W., Kerr, G.R. "The curability of breast cancer." BMJ.
     2: 781-783. 2/10/76.

6.   Hill, D., Todd, P. "A psychological investigation of womens responses
     to the threat of breast cancer and self-detection procedures."
     Australian Cancer Society, 1976.

Cancer Prevention: Responsibilities and Methods of Industry

M. Habs

Institut für Toxikologie und Chemotherapie, Deutsches
Krebsforschungszentrum, Im Neuenheimer Feld 280, 69 Heidelberg F.R.G.

ABSTRACT

Together with the continued development of industry the risk of inducing occupational cancer diseases by pollutants at the working place
increases. Also the industrial pollution of the environment with carcinogenic substances has to be taken into consideration. Already existing hazards can be detected by epidemiological studies and verification of the results in animal experiments. The aim should be to dis-
close possible cancer hazards of new chemical products by means of
biologic investigations and to prevent a cancer risk at the working
place or for the general public by implementing appropriate methods.
At present there seems to be no satisfactory alternative for long-
term animal experiments to predict toxic, in particular carcinogenic
effects. In case of substances with a known possible cancer risk for
man expert groups should decide individually which measures are best
suited to minimize or exclude health risks. Complete exchange of information and cooperation in the field of toxicology are urgently
required to detect possible hazards in time and to shorten the period
between the discovery of a hazard and its world-wide elimination.

KEYWORDS

Cancer prevention - industrial responsibilities - occupational cancer -
cancer in the general population - epidemiology - animal tests -
risk-benefit ratio - legislation - expert groups.

It has been suggested that four out of every five cancers in man have
their origin in the environment and only a small proportion thereof
amounting to less than five percent is so-called occupational cancer
(Clayson, 1967; Preussmann, 1975; Higginson, 1969; Wynder and Gori,
1977).

The evidence for this statement consists of epidemiological surveys
and animal experiments. However, it does not seem to be worthwhile
to argue on the exact percentages of tumors of industrial origin
since at present it is perhaps impossible to establish a convincing
figure and - much more important - intervention against these can-

cers seems possible.

Without any doubt "pseudoexperimental exposures" of workpeople in a number of occupations have proven the existence of industrial carcinogens.

In the last years public has become increasingly interested in the role of industry in cancer prevention. A possible cancer risk from industrial sources cannot only occur at the working place but also for the population via pollution. In the following table chemicals for which carcinogenicity to man or a strong suspicion of carcinogenicity to man has been found are shown.

TABLE 1   Chemicals Known or Suspected to Induce Cancer in Man and Occupational Risk

Chemicals carcinogenic to man	Occupational exposure
Aflatoxin	
4-Aminobiphenyl	+
Arsenic	
Asbestos (crocidolite, amosite, crysotile)	+
Auramine (manufacture of)	+
Benzene	+
Benzidine	+
Bis(chloromethyl)ether	+
Cadmium oxide	+
Chloramphenicol	
Cyclophosphamide	
Chrome (chromate-producing industries)	+
Hematite (mining)	+
Melphalan	
Mustard gas	+
2-Naphthylamine	+
Nickel (nickel refining)	+
N,N-Bis(2-chloromethyl)2-naphthylamine	
Stilbestrol	
Vinyl chloride	+
Soot and tars	+

Out of 21 compounds, for 14 exposure was solely or mainly occupational. Tomatis (1977) reviewed last year the data of 296 chemicals on which the International Agency for Research on Cancer had prepared 12 monograph volumes in the last years. For 145 compounds of these 296 chemicals there was experimental evidence of carcinogenicity. For about 20 of these chemicals production figures are well over 500,000 kg per year and for about 120 compounds that were carcinogenic under experimental conditions he stated occupational exposure.

For years industry was blamed for polluting air and water with chemical carcinogens. However, at least in most of the industrialized countries in the last years a lot of money was spent in order to reduce the environmental burden by known carcinogens of industrial origin. Unfortunately the benefits of the chemical industry have been accompanied by serious accidents as shown in the following table.

TABLE 2   Industrial Cancers: Examples of "Accidents" in the Last Years

Bis(chloromethyl)ether	⟶	Lung cancer
Vinyl chloride	⟶	Haemangiosarcomas
Asbestos and other "fibers"	⟶	Mesotheliomas

These results clearly underline the need for identification of possible carcinogenic hazards from industrial origin.

Retrospective epidemiological studies in combination with monitoring of harmful compounds have identified most of the known oncogenic occupational agents. These investigations help to identify already established hazards and sometimes allow to quantify the impact on human health. In the past results from those studies were a basis for preventing further hazards for the workmen or the general population. In most circumstances waiting for human evidence of carcinogenicity means accepting a continuation of human exposure to possible carcinogenic compounds. Therefore, our aim should be to avoid epidemiological evidence for industry-related tumors in man.

Bioassays have to be undertaken to detect the carcinogenic potential of agents to which man is exposed in order to protect human society against hazardous compounds. As a matter of fact all chemical carcinogens - with few notable exceptions - which are shown to be active in man are also active under experimental conditions in animals (Schmähl, 1977). It seems, therefore, prudent to assume that there is a possibility of a carcinogenic effect in man for any chemical that is shown to be carcinogenic in animal tests. It has been established that more than 700 new chemicals with an originally new chemical structure are introduced into industry every year. Bioassays of new products and intermediates for industrial processing should help to identify risks. Development of alternative products and sufficient protection of the general environment as well as for the people living in the working area, including personal hygiene, can help to reduce cancer risks from industrial compounds.

It is beyond the aim of this report to discuss the present state of the testing for carcinogenic potentials. In my opinion today there seems to be no satisfying alternative to long-term tests for possible carcinogenic effects of new compounds (Schmähl and Habs, 1977). Experimental tests with animals are believed to the more relevant, the more they reproduce the conditions of human exposure. On the other hand, if a substance causes cancer in one of the established animal test models it should be considered as potentially carcinogenic to man until it is retested under more sophisticated and appropriate conditions (Schmähl, 1970). Subcutaneous injection, probably the most simple and less expensive long-term test in rodents is often quoted as an example of an unreliable route of administration. IARC compared test results for potential carcinogens after different modes of application. In 15 compounds of 102 chemicals considered the carcinogenic results obtained were false-positive or false-negative if compared to observations after other routes of exposure (Tomatis, 1977). Therefore, it was stated that the subcutaneous route is not much worse than any other route and in any case a lot better than the alternative of not testing new compounds in long-term tests at all. With respect to the extrapolation of animal data to man, in future comparative metabolic studies seem to be increasingly important.

I do not want to comment on the value of short-term tests for pre-
dicting carcinogenic hazards to man. In my opinion as long as they
have a 10% risk of missing the carcinogenic activity of a test compound I would abstain from using these tests as alternatives to long-
term animal models (Sugimura et al., 1976). The value of short-term
tests as prescreening models is yet questionable. If not all newly
developed compounds can be tested adequately further information, as
e.g. the assumed yearly production rate of the chemical, its possible
spreading in the environment, its likely contact to humans etc.,
should be taken into account in order to establish a preference list
for long-term testing.

Comparison of legislation dealing with likely carcinogens in the working environment shows different legislative measures taken with regard to various carcinogens, differences among the legislation of
various countries, and differences in the periods of time between the
discovery of a carcinogen and its legislative regulation. In only a
limited number of the 14 countries that were investigated by Montesano and Tomatis in 1977 there existed a legislation which specifically prohibits the manufacturing of chemicals shown to be carcinogenic or likely to be carcinogenic to man. The legislation does not
cover the same chemicals in the individual countries. In addition,
in only four of 14 European countries considered both the importation
and the manufacture are prohibited. Some chemicals for which carcinogenicity has been proven are still produced in large quantities. Lack
of legislation should not limit the responsibilities of industry in
order to prevent cancer from industrial sources.

From the viewpoint of a scientist it is unacceptable that a carcinogenic risk from a certain compound is restricted by political borders.
Cooperation and exchange of information are necessary to reduce the
periods of time between the identification of a hazard and its ban.
In case of doubtful products we think it more desirable at present
to decide each case separately with the assistance of expert groups
rather than to release automatic regulative mechanisms by a too strict
legislation which from the viewpoint of the scientist are partly in-
comprehensible. The benefit-risk evaluation and considerations on the
tolerable concentrations of pollutants at the working place or in the
environment can only individually be regulated in a suitable way.
Therefore, a close and trustful cooperation between scientists from
the industry and legislative organs is highly desirable.

REFERENCES

Clayson, D.B. (1967). Chemicals and environmental carcinogenesis in
    man. Europ. J. Cancer, 3, 405-415.
Higginson, J. (1969). Present trends in cancer epidemiology. In Proc.
    8th Canadian Cancer Conference, Honey Harbor 1968, Pergamon of
    Canada, Toronto. pp. 40-73.
Montesano, R. and L. Tomatis (1977). Legislation concerning chemical
    carcinogens in several industrialized countries. Cancer Res., 37,
    310-316.
Preussmann, R. (1975). Chemische Carcinogene in der menschlichen Um-
    welt. In Handbuch der allgemeinen Pathologie, Vol. VI,2, part 2.
    Springer Verlag, Berlin-Heidelberg-New York. pp. 421-594.

Schmähl, D. (1970). Entstehung, Wachstum und Chemotherapie maligner
    Tumoren. 2nd ed. Editio Kantor, Aulendorf, F.R.G.
Schmähl, D. (1977). Toxicology in cancer research. Interdisciplinary
    Science Reviews, 2, 4, 305-311.
Schmähl, D. and M. Habs (1977). A critical review of the present state
    of the testing for carcinogenic potentials. In The Evaluation of
    Toxicological Data for the Protection of Public Health. Ed. W. J.
    Hunter and J. G. P. M. Smeets, Pergamon Press, Oxford-New York-
    Toronto-Sydney-Paris-Frankfurt. pp. 59-63.
Sugimura, T., S. Sato, M. Nagao, T. Yahagi, T. Matsushima, Y. Seino,
    M. Takeuchi and T. Kawachi (1976). Overlapping of carcinogens and
    mutagens. In P. N. Magee et al. Fundamentals in Cancer Prevention.
    Tokyo University Press, Baltimore. pp. 191-215.
Tomatis, L. (1977). The value of long-term testing for the implemen-
    tation of primary prevention. In H. H. Hiatt, J. D. Watson and
    J. A. Winston (Ed.), Origins of Human Cancer, Cold Spring Harbor
    Laboratory. pp. 1339-1357.
Wynder, E. L. (1977). Cancer prevention: A question of priorities.
    Nature, 268, 284
Wynder, E. L. and G. B. Gori (1977). Contribution of the environment
    to cancer incidence: An epidemiological exercise. J. Natl. Cancer
    Inst., 58, 4, 825-832.

Cancer Prevention: The Outlook in France

J. S. Abbatucci

Professor of Radiology, Caen University of Medicine, Chief,
Department of Radiotherapy, Director of Centre François
Baclesse, Route de Lion-sur-mer, 14021 Caen Cedex, France

INTRODUCTION

Cancer prevention can be approached in two ways :
- the first consists in identifying environmental elements that are known to be carcinogenic, and eliminating them (primary prevention).
- the second, in identifying tissue lesions likely to lead to invasive cancers, and eradicating them (secondary prevention).

CARCINOGENIC FACTORS

In the industrialized countries, specifically in Europe and in France (Higginson, 1977; Tubiana, 1978; Tuyns, 1970) in particular, it has been possible to group the principle carcinogenic factors into 4 main categories :

TABLE 1. Cancerogenic factors in western Europe

Occupational cancer	< 4 %	
professional (<2 %)		
air or diet pollution (2 %)		Environmental
Tobacco - alcohol	30 to 50 %	factors ∿ 80 %
Diet factors (unbalance, etc...)	30 to 40 %	
Non environmental factors	∿ 20 %	

The first category comprises occupation-related cancers and those linked to respiratory of digestive pollution. This category accounts for 5 % of cancer incidence. Preventive action is the responsibility of society, and, especially, of the industries at fault, and should essentially be implemented by means of regulations and legislation.

Although professional cancer represents less than 2 p. 100 of the total cancer incidence it must be pointed out that this category deserves the best attention for preventive action. There are two main reasons in doing this : the first is that it is the society duty to protect his workers, at any costs. The second is that the professional exposition to the various potentially carcinogenic agents represents a kind of experimental model, since the concentration of these agents are often a

thousand times greater than in the general environment. Thus it can act as a sort
of alarm system which allows taking general preventive measures much earlier.

The second category, which is the most important in our country, is related to tobacco usage and alcoholism, which, together, are responsible for 50 % of all cancers in males. Preventive action here is the responsibility of both society and the
individual.

The third category covers diet-related factors, which are probably responsible for
30 to 40 % of cancer incidence. Epidemiologic and experimental researchers are able
to collect increasingly reliable data, and there is room for hope that they will
succeed in finding preventive measures, but it is, as yet, too early for generalized
action .

The fourth category is related to non-environmental causes such as genetic and
constitutional factors. Some 20 % of cancer cases fall into this category, and at
present no means of prevention is known.

CARCINOGENIC FACTORS AND PRIMARY PREVENTION

In France, our particular concern is with the factors of the 2nd category, that is,
alcohol and tobacco.

Alcohol

Epidemiological studies (Lassérré, 1967) have revealed a marked correlation between
alcohol mortality and cancer mortality in France.

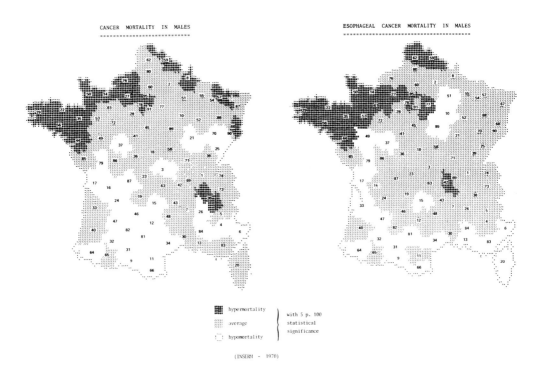

Fig. 1. Alcohol mortality and cancer mortality in France.

This correlation is particularly apparent in esophageal cancers and incidence of
this disease is 3 times higher in France than in the rest of the world. The regions
of Brittany and Normandy are the most afflicted areas with an average rate of 30
per 100.000, with peaks exceeding 60 per 100.000 (Barrellier, 1974; Tuyns, 1973) in
certain places. Epidemiologic research has shown a correlation between this phenomenon and intake of pure alcohol which is accentuated in the case of specific types of spirits, suggesting the presence of carcinogenic substances in the latter.

Preventive action thus consists in informing the public of the risks, collaborating
closely with anti-alcoholic's organizations and, at the same time, undertaking dissuasive action to discourage excessive consumption of alcohol. Sales taxes on li-
quor are one of the ways of doing this, although thus far they seem to have had a
limited effect. A recent law introducing random alcohol tests for drivers may turn
out to play a significantly dissuasive role, if one can judge by the reactions of
restaurant and cafe owners who have claimed a drop in sales.

Finally, another appropriate action is the promotion of research into the presence
of carcinogens in certain alcoholic beverages; their elimination would be an added
help to cancer prevention.

Tobacco

TABLE 2. Estimate of Tobacco Related Mortality in France

Cancers	18.500
Cardiovascular diseases	20.000
Respiratory diseases	15.000
Other	7.500
Total	60.000

A series of studies on tobacco-related mortality in France were summarized by the
Ministry of Health, and the following estimates were given : it would seem that some 60.000 annual deaths can be ascribed to tobacco usage, of which 18.500 are from
cancers.

TABLE 3. Breakdown According to Tumor Location

Cancers related to tobacco usage	Cancer risk for smoker compared with non-smoker	No of annual deaths	No of annual deaths ascribed to tobacco usage
Lung	10	10.000	9.000
Oral cavity	4	1.500	1.000
Pharynx	7	2.000	1.500
Esophagus	4	4.500	3.000
Larynx	10	3.500	3.000
Bladder	2	2.000	1.000
Total		23.500	18.500

Cancer risk is 10 times higher for smokers that for non-smokers in cancers of the lung and larynx, 7 times higher in cancer of the pharynx, 4 times higher for oral cavity and esophageal cancers and 2 times higher for bladder cancers.

These sites account for a total of 23.500 cancer deaths; 18.500 of them, that is, more than three-fourths, could theoretically be avoided by the elimination of tobacco. Total morbidity due to tobacco intoxication costs around 90 millions dollars.

In response of these findings, the French Government launched an extensive anti-smoking campaign, which, if it is to be of any effect, will necessarily be long term. In 1975, the Ministry of Health initiated a number of programs as part of the first stage of a series of operations that are to be implemented in the years to come. Several media campaigns have been launched to sensitize the public, especially on Television. A bill was passed in July 1976 to regulate and limit tobacco advertizing and to safeguard the rights of non-smokers.

The principle lines of action of the anti-tobacco campaign are :

To convince the public of the dangers of tobacco-smoking for the smoker and his environment.

To encourage non-smokers to speak out and to insist on their rights :

TABLE 4. Rights of Non-Smokers - Bill of September 17, 1977 (15 Ministries involved)

Smoking not allowed in :
Rooms for collective use Public schools and colleges Hospitals and sanitary institutions Food stores 50 p. 100 of seats in public transports 100 p. 100 in town transports Lifts

To demystify the glorified image of the smoker.

Two target populations were given special attention : the young, and pregnant women.

A series of polls and surveys adressed to adults and young people between 10 - 17 years of age were conducted to assess the impact and results of this national information campaign. Public reception was found to be excellent and memorisation very high (higher than for any other national interest campaign led to date). Demystification of the image of the smoker has gained amongst the young; the number of smokers in the general population has begun to drop.

Successive polls will be conducted to follow the evolution of the changes in personal behavior and tobacco sales figures. However, a decrease in mortality cannot be expected before the year 2000.

Extensive research into the subject of combined effects of tobacco and alcohol has demonstrated that the carcinogenic effect of alcohol and tobacco is synergic.

Risks of cancer of the mouth and pharynx is 15 x greater for persons who are both heavy smokers and drinkers (Bonneterre, 1976; Rothman, 1972).

Tuyns and co-workers of the IARC (1977) have shown that the combination of alcohol and tobacco results in a much greater increase in the risk of esophageal cancer than would be obtained by a simple addition of the effects of each. This risk is considered as being equal to 1 for a person who does not smoke or smokes less than 9 cigarettes per day and who does not drink or drinks less than 40 g. of alcohol per day; this risk is multiplicated 44,4 times for a smoker of more than 20 cigarettes drinking more than 80 g. of alcohol per day.

Then, it is clear that our preventive action should essentially be focused on combatting the two major factors which are responsible for close to 50 % of cancer incidence in male in France.

Public education and information, with the aid of the necessary psychologic studies, are the two fundamental means to accomplishing this. However, it is equally urgent that this effort be backed-up by appropriate legislation, as is currently being done in our country.

PREVENTION OF CANCER BY ERADICATION OF PRE-CANCEROUS LESIONS

The second aspect of preventive action has not received the same systematic and generalized attention in France as the first, and more satisfactory methods of cancer detection are still to be developed. The Centre François Baclesse, aware of the acute nature of the problem, is in the process of organizing a conference, "Cancer Detection : in search of the best methods" to encourage reflexion on the subjet. The conference, organized under the auspices of the National Federation of Cancer Centers will be held in Caen from April 6-8, 1979.

Prevention, in the true sense of the word, consists in detecting those lesions which are not yet malignant but which, in faire probability, could develop into cancerous tumors.

More broadly, the early diagnosis of invasive carcinomas could also be included in this definition. However, it would seem that preventive action in this direction is only really worth while in the case of curable disease, such as cancers of the breast and uterus, and even then, we cannot be sure that prognosis would be significantly affected (Denoix, 1974). For cancers that are only rarely curable such as tumors of the lung and esophagus, early diagnosis does not, at the present time, seem to obtain better chances of cure; in these cases, it would be better to target the etiological factors as the source of the problem : tobacco and alcohol.

In France today, our efforts to promote cancer detection are generally oriented towards encouraging the general practitioner to a fuller participation in screening programs. There is no doubt that the family physician is in the best position to carry out simple screening procedures during routine check-up; cancer screening in this situation is also much less likely to trigger cancerophobic reactions.

However, this presupposes a well informed physician, and the availability of university-level and graduate courses that would provide him with the training needed to carry out the required procedures. The Ministry of Health has directed the medical departments in all the universities to institute appropriate programs.

Two of the screening procedures falling within the competence of the general practitioner, in addition, of course, to the complete clinical examination, should be given special emphasis : instruction in self-examination of the breast; cervical smears.

Breast self-examination has been recognized as being one of the most effective ways to increase the chances of early cancer detection. The Ministry of Health has published a brochure on the subject, and has also distributed several instructional films.

Instruction in this method should also be given to the family doctor, who has a major role to play in its dissemination.

Cervical smears can also easily be carried out by the family doctor once he has received the necessary training. However, a generalization of this practice would imply a substantial increase in the number of cytologists and technicians, and would thus pose training and organizational problems that are, as yet, beyond our scope.

The Cancer Commission of the Ministry of Health headed by Professor Tubiana, conducted studies on the cost-effect relationship of a generalized screening program for cervical cancers in France (Brunet, 1975); it was estimated that it would take 15 years for the effectiveness of the program to compensate for the costs incurred in its implementation.

In the meantime, until a program of this nature can be envisaged - if indeed, it is found to be worth while - the Ministry of Health has published a brochure for young couples planning to get married, in which future brides are urged to have cervical smears as part of the general medical check-up required for the delivery of the prenuptial certificate which was made mandatory by Ministerial decree in March, 1978.

A recommendation is now beeing distributed to all the collectivities which possess a medical department, such as factories, farmers associations, universities, etc... to make sure that a gynecological examination is performed every 5 years at least.

It must be reminded that it is also of usual medical practive to check the cervical smears before every prescription of oral contraceptive and at periodic times thereafter.

CONCLUSION

As it can be seen, priority is given to primary cancer prevention in France. Current epidemiologic studies, such as those underway at the IARC, amply demonstrate the enormous etiological importance of tobacco and alcohol usage, which, together, are responsible for close to half of the cancers occuring in Western Europe, and in France in particular.

Special attention is also focused on detection of pre-cancerous lesions of the cervix. But, systematic screening for early cancerous lesions, for which we are still to find the best methods, is clearly relegated to second place, and all the more so because of the heavy financial investments involved in the setting up of programs whose efficacy is yet to be demonstrated.

Clearly, public information and education must be accorded top priority in preventive programs, and this action should be backed-up by appropriate legislative measures, the fight against cancer is, first and foremost, a matter of both personal and social responsibility.

REFERENCES

Barrellier, M.T. (1974). Le cancer de l'oesophage en Basse-Normandie. Essai d'étude de pathologie géographique. Thesis, Caen.
Bonneterre, J. (1976). Alcool, tabac et cancers. Revue Générale et bibliographique. Thesis, Lille.
Brunet, M. (1975). Dépistage du cancer du col de l'utérus. Monographie Santé Publique I.N.S.E.R.M., Paris.
Denoix, P. (1974). Prévention et dépistage des cancers. Rapport de la Commission du Cancer, Ministère de la Santé.
Higgison, J., and C. S. Muis (1977). Détermination de l'importance des facteurs en-

vironnementaux dans le cancer humain : rôle de l'épidémiologie. Bull. Cancer,
64, 365-384.
Lassérré, O. and co-workers (1967). Alcool et cancer. Etude de pathologie géographi-
que portant sur les départements Français. Bull. INSERM, 22, 53-60.
Rothman, K. ans A. Keller (1972). The effect of joint exposure to alcohol and tobac-
co on risk of cancer of the mouth and pharynx. J. Chron. Dis., 25, 711-716.
Tubiana, M. (1978). Cancer et environnement. To be published.
Tuyns, A. J. (1970). Cancer of the esophagus : further evidence of the relation to
drinking habits in France. Int. J. Cancer, 5, 152-156.
Tuyns, A. J., and G. Massé (1973). Le cancer de l'oesophage en Ille-et-Vilaine.
IARC Internal Techn. Rep. 73/003.
Tuyns, A. J., G. Pequignot, and O. M. Jensen (1977). Le cancer de l'oesophage en
Ille-et-Vilaine en fonction des niveaux de consommation d'alcool et de tabac.
Des risques qui se multiplient. Bull. Cancer, 64, 45-60.

Detection: Mass Screening and High Risk

A. B. Miller

NCIC Epidemiology Unit, University of Toronto, McMurrich Bldg., Toronto, Ontario M5S 1A8, Canada

ABSTRACT

In Canada the current approach to breast screening is that further evaluation is required. Priority must be given to the reassessment of benefit from mammography and physical examination in women age 40-49 and in women over the age of 50 an assessment of the independent effect of mammography. Current knowledge on high risk groups does not permit adequate discrimination between women at low and high risk. All women age 40 or more, therefore, have to be regarded as of high risk and potentially eligible for screening.

For cancer of the cervix we now have evidence of reduction in mortality attributable to screening. A Task Force has recommended that all sexually active women age 18 or more should be encouraged to enter a screening programme and examinations subsequently scheduled according to whether they are "at-risk" or in the "high risk" sub-group. Although cancer of the cervix is not as important a cause of mortality as it used to be, screening from an early age may prevent a future increase in mortality.

Breast neoplasms, Carcinoma in situ, Cervix neoplasms, Cytodiagnosis, Cytology, Mammography, Mass screening, Public health.

BREAST CANCER SCREENING

In Canada there is increasing recognition that the mere fact that a cancer is discovered by some sort of approach to early detection or screening does not necessarily mean that the individual concerned has been benefited. Although this is a difficult concept to accept for many clinicians there is a basis for concern over the fact that some screening programmes may only succeed in prolonging the period of observation of a case and may even in some instances bring to light disease which would have remained undiagnosed, thus increasing the total of morbidity. In Canada, therefore, we are examining very carefully the evidence for the efficacy of mass screening, being well aware that even in a relatively rich country our resources are finite and dollars spent on mass screening are not, therefore, available for other health or possibly more important community directed projects. These problems are well illustrated by the two sites we are considering today.

In Canada breast cancer is the most important cancer in women and indeed is the most important cause of death from any cause in women aged 35-54. Thus, if anything, we have a greater incentive to launch mass screening programmes than in Czechoslovakia where breast cancer is the second most important cancer in women. Over the years there has been an increasing tendency, led by the public education programme of the Canadian Cancer Society, to encourage women to present early to their physician if they discover an abnormality in the breast. The effect of this is difficult to evaluate particularly in a situation where the mortality from cancer of the breast has been stable for the last thirty years at least (Health and Welfare, 1976). In areas in North America where cancer registration data has been available for many years, there is evidence of increasing incidence of breast cancer particularly in post-menopausal women (Cutler, Christine and Barclay, 1971; Barclay and others, 1975; Grace, Gaudette and Burns, 1977). Although this, in conjunction with stable mortality rates, has been interpreted as evidence of increasing efficacy of treatment or the impact of earlier diagnosis, it is indeed possible that the process I spoke about earlier in relation to screening may be affecting our approach to the diagnosis of breast cancer and that in fact what we are seeing with increasing incidence is the impact of changing diagnostic practices.

In 1974, an Ad Hoc Committee of the Canadian Association of Radiology recommended that breast cancer screening should not be adopted as a public health policy in Canada but that the National Cancer Institute of Canada in collaboration with Health and Welfare Canada should develop appropriate investigations to evaluate its impact (Leger and others, 1974). In spite of this, largely through publicity crossing our extensive border with the United States, physicians and in some instances entrepreneurs have promoted the use of mammography not only for diagnosis but also for the examination of asymptomatic women. This policy has come under attack because of its expense, because of the lack of proof of efficacy in women under the age of 50 and because of fears of radiogenic hazards of mammography. For this reason, the health care insurance commissions are increasingly moving to decline payment for such services in the absence of defined indications.

Currently the Canadian Cancer Society in Collaboration with the College of Family Physicians of Canada is promoting the use of breast self-examination throughout the country. Population surveys have indicated that although many women are aware of the need to perform breast self-examination, the majority do not know how to carry out the examination correctly. It is obvious that family physicians have a major role to play in teaching women the correct approach. Fears have been expressed that this approach may increase the extent to which benign abnormalities are biopsied particularly in younger women without necessarily having any effect on malignant disease. Unfortunately at present, there are no plans for evaluating this as a public health procedure.

Nevertheless, the evidence on the efficacy of mammography combined with physical examination in the Health Insurance Plan Study in New York in women over the age of 50 (Shapiro, 1977) and increasing evidence from the U.S. Breast Cancer Demonstration Detection Projects that mammographic screening produces a reasonable yield of early disease, (Working Group, 1977) at least in terms of its ability to detect cases, encourages the hope that breast cancer screening may make a substantial impact on reducing mortality from the disease. A number of investigators, therefore, have collaborated in designing a large scale controlled clinical trial to evaluate the independent effect of mammography in women over the age of 50 and the efficacy of screening by mammography plus physical examination in women under the age of 50. Because of the high costs of this study it is not yet known whether or not support will be obtained. However, in its absence both the National Cancer Institute of Canada and Health and Welfare

Canada have declared themselves as being opposed to the wide spread adoption of public health screening practices (Miller, 1977).

Our knowledge of the epidemiology of breast cancer does not unfortunately enable us to discriminate effectively between women at high and low risk for breast cancer. Indeed in many respects it is apparent that in our population, once women reach the appropriate age group, they must be regarded as at high risk particularly in comparison to the risks in other countries. Research, however, is still proceeding in the hope that we may eventually be able to distinguish women who are at high risk and possibly restrict our screening approaches to them.

SCREENING FOR CANCER OF THE CERVIX

For cancer of the cervix, Canada has been particularly active especially with the pioneer programme in British Columbia which commenced in 1949 and which became population wide with the help of the local division of Canadian Cancer Society towards the end of the 1950's (Fidler, Boyes and Worth, 1968). The Canadian Cancer Society has actively encouraged women across the country in the last decade to attend their physicians for regular pap smears and we now have evidence that the programme has indeed contributed to the on-going reduction in mortality from cancer of the uterus which has been observed in Canada for some years (Miller, Lindsay and Hill, 1976). The evidence for this was assessed by a special federal provincial task force on screening for cancer of the cervix which made specific recommendations on the future conduct of the programme, designed to concentrate screening on women at high risk as evidenced by their exposure to recognized risk factors and the extent to which abnormalities were discovered on smear (Task Force, 1976). These recommendations were as follows:

1. Initial smears should be taken on all women over the age of 18 who have had sexual intercourse.
2. If the initial smear is satisfactory and without atypia, a second smear should be taken about a year later.
3. Providing the initial two smears and all subsequent smears are satisfactory and without significant atypia, further smears should be taken at approximately 3-year intervals until the age of 35 and thereafter at 5-year intervals until the age of 60.
4. Women over the age of 60 who have had repeated negative smears may be dropped from a screening programme for squamous cell carcinoma of the cervix.
5. Women who are not at high risk should be discouraged from having smears more frequently than is suggested above.
6. Women at continuous high risk should be screened at least once a year.

The Task Force carefully defined what is meant by "risk". In practice the "at-risk" group for cervical cancer that should be kept under surveillance are all sexually active women between the ages of 18 and 60 who have not had a hysterectomy for benign disease with complete removal of the cervical epithelium.

Smears are largely taken by family physicians though it is recognized that under some circumstances it is appropriate to use nurse practitioners for this examination providing they have been appropriately trained, as are utilized in Peru.

In general, an approach to screening through factories as in China is not encouraged mainly because the proportion of the Canadian women employed continuously in one particular type of occupation is small, there being high mobility in and out of the work force. Thus it is far more appropriate to base a screening programme on family physicians. However, with increasing experience, as in China, there has been a trend to more conservative treatment of lesions discovered on screening with an efficient cone-biopsy generally being regarded as being sufficient therapy for carcinoma in situ providing adequate post treatment cytological surveillance can be ensured. In addition, for the earlier lesions, particularly the various grades of dysplasia identified by cytology, there is increasing tendency to develop special clinics where colposcopically directed biopsies and treatment with careful cytological control are carried out. With an increasing tendency for lesions to be found in young women, presumably because of the changing sexual mores of our younger population, it is important that such conservative approaches to treatment should be encouraged. In British Columbia colposcopy clinics have now been set up in various parts of the province to ensure the availability of this technique to the total population while in most urban areas in Canada colposcopic consultations are now available.

It is recognized that with diminishing mortality carcinoma of the cervix is not as important a condition as it used to be. Indeed it is now sixth in the list of female cancers as a cause of premature mortality in Canada. However, in the light of the frequency of detection of abnormalities in younger women it seems possible that were it not for our screening programme we would already be beginning to see an increase in disease in the young. Indeed there have already been isolated reports of this in populations which have not been adequately screened (Yule, 1978). It thus seems necessary to continue our programme but ensure it is efficient and directed to those at greatest need in order to ensure the greatest impact. Providing this can be achieved, cost benefit calculations confirm that screening for cancer of the cervix can be regarded as an efficient and important public health approach to the control of the disease (Miller, 1979).

REFERENCES

Barclay, T.H.C., Black, M.M., Hankey, B.F. and Cutler, S.J. (1975). The
    increasing incidence of breast cancer in Saskatchewan. Proceeding XI
    International Cancer Congress Florence 1974, Vol. 3. Excerpta Medica,
    Amsterdam. pp. 282-288.
Cutler, S.J., Christine, B. and Barclay, T.H.C. (1971). Increasing incidence
    and decreasing mortality rates for breast cancer. Cancer, 28, 1376-1380.
Fidler, H.K., Boyes, D.A. and Worth, A.J. (1968). Cervical cancer detection
    in British Columbia. J. Obstet. Gynaec. Brit. Cwlth., 75, 392-404.
Grace, M., Gaudette, L.A. and Burns, P.E. (1977). The increasing incidence
    of breast cancer in Alberta, 1953-1973. Cancer, 40, 358-363.
Health and Welfare Canada (1976). Cancer patterns in Canada, 1931-1974.
    Bureau of Epidemiology, Laboratory Centre for Disease Control, Ottawa, p.
    151.
Leger, J.L., Naimark, A.P., Beique,R.A., McFarlane, D.V., Miller, S. and
    Miller, A.B. (1974) Report of the "ad hoc" Committee on mammography. J. Can
    Assoc. Radiol, 25, 3-21.
Miller, A.B. (1977) Present Status of Breast Cancer Screening. Canad. Med.
    Ass. J., 117, 845-846.
Miller, A.B. (1979) An Evaluation of Population Screening for Cervical
    Cancer. In. D.V. Coleman and L. Koss (Eds), Diagnostic Cytology in Modern
    Clinical Practice, Butterworths, London, In Press.
Miller, A.B., Lindsay, J. and Hill, G.B. (1976). Mortality from cancer of the
    uterus in Canada and its relationship to screening for cancer of the cervix.
    Int. J. Cancer, 17, 602-612.
Shapiro, S. (1977). Eivdence on screening for breast cancer from a randomized
    trial. Cancer, 39, 2772-2782.

Task Force appointed by the Conference of Deputy Ministers of Health (1976)
    Cervical Cancer Screening Programs. Canad. Med. Ass. J., 114, 2-28.
Working Group (1977). Report of the working group to review the NCI/ACS
    Breast Cancer Detection Demonstration Projects, submitted to the Division of
    Cancer Control and Rehabilitation, NCI.
Yule, R. (1978) Mortality from Carcinoma of the Cervix. Lancet, 1, 1031-1032.

Detection: Mass Screening and High Risks—Cervical Cancer

Kazumasa Masubuchi

*Chairman, Department of Gynecology, Vice-Director, Cancer Institute Hospital,
Kami-Ikebukuro, Toshima-ku, Tokyo 170, Japan*

The reaction to the speakers is as follows:

MOBILE UNIT

I should like to explain first about mass screening by mobile units.

For the detection of cancer in the people living in remote area, a mobile unit for
mass screening of stomach cancer was developed in Japan in 1960, and a mobile unit
for the detection of cervical cancer was put into practice in 1962. Mobile units
for cervical cancer detection mainly use cytological examination, but some units
are equipped with colposcope.

There are three methods in mass screening for cervical cancer (Table 1); one is for
examinees to come to the detection center or to gynecologist's clinics or offices,
the other for a mobile unit to visit the people where they live, and another one is
the self-irrigation smear method. Ratio of these three methods during 1972 to 1976
showed that over one-half of examinations were made by the mobile unit, but examinations at the detection center and/or gynecologist's office are beginning to
increase. No emphasis is made on the self-irrigation method.

TABLE 1   Method Performed for Mass Screening of Cervical Cancer

(Japan Cancer Society: 1972 - 1976)

Year	by Mobile unit		at Detection center		at Gynecologist's office		by Self irrigation	
	No.	%	No.	%	No.	%	No.	%
1972	767,242	72.9	68,834	6.5	166,108	15.8	49,871	4.8
1973	851,676	68.8	161,984	13.1	169,425	13.7	53,982	4.4
1974	932,704	64.7	136,406	9.4	304,113	21.1	69,470	4.8
1975	985,908	63.4	151,665	9.7	347,778	22.4	70,265	4.5
1976	1,033,830	63.5	154,618	9.5	375,518	23.0	64,813	4.0

K. Masubuchi

Examination by the mobile unit is an effective means for poor people and for those
who are not anxious to receive examination. At present, there are 100 mobile cars
for cervical cancer detection in Japan. Another significance of a mobile unit is
its contribution to public education about cancer. Man-power required for the management of mobile units is now at the limit in Japan, but the value and significance of examinations by a mobile unit is fully understood. Under such a circumstance, examination in institutions and other facilities must be increased and for-
tified.

Detection rate of cervical cancer by the mobile unit is about 0.2% and majority of
it has been carcinoma in situ (Table 2).

TABLE 2 Results of Mass Screening for Cervical Cancer by Mobile Unit
(1966 - 1977, Japan)

Year	Total no. screened	Cancer detected No.	%
1966	126,603	412	0.32
1967	172,968	392	0.22
1968	305,507	687	0.22
1969	538,714	1,069	0.20
1970	748,377	1,516	0.20
1971	794,616	1,463	0.18
1972	905,207	1,824	0.20
1973	1,216,938	2,339	0.19
1974	1,452,528	2,498	0.17
1975	1,524,944	2,570	0.17
1976	1,675,243	2,746	0.16

Number of death from cancer of the uterus and death rate per 100,000 female population have decreased markedly in recent years in Japan (TABLE 3).

TABLE 3 Death from Uterine Cancer in Japan (1950 - 1977)

Year	No. of death	Per 100,000 female population
1950	8,356	19.7
51	8,197	19.0
52	8,061	18.4
53	7,638	17.2
54	7,763	17.2
55	7,289	16.0
56	7,343	16.0
57	7,144	15.4
58	7,105	15.2
59	7,099	15.0
60	7,068	14.9
:	:	:

— Continued to next page —

— Continued —

Year	No. of death	Per 100,000 female population
1950	8,356	19.7
⋮	⋮	⋮
61	6,964	14.5
62	6,940	14.3
63	6,940	14.2
64	6,936	13.6
65	6,689	13.4
66	6,667	13.2
67	6,668	13.1
68	6,610	12.9
69	6,523	12.6
70	6,373	12.1
71	6,194	11.7
72	6,326	11.7
73	6,052	11.0
74	6,142	11.0
75	6,068	10.7
76	5,877	10.3
77	5,688	10.3

CYTOLOGY LABORATORY

The fundamental requisite for mass screening is to have a reliable quality of cytology laboratory and to have a sufficient quantity of such laboratories. In Japan, a system has already been established that the Japanese Society of Clinical Cytology can authorize cytotechnologists and cytopathologists, and cytology laboratory is to be constituted of these authorized staff. The International Academy of Cytology carries out International Registry Examination of cytotechnologists, and Japan and U.S.A. have the largest number of cytotechnologists, CT(IAC). It is hoped that this system would be extended to all the countries of the world.

HIGH-RISK FOR ADVANCED CERVICAL CANCER

I would like to mention additionally about the high-risk group. In Japan, the number of invasive cervical cancer has been decreasing in recent years, and carcinoma in situ is found in about one-half of cervical cancer cases. On the other hand, stage III and IV advanced cases are still found, and these patients are mostly in 60s, 70s, and 80s or over. Consequently, it is extremely important to include aged women of over 60 years as subjects for mass screening.

ADENOCARCINOMA OF THE CERVIX IN VIRGIN WOMAN

Common occurrence of cervical carcinoma is in married woman. But adenocarcinoma of the cervix does occur even in virgin woman. This fact should be kept in mind at the public education program.

CURED CANCER ASSEMBLY

In connection with public education on cancer, it is most effective to demonstrate patients cured of cancer. Actual demonstration of Cured Cancer Assembly was taken place at the Ninth International Cancer Congress held in Tokyo in 1966. This Assembly of Cured Patients was started 18 years ago, and an 18th Annual Meeting was held in July, 1978.

It is strongly hoped that this kind of assembly of cured cancer patients should be organized widely for the purpose of public education of cancer.

REFERENCES

Masubuchi, K. (1966). Voluntary organization for cancer in Japan. Proceedings of Panel on Voluntary Organizations, 9th International Cancer Congress. U.I.C.C. pp. 25-35.

Masubuchi, K. (1969). Uterine cancer control in Japan. Proceedings of World Conference on Cancer of the Uterus. American Cancer Society. pp. 41-45.

Sagara, S. (1977). Report on the mass screening of cancer of the cervix in Japan. Proceedings of 8th symposium on mass screening of gynecologic cancer. Japan Cancer Society. pp. 3-9.

Prevention and Treatment of Carcinoma of the Cervix Uteri in the Shanghai Area

Shangahi Coordinating Group for Carcinoma of the Cervix Uteri

INTRODUCTION

In less than 10 years after the establishment of the present Government, owing to the active measures undertaken in relation to control of communicable and infectious diseases, to improvement in living and working conditions and raising the living standards and health status of the population in general — as a result of these measures, malignant diseases became around 1958, a major health problem for us medical workers in China.

In the Shanghai Area, this trend has been especially visible thru a study of the vital statistics for this city of about 10 million population. The annual death rate, due to malignant diseases in 1958 was listed second and in the recent 2 years, it was placed above the cardio vascular diseases.

Shanghai is an industrial city with an important sector of textile weaving factories. There are approximately some 300 thousand female workers involved in the textile industry. Mass screening and prevention work in the cancer campaign in Shanghai was first initiated in 1958 amongst mainly this large female population in the textile factories, a population more or less "stationary" and easy to organize for carrying out the mass screening.

We now report here the results achieved from these yearly screenings of the textile women workers in relation to the incidence of Ca cervix uteri.

METHODS OF CARRYING OUT THE WORK AND RESULTS ACHIEVED

Three stages could be described:

First stage. This stage is from 1958 to 1969. The mass screening started in 1958; the total number of cases examined varied yearly from around the 35 to 40 thousand. The usual attendance rate was 70-80%. The age of the cases examined varied between 20 to 54; at age 55 the women workers are retired.

At this first stage the results showed already a marked decrease in prevalence rate; viz: 1958=127.9/10^5, 1969=46/10^5.

Second stage. Beginning from 1969, a new policy was adopted concerning the treatment of cases showing abnormal cytological smears. While in the previous stage, only cases detected and diagnosed Ca in sites or invasive carcinoma are treated, in this present stage more attention is paid to cases detected and diagnosed cervicitis or cases showing cellular atypia. On the assumption that cervicitis and cellular atypia are precursors of malignancy or prone to malignant degeneration, active treatment was instituted for these cases.

As a result of these measures, the prevalence rate in 1969 of 46/10^5 dropped further down to 26.5/10^5 in 1974.

Third stage. In this stage, there is an extension in the scope of cases examined. In previous two stages, the work was carried out mainly amongst the female population of the textile factories. As already mentioned, the women factory workers examined every year numbered around the figure of 35 to 40 thousand from 1958 to 1972.

In 1973, it was decided to enlarge the population to be examined by inclusion of (a) retired factory workers, (b) workers in other factories outside the textile industry, (c) ordinary housewives, (d) peasant worker living in the agricultural suburbs of Shanghai, and (e) women civil service workers.

The amount of women population examined yearly resulting from this new policy jumped from the 35-40 thousand to over the million mark. This work on such a scale was made possible thru accumulated experience in field work organization, thru increased number of medical and paramedical staff, including the equivalent of "barefoot" doctors of the factories and of community health centers.

As to be expected, further decrease in the prevalence rate is noted for the subsequent following years.

The mean annual incidence of 1968 to 1972 was 40/10^5 and of 1973 to 1976 was 16.7/10^5.

It is confidently hoped that this yearly mass screening in conjunction with health education related to sex hygiene will ultimately place the incidence of carcinoma of cervix uteri well down on the list of malignant diseases. It was listed first in 1958 and by 1975 it has dropped to fourth place. Already there is now practical elimination of late stages Ca cervix in women of the Shanghai textile factories.

RELATION BETWEEN CERVICITIS, CELLULAR ATYPIA AND OTHER FACTORS IN CERVICAL MALIGNANT CHANGES

A well controlled study on this problem was carried out by one unit of the Shanghai Coordinating Group, the 2nd Textile Hospital, 400 cases of Ca cervix uteri were analysed.

viz: Ca in situ   122 ⎫
      Invasive Ca   205 ⎪
      Stage II   47 ⎬ 400
      Stage III   3 ⎪
      Stage Undetermined   19 ⎪
      Adenocarcinoma   4 ⎭

Youngest patient was 28 and oldest 73 years. The average age for

          Ca in situ   46.5 years
          Invasive Ca   43.5
          Stage II   46.6

It will be noted that the average age for Ca in situ cases is above
the one for Invasive Ca — which is not the usual finding in routine
clinical cases analysis. This fact can be explained that in the
population receiving yearly mass screening, the detected Ca in situ
cases are radically treated and thus, relatively speaking, there will
result a decrease in the number of cases developing invasive carcinomas. This group of 400 Ca cases is compared to a control group of
400 apparently healthy women, also textile factory workers, of equivalent age, environmental and living standard conditions.

The importance of such factors are analysed such as (1) cervicitis,
(2) leucorrhea, (3) trichomonas infection, (4) vulvar pruritus, (5)
age of menstruation onset, (6) age at marriage, (7) age of first
pregnancy, (8) time of resumption of sexual activities after pregnancy, (9) use of various contraceptive measures, (10) phimosis,
(11) alcohol and smoking. The conclusions are practically similar
to those studies already published.

The conclusion from this study of 400 cancer cases of cervix uteri
show definitely that elimination of chronic infections in the cervix
and other excessive local irritations (biological or otherwise) will
markedly decrease the incidence rate of this disease. That hospital
gave the following figures to show the results achieved. From 1958
to 1977, a duration of 20 years of screenings yearly and treatment
of cervical lesions detected in a large population of women textile
workers, the prevalence rate of $136.09/10^5$ in 1958 was reduced to
$9.49/10^5$ in 1977, and the incidence rate in 1958 was $31.34/10^5$ reduced to $4.91/10^5$ in 1977. This survey also reported that for the
3 years 1975 to 1977 no late stage Ca cervix was found.

Concerning the relation of cellular atypia to cancer, the following
report may be interesting. One gynecological clinic in Shanghai reported that for the years 1972 to 1976 they had detected 64 cases of
cervix with cellular atypia. 51 of the 64 cases received treatment
whilst the remaining 13 had refused or neglected the treatment. A
follow-up for one year revealed that none of the treated cases showed
any sign of malignancy changes on cytosmear whilst 3 of the untreated
had cytosmears with presence of cells showing malignancy characteristics.

IMPROVING THE DIAGNOSTIC ACCURACY OF CYTOSMEARS IN MASS
SCREENING

Fluorescent dyes' affinity to fix on cells with malignant changes
has been used to help increase diagnostic accuracy of cytosmears.

The following figures are given as reference. 5,241 cervix examined
using the fluorescent dye, 4,444 showed no dye fixation and the cytosmears are also correspondingly negative, the remaining 797 cases
which showed dye affinity, 79 cases were diagnosed invasive carcinoma, 147 cases carcinoma in situ, 429 cases cervical cell atypia,
142 cases infection.

TREATMENT METHODS

For the management of non-malignant lesions such as cervicitis and
cervical lesions with cellular atypia, cryotherapy and laser irradia-
tion had been used in some cases with satisfactory results. For
early carcinoma, it is still too early to judge on their suferiority
over other classical methods (surgical and ionising radiations).
The same remarks are made concerning the use of herbals either in
topical applications to cervix or per os.

The Shanghai Group has also attempted to classify Stage I carcinomas
into 4 subgroups according to the extent and size of lesion on the
cervix. This classification is aimed at proposing the extent of the
surgical excision in parametria and vagina according to the subgroup,
hoping thus to minimize the trauma of postoperative sequelae and yet
obtaining the same survival rates as in more extensive operations.

The 5- and 10-year survival rates of surgically treated Ca cervix
cases (1.417 for 5 years and 676 for 10 years) are given in Table 1
and Table 2.

CONCLUDING REMARKS

It is an accepted medical axiom that prevention is better than cure,
and this truth is doubly more important in relation to malignant
diseases. Despite the fact that treatment of invasive carcinoma of
cervix uteri by radiation or by surgery could give a relatively high
percentage of 5- and 10-year survival rates, yet prevention of the
disease thru periodic screening and elimination of cervical lesions
presumed precancerous should be a primordial concern in the campaign
against this cancer. The Shanghai Coordinating Group, which includes
the medical and paramedical staffs of many hospitals and clinics,
has consistently carried out large mass screening of the women workers of the textile factories and of women in many other sectors.
This uninterrupted mass screening spanning now over 20 years has
resulted in a remarkable lowering of the incidence rates of both Ca
in situ and invasive Ca of cervix uteri.

The motto adopted by the Shanghai Group is: First step is eradication of late cases, then of early invasive cases and ultimately
eradication of even the carcinoma in situ lesions.

TABLE 1 The 5-year survival rate of surgically treated cases of carcinoma of cervix uteri

Stage	No. of cases treated	No. of cases followed	Lost to follow-up	5-year survival cases	No. of deaths			Relative survival rate (%)	Absolute survival rate (%)
					Death due to carcinoma of cervix	Death due to other cases	Cause unknown		
I₁	632	632	0	627		5		99.21	99.21
I₂	232	228	4	223	2	3		97.81	96.12
I₃	237	231	6	223	6	1	1	96.54 (98.34)	94.09
I₄	195	190	5	177	10	2	1	93.16	90.71
II early	109	105	4	81	23	1		77.14 (73.55)	74.31
II late	12	12	0	8	4			66.61	66.67
Total	1,417	1,398	19	1,339	45	12	2	95.78	94.5

TABLE 2 The 10-year survival rate of surgically treated cases of carcinoma of cervix uteri

Stage	No. of cases treated	No. of cases followed	Lost to follow-up	10-year survival cases	No. of deaths			Relative survival rate (%)	Absolute survival rate (%)
					Death due to carcinoma of cervix	Death due to other causes	Cause unknown		
I_1	261	261	0	256		5		98.08	98.08
I_2	149	148	1	142	2	4		95.95 ⎫ 95.91	95.32
I_3	130	128	2	122	4	2		95.31 ⎭	93.85
I_4	77	75	2	67	7	1		89.33	89.01
II early	55	53	2	34	19			64.15 ⎫ 63.15	61.82
II late	4	4		2	2			50 ⎭	50
Total	676	669	7	623	34	12		93.12	92.16

Rehabilitation

Ramon Paterno

President, Philippine Cancer Society, Inc.
Director, Cancer Detection & Diagnostic Center,
Chairman, Dept. of Radiology, Our Lady of Lourdes Hospital and
Singian Memorial Hospital

ABSTRACT

The problems and difficulties that are encountered by a voluntary non-govern-
ment organization in a developing country like the Philippines in setting up
a program of Rehabilitation for Cancer Patients are presented.

Most important among these are loss of **contact** with Cancer survivors whose
exact number is not known; and unwillingness of survivors to publicize their
disease.

Recommended remedies are more thorough follow-up of Cancer patients discharged from hospitals; and public education, to change the people's
attitude toward Cancer.

I bring you greetings from the Philippines in Southeast Asia; in particular,
from the Philippine Cancer Society. The Philippine Cancer Society, as most
of your Cancer Societies, is a voluntary, non-profit, socio-medical, non-
government organization. (In the first place, warmest congratulations to Ms.
Timothy, Drs. Volpio and Shannon, for their excellent presentation).

As a developing country, the Philippines has many priorities over Cancer.
Infectious diseases like pneumonias, pulmonary tuberculosis, gastro-
enteritis, are still taking a very heavy toll on our population. However,
lately great progress has been made, and more is expected.

In a country whose population is now placed at 44,000,000 spread over 7,083
islands, speaking 123 different dialects, the average life span has been
raised from 52 to 58 years in the last decade. And naturally, the cancer
menace is definitely on the increase. (Cancer now ranks No. 5 as most
common cause of death; after pneumonias, tuberculosis, cardiac and vascular
diseases).

Rehabilitation of Cancer patients, is not yet a developed movement in our
part of the world. Generally, rehabilitation of Cancer patients is included
in the general rehabilitation units of our Hospitals and Medical Centers,
but cancer cases are referred to them only in specific instances. For

example, for artificial limbs after amputations, etc.

We are grateful to the UICC for focussing our attention on this matter,
prompting us to take the first steps. Incidentally, the UICC has done the
same thing for us, regarding undergraduate cancer medical education in Asia,
and the anti-smoking campaign, by sponsoring highly successful workshops.
These were held during the 3rd Asian Cancer Conference of the Asian Federation of Organizations for Cancer Research and Control, which was hosted by
the Philippine Cancer Society in Manila, in late September, 1977.

What are our main problems in Cancer Rehabilitation?

Firstly, most cases of cancer are still diagnosed late. This, in spite of
our efforts at public and professional education, aimed mainly at early
detection. So that we feel our survival figures are low. But we have no
exact figures because follow-up is inadequate.

A big proportion of our people still believe that a diagnosis of cancer
especially in internal organs, is practically a sentence of death. 40 or
50 years ago, the family used to say, "Gosh, he has PTB". Now, the reaction
is "Thank God it is only TB and not Cancer".

Because of above-mentioned priorities, we still have no Government or
Private Centralized Cancer Hospital & Research Center. Government, however,
is really exerting efforts to expand its National Cancer Control program to
a national scope, within the limits of available resources, by efforts to
incorporate a Cancer Unit in existing Regional General Hospitals.

Secondly, the Philippine Cancer Society runs a Central Tumor Registry, which
collects Cancer statistics from qualified Hospitals. A requirement of the
International Association of Cancer Registries which has accepted ours, is
to enter only proven cases of Cancer - so that our figures are necessarily
for the moment limited to urban centers, leaving rural areas uncovered.

However, even in these qualified hospitals, our records lose track of the
cancer patients upon discharge. Follow-up has been deficient. We have
taken measures to remedy this situation - by instituting a program of more
thorough home follow-up of discharged cancer patients, as well as a periodic
review of government vital statistics records,to tally with our own.

Thirdly, our people in general are not yet quite ready to acknowledge
publicly that they have, or have had, Cancer. This is true even of
survivors.

Mastectomies, for example. We have quite a number. Sometime in 1975 Mrs.
Teresa Lasser came over personally to Manila, thru the good offices of the
American Cancer Society, to start a Reach to Recovery program. We arranged
lectures and demonstrations in the main teaching Hospitals, and she left us
literature, prosthetic samples, etc.

The movement did not advance much. Well-to-do patients are taken care of
by their private physicians, and do not care to advertise their mutilation
in public. Indigent patients, on the other hand, in the experience of
Hospital Social Services, accept their amputation stoically. Typical is one
saying, "A shawl over my shoulders and folded across my chest, will hide the
defect."

So it has been difficult to find a volunteer an actual mastectomized patient, much less a group, to form the core of Reach to Recovery Program. Social Workers and volunteers we have many, but the effectiveness of the program seems to hinge on the volunteer being a mastectomized patient. As Mlle Timothy says, nobody can realize the anguish, until she has actually undergone the operation.

Laryngectomees very seldom we meet. Our CTRP records 422 cases of cancer of the larynx, from a total of 32,500 cases, collected from June 1968 to May 31, 1977 (9 years or 1.29%.) Of these, 103 or 24% underwent laryngectomy, either by itself or in combination with radiation and/or chemotherapy. The laryngectomees have an estimated 5-year survival rate of about 38%.

Ostomies are fairly common but also taken care of individually.

Regarding the question - should the patient be told that he has Cancer? As a radiologist, it is practically a daily experience to be cautioned by the relatives, "Doctor if you find anything like Cancer, please do not tell the patient - it will kill him." We take our cases individually, and act as we judge best in each particular case, altho I personally believe he should be told.

Recapitulating - from the point of view of a developing country like ours:

(1) We have a crying need for a National Centralized Cancer Institute or a Comprehensive Cancer Center, to provide facilities for treatment and research, and to coordinate the national effort. Preferably to be run by Government, as private enterprise has limited resources.

We have an abundance of excellent, fully qualified oncologists trained abroad. Coming home, they either have to become general practitioners, or general surgeons, to survive. Or go back abroad, for more satisfying and remunerative use of their acquired skill and training. This is what we call the "brain-drain".

We are not yet quite used to the concept of multidisciplinary approach to treatment of Cancer cases. Professional competition is quite acute, and private paying patients are kept private.

However, in Government National Regional and Provincial Hospitals, and in some teaching hospitals, for indigents, many already have a Tumor Board, of different disciplines. A National Cancer Institute or Comprehensive Cancer Center, should hasten this phase of professional education.

(2) In the meantime, more thorough follow-up of Cancer patients is absolutely necessary, after their discharge from hospital. As I said before, we have taken the initial steps in this direction, thru home follow-up, since this rehabilitation session was announced to us by the UICC a year ago.

(3) Public Education is also necessary to teach our people that Cancer is not a fatal nor a "shameful" disease..

With improved facilities and more thorough follow-up, we can expect a greater number of survivors surfacing, who can be organized into Rehabilitation clubs, to help each other and boost each other's spirits. To imbue them with a spirit of service to their fellow sufferers and serve as examples that Cancer can be cured or at least controlled.

A corollary to this is the placement of Cancer survivors in useful and gain-
ful occupations. Businessmen to be approached, and asked to help place them
in temporary jobs, less strenuous than formerly, for the duration of remission. Many of these survivors are fully qualified and valuable, and good
for many more years of useful service.

We believe therefore that all this evolution is a matter of time but we are
inspired to action by UICC sessions like this, to accelerate the pace of
this change towards more effective complete care of Cancer patients.

Thank you.

Rehabilitation: Psychological and Physical
—Finnish Experience

Niilo Voipio

The Cancer Society of Finland

When we speak of the rehabilitation of cancer patients, a basic condition for success in this as in any other form of rehabilitation is that the patient himself or herself can be activated into efforts to promote rehabilitation. In the case of the cancer patient, a very important role is played by the question of whether the patient should be aware of the nature of his disease. As far as I know, the old manner of thinking is still adhered to in many countries - that is, that the cancer patient should not be informed of the diagnosis. This conception is based on the idea that the knowledge of an advanced, often incurable disease will depress the patient and thus make treatment difficult. We begin from quite a different footing when the patient is told the nature of his disease while appealing to ever improving results of treatment: that is, to the fact that between 30 and 50 per cent of all cancer patients can be cured, and as many as 80 to 95 per cent of the cases detected at an early stage.

By telling the patient the right diagnosis, it is easy to motivate the patient to accept even radical treatment which lead to a curative end result though causing permanent injury. Where the general level of education is high, the public is already beginning to be aware of the fact that contracting cancer by no means amounts to an immediate death sentence. Consequently, the patient who contracts cancer and gains awareness of his or her illness will become oriented towards planning for the future months and the future years that he must cope with after the end of hospitalisation.

Where the level of education is high, laymen too - upon comprehending the nature of the treatment - are pretty well aware of what kind of disease is involved. The confidence between patient and doctor will falter if the patient is unable to believe that he has been told the whole truth without reservation. If, at the very beginning of the treatment, as soon as the diagnosis has been confirmed, a relationship of confidence has been established between patient and doctor, the same confidence will assist rehabilitation and will be a basis for its motivation.

These are the basic ideas that have been the motivating force for
the Finnish Cancer Society in printing a specific series of guide
brochures - one about each of the most common forms of cancer -
which are distributed by hospitals, according to the case, to re-
leased patients. The brochure has instructions concerning rehabilitation, information about financial and social support
obtainable from the community, and directions on steps warranted
by the occurrence of symptoms suggesting relapse, etc.   These
booklets also carry a report on diet and instructions concerning
the terminal stage.

The previous bad reputation of cancer had the result that cancer
patients tried to conceal the nature of their illness from out-
siders.   However, it was not possible for every patient to do so,
particularly after the termination of treatment.   The most typical
of these groups is that of patients with laryngectomies.

Starting from the idea that bringing together such fellows in ad-
versity could be encouraging and could, in particular, help the
patient's family when it meets other families in which a member
has had a laryngectomy, the Finnish Cancer Society proceeded to
experiment with the psychological rehabilitation of laryngectomy
patients by means of activities within a society of their own.
In 1962, which is 16 years ago, a society of the sort was
established, with its objective being to teach people with laryngectomies how to speak again by means of air taken into the oeso-
phagus, to provide general rehabilitation for them, to have the
aids needed by them included among aids totally financed by the
government, and to get them and their families adjusted to the
new situation.

Othologists soon noticed that laryngectomy patients who had
learned to speak well provided excellent encouragement for patients
in hospital who were being prepared for laryngectomy and were
excellent instructors in speech exercises begun immediately after
the operation.

In Finland, with its population of 4.7 million and its total of
1,500 to 2,000 living patients with cancer of the larynx, the
society of laryngectomy patients has been able to accomplish just
about all the targets it originally set itself.   It also has its
own centre for rehabilitation leaves and courses, on the shore of
a lake, where patients meet for annual courses in groups of
50-100 usually with wives and children, for the purposes both of
speech exercise and general rehabilitation as well as training
for adjustment.

The experience from the work of the society for laryngectomy cases
encouraged the Finnish Cancer Society to found a general association of cancer patients too.   This was done in 1971.   The idea was
that the persons with laryngectomy were a unique group to such an
extent that it could continue as a separate entity.   However, the
distribution of other cancer patients into subdivisions was regarded as being unnecessary and actually undesirable.   It is good
that persons whose prognosis may be worse should be able to take
part in the same association as those whose prognosis, generally
speaking, is quite good.

In the same manner as the society for laryngectomy patients, this general society of cancer patients proceeded to promote the granting of statutory social benefits on the same grounds as they were granted to other disabled persons. It also took up rehabilitation and adjustment training.

Organisationally, the association of cancer patients works with the support of the divisions of the Finnish Cancer Society, and frequently in such a manner that the central town of the division has premises for meetings and rehabilitation specifically for the sub-section.

Mainly for the purpose of the early diagnosing of cancer, the Finnish Cancer Society also maintains cancer detection stations but has linked these with social counselling, after-examinations and rehabilitation units intended for cancer sufferers. The rehabilitation is both physical, with conventional devices, and psychological - to include even legal advice.

It has been possible to provide adjustment training courses, trips abroad, excursions within the country and joint evening events for these patients too.

The activities of the cancer victims' own association has led to an increasingly open attitude towards cancer, and to the spreading of the view that cancer is just one disease among many. At the same time, the fact that patients treated dozens of years ago and now free of symptoms can publicly declare themselves to be cancer cases tends to show that cancer is a chronic disease that is exceptional in the sense that it is possible to recover from it completely. In this way the work of the patients' association serves the general health education objectives of the Cancer Society.

Rehabilitation of Laryngectomees in Israel

E. Shanon

Israel Cancer Association, Dept. of Otolaryngology, Ichilov Medical Center and Sackler's School of Medicine, Tel-Aviv University, Israel

ABSTRACT

This article describes the functional organization of rehabilitation of laryngectomees in Israel. Results of a retrospective study on 146 laryngectomees are presented. Both physical and psychological aspects of rehabilitation are analyzed. Speech proficiency correlated positively with optimistic and realstic outlook and with continued employment. 15% of the patients presented moderate or marked symptoms of depression and additional 23% of the group faced difficulties in social readjustment. Special problems were posed by women, old people and Arab laryngectomees. Pertinent data from the literature are briefly reviewed and some recommendations are suggested.

KEYWORDS: laryngectomee, esophageal speech, rehabilitation, motivation, realism, depression, psychology.

INTRODUCTION

The problem of rehabilitation of laryngectomees in Israel should be viewed in the proper perpective. In a country with a population of 3.2 million there are about 100 new cases of cancer of the larynx diagnosed yearly, 93.9% men and 6.1% women. One half of these patients receive radiotherapy, 38% are treated by laryngectomy and 12% by conservative laryngeal surgery.

Up to 1960 rehabilitation was limited to speech instruction given by untrained laryngectomees or by speech therapists. in 1960 the first center for rehabilitation of laryngectomees was set up in Tel Aviv. This represented a joint project sponsored by the Israel Cancer Association, the Bnei-Brith lady volunteers and an otolaryngologist. Additional, smaller centers were set up in the other cities.

FUNCTIONAL ORGANIZATION OF THE REHABILITATION CENTER IN TEL AVIV

The yearly enrollment varied from 18 - 22 new patients over the period of the past seven years. Two bi-hourly sessions took place evey week. The average attendance ranged from 15 - 20 patients per session. Instruction was provided on an individual basis for new

pupils and in small classes for beginners, moderately advanced
speakers and those using an electrolarynx. The rehabilitation team
comprised a senior speech pathologist, three speech clinicians, a
social worker and lady-volunteers who fulfilled the functions of
administrators, hostesses and non-professional socio-economic and
vocational advisors. Up till now sporadic help of a psychologist
was available. However, efforts are made to include a rehabilitation
psychologist as a permanent member of the team. The Israel Cancer
Association provides the premises, the budget, coordinate the various
disciplines, stimulates and supports research and ensures the general
administration.

EVALUATION OF THE REHABILITATION STATUS OF 131 LARYNGECTOMEES

A. Physical Factors

Retrospective assessment of 146 laryngectomized patients was based on
questionnaires and personal interviews. Adequate data were obtained
on 131 patients. The original group of 146 subjects comprised 137 men
(94.5%) and 9 women (5.5%). The majority of the patients (67%) were
50-65 years old. 23 patients (16%) were 40-49 years old and 24 (17%)
were more than 65 years of age. No specific ethnic predilection in
the incidence could be observed. 91% of the group were Jews and 9%
Arabs.

Medical records included personal data, the type of surgery, details
on radiotherapy and the status of the tracheostoma.

Multiple physical traits were evaluated: hearing function, discrimination of post-laryngectomy speech, oromotor function, dental
status, sense of smell, and structure and function of the neoglottis.
Electromyographic study of the neoglottic muscles was conducted on
twelve patients (Arlazoroff and co-workers, 1968, 1972).

The study of habits referred mostly to smoking, drinking and sucking
candy. 95% of the subjects smoked before surgery and 30% continued to
do so after the operation. Alcohol drinking was confirmed to 6.1% of
the subjects before the operation and to 2.2% after the operation.
None of the patients reported eating sweets as a habit before laryngectomy, but 40% acquired this habit following surgery. Sweets appear
to be a substitute for cigarettes.

The quality of esophageal speech was graded as good in 25% (32 subjects), adequate in 36% (47 subjects), fair in 25% (33 cases) and
poor in 14% (19 cases). No significant correlation was noted between
speech proficiency and educational level, occupation and economic
 status. Women, older people and Arab patients did poorly and their
problem will be considered under a separate heading.

In 44% of the patients the onset of speech was observed within one
month of training and in additional 30% of the patients within two
months. Somewhat superior early results were observed among patients
of oriental background who did not reject belching as an unaesthetic
act. Good esophageal speech was acquired by 48% of the patients
during the first three months of rehabilitation; 5% learned to
speak well in six months, 3% in nine months and 5% in mor than a year.

Regular attendance in the center was reflected in the attained speech proficiency. 43% of good esophageal speakers were regular attendants but only 11% of the non-regular attendants achieved good speech. Lack of interest was indicated as the main cause of inattendance. It should be pointed out that these subjects not only failed to achieve adequate communicative and socio-economic rehabilitation but they also presented the most prominent emotional problems.

Special measures deemed appropriate in individual cases. These included hearing aid fitting, auditory training, dental prosthesis, dilatation and physiotherapy of the cricopharyngeal muscles (weight-lifting and Valsalva's manoeuvre), neck, shoulder and jaw exercises, smelling exercises and care of the tracheostoma.

B. Psychological and socio-economic factors

In the group of 131 patients studies 20 (15%) appeared withdrawn and depressed. This was the impression gained by the rehabilitation team rather than a professional psychiatric diagnosis. 13 of these 20 patients had poor esophageal voice, 5 fair and only 2 acquired good speech. 13 subjects ceased to work following the operation and 8 were supported by social welfare. The majority of the subjects in this group displayed lack of hope for rehabilitation and frequently refused to cooperate in the program.

Additional 30 patients (23%) had difficulties in social readjustment associated with emotional problems.

The question arose whether a positive correlation exists between strong family structure and social adjustment. Family ties are usually stronger among Oriental Jews than among those of European origin. However, the group of 50 patients who showed psychological disturbances was almost equally divided between these two groups. Strong family ties do not appear adequate in providing support to a laryngectomee during the difficult period of rehabilitation. Outside help deems necessary.

Continued employment was recorded in 63% of the patients. 20% changed the place of their work and 17% retired. Continued employment correlated positively with the acquisition of esophageal speech as well as a realistic and optimistic rehabilitation outlook. The usual cause of a change of work was the search for a lighter type of occupation, rather than a communicative problem.

The economic status remained unchanged in 46% of the laryngectomized patients. It was seriously impaired in 27% of the patients (who either retired or changed the place of work) and moderately reduced in the remaining 27%.

During the first three postoperative months low morale and depressive reaction may prevail. However, if these persist for a longer period of time one should attempt to differentiate between compensatory neurosis (associated with the wish to gain material compensation because of the handicap), depressive reaction, psychosis of various

types and grades which may progress to psychotic depresseion, and
senile psychosis. The boundaries between these different conditions
may be vague.

The diagnosis of a depressive reaction should be made as early as
possible. Suggestive symptoms are insomnia, lassitude, anorexia,
loss of power to concentrate and to decide, lack of interest,
social withdrawal, crying spells, untidiness and the wish to die.

Our study lacked a presurgical assessment of the personality and
thus it is difficult to determine whether the diverse psychological
reactions reflected the antecedent status or were the results of the
medical therapy.

SPECIAL PROBLEMS

Older laryngectomees faced special rehabilitation problems, due to
less faith, less hope and less motivation as well as impaired
hearing function, discrimination and oromotor function and a delayed
onset of training caused by a longer time required to recover
physically.

Women laryngectomees comprised nine subjects whose ages ranged
from 50 - 60 years. Eight were Jewish and one was Arabic. Seven
worked as housewives and two as factory workers. Only five attended
the Center. Of these - two did so on a rather irregular basis. Most
female patients expressed aesthetic objection to esophapgeal speech.
Only one patient acquired good speech and four acquired fair speech.
Poor speech and lack of speech were associated with social withdrawal and depression.

Arab laryngectomees, 13 in number, lived in diverse parts of the
country. Only two patients attended classes regularly and these two
only acquired good esophageal speech. The main problems of this
group of patients were language and geographic distance from the
Center.

CURRENT TRENDS AND PROPOSALD FOR THE FUTURE

For more than one hundred years since the performance of the first
laryngectomy by Billroth in 1873 (Gussenbauer, 1874) rehabilitation
of laryngectomees was focused mainly on the acquisition of speech
(Damtse, 1958; Gardner, 1971; Snidecor, 1962). However, it became
apparent that emotional and other factors play a significant role
and are intimately related to speech restoration (Haase, 1960;
Hunt, 1964; Murphy, 1964; Nahum, 1963; Pitkin, 1953; Shames, 1963;
Stall, 1958). A profile of personality traits which would favour a
successful development of esophageal speech could not be adequately
defined on the basis of retrospective evaluation. Greene (1974)
and Snidecor (1957) recommended a presurgical assessment of the
emotional status. Ideally this should be completed before the
patient is aware of the serious implications of his persistent

hoarseness. Such data, not available as yet may help to individualize the methods employed to convey to the patient the implications of his illness and of the required operation. Additional progress during the preoperative phase of rehabilitation may be expected in an organization of active involvement of rehabilitated laryngectomees and in expert counseling of the family.

Postoperative rehabilitation is based on individual initiation of the laryngectomee into the new world of speech, and later _ on the principle of group therapy and a multidisciplinary team approach. The need of a rehabilitation psychologist is felt in many centers. His task would include not only professional advice in selected cases, but also education of members of the team in the nature of the "normal" postlaryngectomy depression and the early symptoms of a reactive depression of a more serious nature. The wide sphere of the emotional problems associated with laryngectomy has yet to be explored in depth. The acquired knowledge should constitute part of a comprehensive educational program for the family, employers, work associates and the public at large. The sexual problems of laryngectomees deserve further research which may improve marital and family interactions. Greene (1947) and Bisi and Conley (1965) as a loss of sexual attractiveness or castration.

Gardner (1966) has studied extensively the special problems of rehabilitation posed by women. Some of these problems still await adequate solutions. Older patients, those physically disabled or hard of hearing also require individualized solutions.

Goldberg (1975), and Goldberg and Bigwood (1975) studied the vocational and social aspects of rehabilitation of laryngectomees. Realism, optimism about the future and a strong desire to resume productive rehabilitation were found to correlate positively with social and vocational rehabilitation, as well as with the acquisition of speech. This work calls for research on the statues for protection of handicapped employees.

Although criteria of esophageal speech proficiency have been defined (Hunt, 1963; Wepmand and co-workers, 1953), it appears beneficial to establish internationally approved criteria of an index of total rehabilitation of laryngectomees. Such an index would encompass the full range of rehabilitation aspects - vocal, vocational, economic, emotional, cosmetic, physical handicaps, social integration and family interaction.

Finally, further progress may be expected in the field of neurophysiology of the neoglottic muscles and in advances in electronic and surgical methods of restoration of the voice.

REFERENCES

Arlazoroff, E., E. Shanon and M. Streifler (1968). Electromyographic
     activity of the neoglottic muscles in laryngectomees.
     Harefuah, 74, 129-130.
Arlazoroff, A. and co-workers (1972). Observations on the electro-
     myogram of the esophagus at rest and during Valsalva's
     manoeuvre. Electroenceph. Clin. Neurophysiol., 33, 110-112.
Bisi, R.M. and J.J. Conley (1965). Psychological factors influencing
     vocal rehabilitation of the post laryngectomy patient.
     Ann. Otol. Rhinol. Laryngol., 74, 1073-1078.
Damsté, P.H. (1958). Oesophageal Speech after Laryngectomy.
     Boekdrukkerig Vorheen Gebroeders Hoitsema, Groningen.
Gardner, W.H. (1966). Adjustment problems of laryngectomized women.
     Arch. of Otolaryng., 83, 31-42
Gardner, W.H. (1971). Laryngectomee Speech and Rehabilitation.
     Charles C. Thomas, Springfield Illinois.
Goldberg, R.T. (1975). Vocational and social adjustment after
     laryngectomy. Scand. J. Rehab. Med., 7, 1-8.
Goldberg, R.T. and A.W. Bigwood (1975). Vocational adjustment after
     laryngectomy. Physical Med. and Rehab., 56, 521-524.
Greene, J.S. .1974). Laryngectomy and its psychological implications.
     N.Y. State J. Med., 47, 53-56.
Gussenbauer, C.V. (1874). Ueber die erste durch Th. Billroth am
     Menschen ausgefuehrte Kehlkopf-Extirpation und die Anwendung
     eines kuenstlichen Kehlkopfes. Arch. Klin. Chir., 17, 343-356.
Haase, H.J. (1960) Psychologie und Psychopathologie Kehlkopfextir-
     pierter. Fortschr. Neurol. Psychiat., 28, 253-273.
Hunt, R.B. (1964) Rehabilitation of the laryngectomee. Laryngoscope,
     74, 382-295.
Murphy, G.E., A.L. Bisno and J.H. Ogura (1964). Determinants of
     rehabilitation following laryngectomy. Laryngoscope, 74,
     1535-1549.
Nahum, A.M. and G.S. Golden (1963). Psychological problems of laryn-
     gectomy. J.A.M.A., 186, 1136-1138.
Pitkin, Y.N. (1953). Factors affecting psychological adjustment of
     laryngectomized patients. Arch. Otolaryng., 58, 38-48.
Shames, G.H., J. Font and J. Mattews (1963). Factors related to speech
     proficiency of laryngectomees. J. Speech, Hear. Dis.,28,
     237-287.
Snidecor, J.C. (1962) Speech Rehabilitation of the Laryngectomized.
     Charles C. Thomas, Springfield Illinois.
Snidecor, J.C. (1975). Some scientific foundations for voice resto-
     ration. Laryngoscope, 85, 640-648.
Stall, B. (1958) Psychological factors determining the success and
     failure of the rehabilitation program of laryngectomized.
     Ann. Otol. Rhinol. Laryngol., 67, 550-557.
Wepman, J.M. and co-workers (1953). The objective measurements of
     progressive esophageal speech development. J. Speech, Hear.
     Dis., 18, 249-250.

The Welfare of the Patient with Cancer and his Family

Antoinette L. Pieroni

Sidney Farber Cancer Institute, 44 Binney Street, Boston, Massachusetts

ABSTRACT

There are some differences between a child who has cancer and an adult patient,
but there are also many similarities as to concerns and fears. Families have to
learn to live with the knowledge of the diagnosis of cancer and learn to cope
with it and all of its ramifications. The social worker is the one person on the
health team who can coordinate the concerns and assistance by meeting the patient
and his family, supporting them through the treatment period, and helping the
family after the death of the patient. Finding solutions for practical matters
such as lodging, home care, and financial assistance must be attended to first.
The family is then ready to receive emotional and supportive help. This is done
in case work interviews and in groups. The financial burden can be enormous for
all families. More comprehensive financial assistance must be provided in the
United States for hospitalizations and care after discharge. The pediatric
patient is cared for by his parents and the community, whereas the adult patient
has fewer support systems. The hospice, as it is known now, is better adapted
for the adult patient. Hostels for the pediatric patient in the United States are
now becoming available.

Communication between the physician and the patient and his family must be honest
and open, for better understanding leads to better communication within a family.
The entire health team must know the patient well, be honest, concerned, and
sincere so that it can give the best medical and emotional care possible.

KEYWORDS

patient with cancer, social worker, case work and groups, emotional and supportive
help, finances, hospitalization, home care

TEXT

As a social worker, I was pleased to read that each of the three preceeding authors
showed concern for the emotional adjustment of the patient, the care facilities,
and for the financial burden borne by the family of the patient. I would like to
comment on these concerns from my experience in Massachusetts, which has been
exclusively in pediatric oncology. While there are some differences in dealing
with a family of a child who has cancer as opposed to a family of an adult patient
with cancer, there are also many similarities as to concerns and fears.

As Professor Garcia-Orcóyen has stated, the patient has the right to respect, dignity and compassion. The initial impact of the diagnosis is primarily borne by the family, for a great deal of anxiety arises from guilt, fears and frustrations, and questions that may or may not have answers. In addition, the possibility of inadequate financial resources is always a threat.

Welfare has come to mean financial aid by government agencies while the basic meaning of the health, happiness, comfort, and well-being of the individual has been lost.

Every family is so devastated by the word "cancer," that it becomes immobilized for a period of time. The members of the family do not dare talk of the fears and frustrations, and find it easier to hide behind facts and practical matters such as housing, costs, treatments, etc.

The first rule of case work is to begin where the family is, so we, in the Social Service Department of the Sidney Farber Cancer Institute, meet each new family. Our first task is to establish a relationship with the family and patient which can be continued throughout treatment, and with the family after the death of the patient. We begin by obtaining factual information, for it is an effective first step in establishing a working relationship. In this process we are doing our initial psycho-social assessment as well. The facts give us a picture of the patient in his or her environment, but of much more importance is the way the information is given—the tone of voice, the facial expression, the affect and mannerisms. It is these that give the experienced worker a clue as to how the family has coped with crises in the past and might cope with the diagnosis and all of its ramifications in the months or years to come.

The social worker then asks what the physician has told them, what the patient knows about the diagnosis, and what thoughts he has expressed, for it is important to know what was heard and how it was interpreted, and to begin immediately to clarify misconceptions. This requires close rapport between the physician and the social worker since the worker must know what the physician has said. From this evaluation, the worker is able to work out an individualized plan for helping the patient and the family through this initial period of crisis by making suggestions for coping with all this new information, by giving continuous support, and by working together with the other members of the health team.

Since experience has taught us that practical matters must be attended to first, we help a family find solutions for their immediate needs such as lodging, travel, home health care and financial assistance. The hostel system as described by Dr. Holland is certainly an immediate answer to both the lodging and part of the financial questions. I do not know of such a program in the United States for the adult patient, but the McDonald Corporation (famous for its hamburgers and milk-shakes) and the National Football League have started such a program for children. We, in Boston, will have a Ronald McDonald House next April. It will house 25 people, have a community kitchen, living room and play areas available not only to the patient and a parent, but also for a family while visiting the hospitalized child. It will have a home-like atmosphere where a family can be together and where many families can support each other. In the United States, financial assistance can be obtained from government agencies on the federal, state, county and local levels, as well as from some private agencies. Monies coming from the federal government are uniform throughout the country, but eligibility for benefits can differ greatly from state to state due to the autonomy of statehood and to the tax structure of the individual state. National Health Insurance is being more seriously considered and debated. Most private agencies are structured to provide counselling to individuals and families rather than to provide financial assistance. A few exceptions are organizations such as the American

Cancer Society and the Leukemia Society of America. In addition, private trust funds sometimes may be found to assist with specific needs such as prostheses, travel money for treatment, etc. In the United States hospital costs can be either partially or fully paid for, through government funds or private insurances, but our nursing and convalescent homes are expensive and for the most part are not geared to the special emotional needs of the cancer patient.

Once some of the pressing practical matters have been taken care of, patients and their families are ready to discuss their anxieties or emotions. The focus of the health team should be to help the family live as normal a life as possible-- whatever might be normal for <u>that</u> <u>individual</u> family, without imposing standards that are <u>foreign</u> to that family. The well-being of all the individuals involved in or affected by the diagnosis of cancer is most important. It is what Dr. Farber called Total Care -- that is: the concern for the entire family given by all the members of the team. It is often the social worker who can coordinate this concern.

Hospitalization can be a frightening experience. It means separation from loved ones and familiar surroundings. It means treatment that can be painful, procedures that can be unpleasant and annoying, surgery or radiation therapy that can be traumatic. The patient has every right to have as full an explanation of the diagnosis and treatment as possible. The physician must spend time to talk with the patient to know him as a human being, his fears, his likes and dislikes so that he can give the information in as meaningful a manner as is possible to the individual patient. The parents of a pediatric patient must also have this information and understanding if they are to give emotional support to their child. A parent or spouse will need to know how to cope with the inevitable changes in family living. Siblings, especially those of a pediatric patient, should be involved from the beginning of treatment - to ask questions and to express their feelings of fear, jealousy, guilt, and resentment. Better under- standing leads to better communication and closeness within the family. Families of pediatric patients are often closer and more involved than those of adult patients, for siblings are still in the household. Aunts, uncles, grandparents and neighbors show more concern for a child. The lives of school personnel and classmates are affected by a child's illness, as well as the lives of employers and fellow employees of the parents.

Because of the heterogenous population in the United States, the social worker has to be sensitive to the ethnic, cultural, add=tudinal and emotional differences of each family, and to the changes that occur throughout treatment. The social worker should be sensitive to the attitudes within a family. She should work with the strengths and help strengthen the weaknesses, for as Professor Garcia-Orcóyen quoted Dyk and Sutherland, "the atmosphere prevailing in the family during the illness will always depend upon the relationship which existed before." I would like to add that we can try to help change the atmosphere if it needs to be changed.

On most pediatric units, the mother, in particular, is allowed to stay with the child, bathe him, feed him and help him with his medical care. These acts preserve her role as mother, give her status and help her be less jealous of other females who are caring for her child. Visiting hours are liberal, visitors are not usually restricted and siblings are allowed to visit at least in the garden or in the lobby. There is usually a play room or activities center supervised by a trained person where the children play together, talk freely in an informal setting, and generally socialize. The return home is relatively tolerable because the family has had the experience of actively taking care of the patient, and the family is reassured that any member of the health team is only as far away as the telephone. There is time and opportunity to help the pediatric and adolescent patient with his feelings of inadequacy, loss of self-esteem, of "being different." The environment of our pediatric unit also allows for parents to get to know each other, and for parents to meet in groups with the social worker where they support each other. We, in pediatric social work at the Sidney Farber Cancer Institute, conduct several parents' groups. There is a daily morning group in the clinic where parents discuss their concerns and exchange ideas. Parents also meet with us in the hospital two afternoons a week. These sessions are intense, for the family is in crisis. One evening a month parents meet with us and a physician to discuss medical information. Because these groups have been so successful, we now have a group for parents whose children have died. They hear each other better than they hear us professionals, and they are not afraid to discuss any subject, because they know they are all facing the same crises. Our adolescents have their own group and look forward to sharing feelings and daily events with peers going through the same miseries.

It is more difficult for adult patients to share feelings and experiences, for the focus is on themselves whereas the focus of parents' groups is on the child. For some strange reason adult hospitals have many more restrictions as to meal times, visiting hours, number of visitors and freedom to inter-relate. Transition to home is anxiety provoking because up to now the adult's family has rarely been allowed to care for the patient, to touch him, to have the freedom of talk that comes with privacy. Going home means a more normal way of living, of staying up late to watch television, of being a part of the family in the kitchen, around the dining table and in the bedroom. It is at home where the patients may first come to understand fully what his diagnosis means, and how to cope with adjust-ments and adaptations necessary for survival, such as ostomy irrigation. All family members should be encouraged to become involved and help the patient become as self sufficient and independent as possible. Family bonds can thus be strengthened. More patients and more families are asking that the patient be permitted to remain at home as long as possible and even die there. This requires coordinate planning for home care involving physicians, nurses, social workers and ancillary personnel. There are many agencies providing home care, from the home-maker who helps with house work and meals to the home health aide who can give nursing care to the patient. This alleviates the total burden of the care of the patient from the family. This service is not free, and our goal should be to work for funding for this service.

Dr. Cole described to us the meaning of the hospice. Patients need not return to a hospital with its rigidity, restrictions, indignities and frightening life-prolonging measures. It is a valuable alternative to hospital or home care. The hospice is an ideal setting in which groups could be therapeutic -- groups for patients, patients and family, and for staff to share their fears and their feelings. There are several hospices already in the United States which are serving as models for many more. At the Sidney Farber Cancer Institute, a committee is discussing the feasibility of having one for adult patients within the Institute. This would mean that medical care with all its technicalities would be close if needed. Because the care and nurturing of the pediatric patient is done by the mother, the hospice does not seem as important for that patient group.

It has been a long time in coming, especially in the United States, but we are beginning to harmonize our care of the very ill and terminal patient. We are not afraid to share our feelings, to give of ourselves, and to laugh and cry.

In helping our patients adjust to a prolonged life or face the terminal stage of their illnesses, we must be factually and emotionally honest with them and their families, with ourselves, and with our co-workers. We must understand our patients as individuals. We must know them as people and we must respect them.

When a good relationship has been formed and a family can trust the oncology team, the family can learn to live with the knowledge of the diagnosis, the treatment becomes tolerable, and the family can support the patient all the more. We can do our best, only if we are honest, concerned, and sincere.

Bienestar del Paciente y su Familia

Jesús García Orcoyen

Vice-Presidente de la Asociación Española Contra el Cáncer, Madrid, Espana

A) ATENCION A LA FAMILIA DEL PACIENTE DE CANCER:

El paciente de cáncer no es solamente un ente orgánico enfermo, sino que constituye una individualidad humana situada en un entorno -
familiar, social y económico peculiar a cada caso.
De la misma manera que es preciso individualizar su terapeútica, el
médico tiene también que individualizar su conducta frente al paciente y su entorno.
En la mayoría de los casos el impacto inicial de un diagnóstico con-
firmado, se ejerce predominantemente sobre la familia creando un -
clima de ansiedad que se refleja inmediatamente en la demanda al médico, de una información sobre las posibilidades terapeúticas, las
espectativas de curación o supervivencia en muchas ocasiones la exi-
gencia económica que su asistencia pueda representar.
Este último aspecto, en la actualidad en numerosos paises ha sido -
superado mediante la cobertura económica de los seguros sociales. -
Pero incluso en muchos de estos paises, todavía existen sectores -
que no alcanzan dicha cobertura, en los que no dejan de plantearse
a las familias la preocupación económica.
En relación con el diagnóstico, y el grado de evolución del proceso,
pueden contemplarse una extensa gama de situaciones, desde aquella
en la que, no puede ofrecerse un tratamiento efectivo, y en la cual
la carga de su asistencia, recaerá en gran medida en la familia, -
hasta aquellos en los que pueda plantearse un pronóstico favorable
con una terapeútica adecuada.
La familia debe de conocer todo aquello de que razonablemente pueda
informar el médico, teniendo en cuenta que tanto en este aspecto como en el del pronóstico, el médico se mueve siempre en un terreno -
incierto. Creo que aun en el caso de peor pronóstico, el médico debe ofrecer a la familia, la posibilidad de recurrir a todos aquello
medios que ofrezcan posibilidades al menos de aliviar al paciente.
En algunos sectores a los que nos hemos referido anteriormente, todavía la base social y económica del paciente y su familia juega un
papel importante en cuanto a las posibilidades asistenciales y este
es un aspecto desgraciadamente vigente en nuestros dias en numero-
sas comunidades.
Como ha dicho GOUGH-THOMAS, para que el tratamiento sea realmente -

efectivo debe encontrarse el medio de alcanzar una seguridad finan-
ciera y desplazar ansiedades familiares evitables.
Por ello la Asociación Española Contra el Cáncer, en sus primeros -
25 años de existencia, ha dedicado un gran esfuerzo a los aspectos
relacionados con la asistencia a pacientes de escasa capacidad económica.
Para cumplir sus fines, por una parte ha dotado a hospitales y centros de diagnóstico de equipos para su labor y por otra, a través
de un servicio social, ha orientado y respaldado económicamente la
asistencia de aquellos pacientes que lo necesitaban.
Âsi ha invertido mas de 200 millones de pesetas en equipos de Cobal-
toterapia (19) sustancias radioactivas, equipos de diagnóstico, etc
y ha atendido a mas de 200.000 pacientes pagando su hospitalización
y tratamiento, liberando con ello al menos, de la angustia económica a pacientes y familiares.
Hoy dispone de Centros Regionales propios en Sevilla, Zaragoza, Va-
lencia, Coruña, Barcelona (en construcción) y numerosos centros de
diagnóstico. El conocimiento de esta realidad por la población, ha
dado lugar a una respuesta de apoyo, mas acusada en los sectores -
mas débiles, que se refleja en la marcha de una recaudación voluntaria que pasa de 27.000 pesetas en 1953 a 350.000.000 de pesetas
en 1977.
Aun siendo los aspectos asistenciales hospitalarios muy importantes
para la familia del paciente, son más decisivos aquellos que se re-
fieren a las atenciones extra-hospitalarias, en el propio domicilio
del paciente, bien en un proceso de rehabilitación, o cuando es necesario desgraciadamente en una fase terminal a veces prolongada.
Es en esta situación en la que juega un importante papel la familia
del paciente, constituyendo siempre una primera interrogante, la de
cual va a ser la actitud de la familia ante la nueva situación, que
puede ser muy exigente desde el punto de vista no solamente emocional, sino de posibilidades personales y económicas.
Cuando el paciente se incorpora a la vida familiar en condiciones -
de reanudar su vida habitual, tras un breve periodo de recuperación
(nuestra experiencia se refiere principalmente al carcinoma genital
en la mujer), los pequeños problemas de atención por parte de la familia se superan facilmente.
Otro es el problema mucho más complejo, cuando las consecuencias de
un tratamiento, supone nuevas situaciones, como la presencia de un
ano iliaco, o deviaciones urinarias, que requieren atenciones espe-
ciales, y en general desagradables para los familiares.
Como apuntan DYK y STHERLAND, (1956) la naturaleza de las relaciones y su familia durante la enfermedad, serán siempre un reflejo de
sus relaciones con anterioridad a la enfermedad.
Cuando la unión de una pareja en un mutuo cariño y cooperación, el
paciente puede encontrar un apoyo permanente y recibir ayuda y áni-
mo, antes y después del tratamiento y esperar y aceptar los cuida-
dos de la esposa e hijos cuando retorna a su hogar, lo cual contri-
buirá a elevar su moral. Si por el contrario en el seno del hogar,
no existe dicho mutuo afecto y cooperación, poco pueden esperar el
uno del otro, y con frecuencia, la hostilidad mutua en el seno de -
una familia, hará que poco pueda esperarse de ésta, como soporte -
emocional ni como asistencia real al paciente. La irritabilidad del
paciente y sus frecuentes tendencias depresivas en algunos casos, -
pueden también perturbar profundamente la relación familiar, tanto
entre los esposos, como entre éstos y los hijos, para los cuales,
la pérdida de un concepto claro de la autoridad paterna, puede con-
ducir a frecuentes conflictos.

De todo ello se desprende, que aun en los casos mas favorables de -
relación familiar, hay que buscar una solución a los numerosos problemas que se plantean cuando el paciente deja el hospital y se incorpora a la vida familiar, para que tanto aquel, como ésta, reciba
el apoyo necesario, según sus necesidades.
Entran en juego en este momento diversos factores para poder alcanzar satisfactoriamente dicho apoyo, pues aun partiendo de una cti-
tud favorable de la familia en cuanto a su colaboración, dependerá
en gran medida de su nivel socio-económico, de su composición, esposa, hijas, hijos, edades de los mismos y condiciones personales de
trabajo y permanencia en el domicilio.
Las exigencias de limpieza del enfermo y de su alimentación, depen-
derán en gran medida de dicha composición familiar.
Por ello, uno de los aspectos mas interesantes en la atención en el
domicilio, es la irradiación de servicios desde el hospital.
Numerosos ensayos han sido realizados a este respecto en el Reino
Unido, Estados Unidos de Norteamerica, Dinamarca, Dolombia, Austria
Belgica, España y otros paises.
Estas necesidades han sido siempre reconocidas y ya en 1740 surgen
en Reims una organización voluntaria para atender a los enfermos de
cáncer. En 1796 el Dispensario de Boston considera el problema de -
la organización de una asistencia en el domicilio de los pacientes
por considerar que es menos costoso que en el Hospital y que "aquellos que han visto mejores días pueden ser ayudados sin ser humilla-
dos".
Entiendo que el estudio detallado de este aspecto no corresponde, a
este apartado que se me ha encomendado mas que parcialmente y en -
aquella medida, en que la familia del paciente, sobre la que recae
el peso directo de su atención en el domicilio debe ser frecuente-
mente ayudad, por médicos y enfermeras en relación con el Hospital
donde fué tratado el paciente. De no ser así, en sus aspectos médicos y psicológicos, el porvenir del paciente, puede ser poco satis-
factorio.

The Rehabilitation of the Cancer Patient

F. Meerwein

Consultant in Liaison-Psychiatry, Department of Oncology,
University Hospital, Zurich

The rehabilitation of the cancer patient consists of a long mourning process which starts at the moment of the onset of the disease. It takes place, generally, within the framework of the doctor-patient relationship and maybe supported by the patient's family, by special rehabilitation programs as presented at this panel, as well as by group activities or group therapy for both patients and relatives. However, every attempt at rehabilitation of the cancer patient has to be accompanied by an adequate psychological guidance of the patient by the doctor and his team, based upon a deep understanding of the patient's personality and the mental processes brought about by the disease.

Despite the wide-spread opinion that malignancies are purely biological in character and quite independent of psychological influences, it is now known with relative certainty that the course taken by such a malignance can be entirely dependent upon the psychological care that a patient receives. With effective care or counseling, and therefore with a generally positive

emotional condition of the patient, the development of the disease
can be much more favorable than with inadequate guidance and a
resultant lack of inner stability.

It is precisely this psychological management of the cancer
patient, however, which creates a number of problems which are
extremely difficult to solve, as they are often based on factors
specifically connected with the onset and the development of
malignancies. I should like to mention a few of these problems
here:

One is that, although undoubtedly many causal factors are involved
in the development of malignancies, it has often been suspected
that important experiences of loss or the inadequate coping with
aggressive affects in early life may form part of the background
leading up to them. Whereas it used to be the practice, as the
famous 1966 Symposium of the New York Academy of Science, for
instance, to test such a hypothesis mainly by retrospective
investigations, the newer method is to employ a broadly-based
prospective investigation to explore the question, and many of
the results thus obtained have tended to verify this connection.
This means, therefore, that in a cancer patient we can be dealing
with a person who has already had a history of latent depression
and disturbed emotional adjustment.

A second problem is that, as with almost any illness, the development of a cancer is accompanied by a specific fantasy. That
of the cancer patient, however, can be particularly malign in

character. The term "cancer" corresponds with the sign of the
Zodiac denoting a crab, and it is actually true that the cancer
patient frequently has the impression or fantasy of having a
crab-like being inside him which possesses all the characteristics
of a real crab - a primitive, spreading, light-shy, grasping,
pain-inflicting, unpredictable being, reaching voraciously in all
directions, and never relinquishing that which is once within
its grasp but only devouring and destroying it. This particular
fantasy can also be found in perfectly healthy people, even
medical doctors, in a frequently more invidious form than it
takes in actual cancer patients. It gives rise to the well-known
phenomena of lying and denial practiced by patients as well as
by their doctors with such prohibitive effect on the development of
a good supporting doctor-patient relationship, and therefore on
a successful rehabilitation of the patient.

A third problem is the question which arises with cancer patients
more than with almost any other category of patients, namely that
of truthfulness. It is partly the above-mentioned malign fantasy,
which repeatedly gives rise to the idea that half-truths, omissions,
or even lies can protect the patient and thus improve his quality
of life during the illness and contribute to a more successful
rehabilitation. We know today beyond all doubt that the opposite
is true. The less truthful the dealings are with the patient, the
more unsatisfactory becomes the doctor-patient relationship and
the more disturbed the course of the illness. Truth means, to be
sure, not simply a ruthless communication that before one stands

but an imminent and unavoidable death. Truth means talking to
the patient and being able to listen to him, means giving an
answer that the patient can understand and accept, means explanation and conveying an assurance of presence and availability and
therefore of hope. Most patients want to know the truth and ask
to have it. Frequently, however, the request is not directly put,
but somehow veiled, disguised, or in a form of code, and it is
not always easy for the doctor to penetrate this disguise or
to decipher the code.

A fourth problem is depression, a regular and understandable
accompaniment to cancer. Depressions have various causes: a latent
depressive tendency of the pre-morbid personality can, as a result
of the illness, become manifest. The feeling of isolation which
accompanies the illness, or the feeling of social death, can
deepen the depression. Finally, guilt feelings and fear of death
can rob the personality of every conception of life and self, so
that a profound depression is inevitable. It is a mistake which
is to be met with over and over again to believe that hiding the
truth from the patient can prevent the occurrence of these depressions. Again the opposite is generally the case. The more
disingenuous the treatment of the patient has been, the deeper
will be the depression. Depressions in cancer patients should not
and cannot be prevented but must be treated. Openness, readiness
to discuss, presence, care are the best means at a doctor's
disposal in this treatment. Antidepressives can help support the
treatment and contribute to the rehabilitation, but cannot

replace it.

A fifth problem arises in the relationship between the patient
and his doctors and nurses. Envy of the healthy, the feeling of
being left out or avoided, of not having lived one's life, can
often lead to hypersensitivity in the patient. He is easily "hurt",
"insulted", or "wounded" and therefore appears to the people around
him to be a difficult, always dissatisfied person. The cause of
this is not always recognized by the nurses and doctors entrusted
with his care, and he will frequently be regarded by them as
overdemanding and ungrateful, which can lead to profoundly
desturbed relationships between him and the hospital staff.

A sixth problem is that, just as a psychotic illness can involve
the whole family of a patient, so it can often happen that the
family of a cancer patient is also drawn into his illness. Thus
the doctor of such a patient is very often faced with the
necessity of family therapies which can make heavy and unsettling
demands on his time.

A final problem is rehabilitation. Cancer patients often complain
that they have been deserted by their doctors in the rehabilitation phase. It is quite true that especially in relation to
these patients, the medical authority involved tends to regard
his task as accomplished as soon as the malignancy has been
controlled or cured. The patient, who, even after this has been
achieved, still has emphatic need of the support and advice of his
doctor, is then often regarded as a difficult person who ought to

be glad that he is still alive at all and not come making more
demands and complaints to his doctor, who has, after all, other,
more critically-ill patients to whom he must devote his time. It
is probably due to such attitudes that rehabilitation programs in
many places have fallen so far behind. They are especially
important for patients who have been exposed to drastic and dis-
figuring operations such as mastectomies, enterostomies, laryngectomies, etc. But in addition to these, every cancer patient needs
constructive help if he is to fit himself back into the community
from which he came. He is well aware that even after being cured
he will continue to be regarded by his fellow human beings as a
kind of leper or social outcast and will be treated accordingly.
Long after his remission or cure a cancer patient can find himself
in a sort of emotional no man's land, even within his immediate
family, under which he may suffer severely and from which he cannot
free himself without constructive and specialized help. Without
this help, left alone in the rehabilitation phase with such problems
which he cannot deal with effectively, he risks the onset of a
chronic depression which may in all likelihood increase the danger
of a recurrence.

At the Department for Oncology at the Zurich University Hospital
where I am engaged as a supervisor of the liaison psychiatric
services, we have made available for doctors, nurses and patients
the following services:

1. Regular staff conferences including doctors, nurses and
   technicians, focussed on the doctor-nurse-patient relationship

and its problems (Balint-group). The group leader is a training
analyst of the Swiss Psychoanalytic Society.

2. Regular group therapy for patients, given by a specially trained
intern and a social worker.

3. Regular group meetings for relatives, given by two social
workers trained in family therapy.

4. Individual psychiatric consultations for patients, supervised
by a psychoanalyst.

5. Besides these services, patients after laryngectomy or entero-
stomy have the opportunity to attend special rehabilitation
programs for speech rehabilitation (oesophageal speech), stoma
care and so on, combined with therapeutic group meetings and
social activities. Programs such as the "Reach to Recovery" have
been organised in French Switzerland but are lagging behind in
the German Part of the country. All these activities take place
under the auspicies of the Swiss Cancer League. However, we feel
that their success depends largely on the observation and careful
management of the above mentioned psychological factors.

Reach to Recovery

Francine Timothy

European Representative of the American Cancer Society,
3, rue Philibert Delorme, 75017 Paris, France

ABSTRACT

Reach to Recovery is a program created especially to help psychologically and physically the woman who has just has breast surgery.
To accomplish this, Reach to Recovery uses as volunteers only women
who have themselves had a mastectomy and who have overcome the problems which often follow. These volunteers are specially trained
for this delicate role, and they serve as positive proof of the
possibility of complete adaptation. They are there to answer the
questions the patient might hesitate to ask her doctor or her
friends.

REACH TO RECOVERY

I am happy to have this opportunity to talk to you about a very
positive, beneficial program.
Reach to Recovery was created to help the woman who has just had
a mastectomy. She will be faced with practical and psychological
problems of a kind she has probably never had to cope with, and it
is important that she be able to turn to someone who can guide her.
Surely you would agree that the best possible help would come from
a woman who has herself had a mastectomy, one who has successfully
overcome the difficulties which follow this unfortunate operation.
To explain the program very simply, a volunteer, especially trained for this role, visits a newly operated woman at the hospital or
clinic. She is there to answer her questions, because unasked questions take on an importance out of all proportion, and she is there
to serve as an example. She is the only one who can say: "If you
had met me at a party, or at the beach, you wouldn't have suspected
that I have only one breast. The same will be true for you."
We are there to listen, to listen without judging so that it will
be easy for the woman to communicate her doubts and fears to someone who is particularly compassionate because of her own experience. Our role isnt to direct, to say, "Do this, or do that," but
rather to show her we truly understand her distress. It is astonish-
ing to discover that problems which seem insurmountable become simple when they can be expressed to someone. Situations which seem
hepelessly confused often become clear when someone understands.
It is healthy and good for us to sometimes be able to pour out the
emotions which we feel obliged to hyde, even from those closest to

us.
A woman is not accepted as a volunteer for Reach to Recovery until
two years after her operation. This is because it takes time to re-
integrate an image of herself after this radical change. As you all
know, any change in ourselves requires an adjustment period. As an
interesting example of this, a man, who had been very fat explained to me that, even though he had wanted to lose weight, once he
became thin, he felt unconfortable with himself. A part of him
wasn't there anymore, and for a while he missed it. Imagine, then,
the distress of a woman who loses her breast, a visible, tangible
part of her body... the emblem of femininity!
No woman can anticipate the shock of awakening to discover only
bandages there where her breast had been. There are many reactions
after this operation, and the woman herself can't predict her own.
These women play different roles in life, and there are subtle variations in each case.
We explain to the new mastectomy patient that it is salutary to
cry... that we all cried... and that for a while she might have moments of depression. She won't feel frightened or ashamed of these
moments if she recognizes that it is normal and inevitable to feel
a very great sadness at the loss of her breast. The volunteer can
never leave the hospital room saying, "Good, this woman has accepted her mastectomy," because acceptance is something she will do
little by little... each day a little. However, seeing and talking
to someone with whom she can identify, will greatly reassure her
that she too will be able to adapt and find again her joie de vivre.
I admit that is must be almost impossible for a man to understand
why a woman makes such a drama about a mastectomy. I think that it
is probably even impossible for a woman that hasn't had one to understand. A nurse who had just had breast surgery, explained that
in her work she had treated many mastectomees, and that she had always confidently done her best to be of help to them, but now that
it has happened to her, she realised that she had had no real idea
of what a woman would feel under these circumstances. I admit,even,
that one can't always find a logical explaination for so much despair, but even without understanding, we must admit that the facts
are there, many women are profoundly affected. A program like Reach
to Recovery can be of genuine help to them.
I don't want to imply that all women who have a mastectomy have emotional problems, but no one can judge in advance which ones will,
and it seems kind and intelligent to offer the possibility of help
to each one. Of course, there isn't any magic word which can solve
everything, but there are magic words which can solve some things,
and we know most of them. When a patient said, "... and I who loved
art and music so much...", as if, because she now had only one
breast she no longer had the right to live like other people, the
Reach to Recovery volunteer knew what words to use to mend her shat-
tered image.
The most important thing of all, and the most difficult, is the
choice of volunteers who have the necessary qualifications for this
delicate role. She must be capable of total discretion, as she has
a privileged and intimate contact with the patient. The most severe
rule of the program is that the volunteer never, never discusses
any medical questions with her patient. She never makes a visit without the consent of the surgeon, and he must have the assurance that
the person he allows to speak freely with his patient has been carefully chosen, and most carefully trained.
We offer each patient a temporary prosthesis, light weight and wash-

able, which she can use immediately, even while still in the hospital. This is a small gift, but it is of enormous importance to her, as it is essential to her morale that she be able to return home with a normal silhouette.

We fit into the hospital team remarkably well, and I sincerely believe that the volunteer is unique and irreplaceable because of the role she plays as a positive example for the mastectomy patient. Our goal is to about visit all mastectomy patients as a logical part of their treatment. If the doctors and nurses try to sort out the women they feel need a visit from a Reach to Recovery volunteer they might overlook some, because these women often put on an act of courage in front of the medical corps. Also, too often, it is supposed that older women are less disheartened by a mastectomy. I can assure you that one is always too young to lose a breast. A seventy-five years old woman said, "I can't explain my anguish, but I need you."

Reach to Recovery isn't a club, and the volunteer visits the patient only once in the hospital. She leaves her name and address, however, so that the patient can contact her if she has further questions, or if she would simply like to talk from time to time to someone who understands her seemingly paradoxical reactions. We are there to help in any way for as long as she likes after, but the request should come from her.

The newly operated woman easily discovers for herself all of the negative aspects of her situation, but she needs us to convinve her that there is also a positive side. Those of us who have gone through this painful experience know that in overcoming it a woman can become more profound and complete, more feminine in the true sense of the word. If we aren't there to convince the patient that she too will find the unsuspected resources in herself, who else can tell her, and be the example that she can believe?

Surely, before too long, a definitive solution will be found for breast cancer, but while we are waiting for this good news, a program such as Reach to Recovery is necessary. Its action is discreet, dignified and giving... a program of great value, based on mutual respect and sharing.

Programme Relating to Terminal Cancer

M. P. Cole

St. Ann's Hospice, Cheadle, Manchester

ABSTRACT

This paper discusses the development of the care of the terminal patient in Great Britain. It describes the establishment of a hospice by a voluntary organisation and indicates the benefits achieved for the patient nursed in such a hospice. It also stresses the educational aspect that the hospice can afford to medical and nursing personnel.

KEYWORDS

Definition of terminal cancer. Hospice. Problem of home nursing. Special hospital units. Role of nurse. Analgesics. Voluntary helpers. Education.

I am **very** conscious that what I will describe and discuss with respect to Terminal Cancer is set within the context of the social and economic conditions existing in Great Britain today, where for the past 30 years we have had a comprehensive National Health Service. At an International Cancer Congress such as this many countries are represented where conditions may be quite different from those in Great Britain, how terminal care is developing in Great Britain may not seem applicable to those countries but there is one common factor for all and that is the concern for the care of the terminal patient.

Only in the past 10-15 years has serious consideration been given to this subject in Great Britain. When one realises that 3 persons out of 10 will develop cancer, and 2 of the 3 will die of the disease, is it not surprising that until recently little consideration has been given to the care of patients at this stage of their disease. Probably most of us who work in the cancer field are optimists, striving to cure 100% of our patients and give little thought to the terminal state of the patients when we fail. Perhaps we leave them to manage as best they can and do not ask how they manage, who cares for them, or how free of symptoms are their last months or days.

I would define a patient as having entered the terminal state of the disease when there is no prospect of benefit from surgery, radiotherapy, chemotherapy or hormone therapy and who also is deteriorating. There comes a time in a patient's illness when one must take the positive decision that it is useless to pursue active treatment, in fact active treatment might even be harmful, as it could

subject the patient to unnecessary discomfort or suffering without any prospect
of benefit.

Even though patients have entered the terminal stage of the disease there is still
much that can be done for them by ensuring that symptoms are relieved as fully as
possible and that there is skilled, sympathetic nursing care.

Where should these patients be nursed? Most people agree that they should be
nursed at home in their own familiar surroundings among relatives and friends.
supported by the family doctor and visiting nurses. Not only will this be to the
patient's advantage, but also relatives will have the satisfaction that they have
given all possible care to the patient, which can be of comfort to them in the
period of bereavement.

In Great Britain approximately 35% will die at home, 60% in hospital and 5% in
homes or hospices. It is not always possible for the patient to be nursed at
home because some patients live alone without any relatives, even if there is a
responsible relative it may be impossible, purely on economic grounds, for that
person to give up work and nurse the patient, sometimes when relatives have been
nursing the patient they become physically tired or frightened and no longer are
capable of caring for the patient. It can occur also that the patient is young,
married with small children, then the other partner may find it impossible to
nurse the patient, care for the children and keep the home together financially.
Alternative arrangements are then sought. The alternatives are (1) the General
Hospital (2) a terminal care unit attached to a General Hospital (3) an independent home or hospice designed to nurse the terminal patient.

Looking at these alternatives, first the General Hospital. It is true that 60%
of patients dying from cancer, die in hospital. But very often these are the
patients who were admitted before the diagnosis was made, and have deteriorated
so much that it has not been possible to discharge them home, or they have been
admitted with a complication of their malignancy such as a fractured femur, ascites or intestinal obstruction and again it has not been possible to discharge
them home. The patients who have had a slow progression of their disease and
have managed to be cared for at home for a period of time, may find it very difficult to be admitted to hospital when necessary because they have no priority with
the great demand for beds for patients on active treatment.

An alternative solution, recently considered, is to have a special unit for nursing terminal patients within the confines of the hospital. This aspect is being
explored by the National Society for Cancer Relief. It is a charitable organisation set up to help cancer patients in need. In the past it has helped patients
financially by small grants and sometimes by paying nursing home fees for a limited period of time. Recently they have been interested in the possibility of
units – called Continuing Care Units – attached to General Hospitals providing a
small number of beds in which to nurse terminal cancer patients. The building of
these units is financed by the National Society for Cancer Relief but the staffing
and running costs of the units is the responsibility of the hospital and therefore
of the National Health Service. Such a unit would provide beds for these patients
separate from yet part of the hospital, where they can be nursed sympathetically
as long as they should need care. The advantage of such a unit is, that it can
use all the hospital facilities such as the X-ray diagnostic department, phar-
macy, and medical social workers. Two such units have been established.

The third alternative I wish to discuss is the independent homes and hospices.
Independent because they have been established outside the National Health Service
by charitable organisations but often having a proportion of the beds supported
financially by the National Health Service. The concept of the individual hospice

for the care of terminal patients has received a considerable amount of interest, goodwill and financial support throughout the country.

I have been associated with one of these independent Hospices, from the time it was only an idea till now when it has been opened more than 7 years, called St. Ann's Hospice. It was established as a medical and religious foundation to provide skilled and sympathetic nursing care for patients with terminal cancer irrespective of race, creed or money. Prior to its founding, medical opinion was sought as to whether there really was a need for this type of care outside the National Health Service, and it certainly was obvious to those of us in the cancer field that many patients were being nursed in far from satisfactory conditions because of the lack of hospital beds for these patients. A survey established that there was a need to provide about 70 beds in the Manchester area alone for a population of 800,000. It was decided to commence by buying and adapting a previous building, so providing 42 beds. This was a venture in faith, as the money had to be raised entirely by public subscription. An appeal was launched in 1969 for £250,000 and by 1971 the money had been realised. It came from individuals, organisations, business concerns, many fund raising efforts but also included a gift of £50,000 from the National Society for Cancer Relief. In 1971, when it was ready to admit patients, the National Health Service entered into an agreement to pay for the upkeep of 20 beds, out of a total of 42, later the National Society for Cancer Relief undertook to support 5 beds, this left a total of 17 beds to be supported by public subscription as no charge is made to any patient. The running cost of a bed per week is £100. Such has been the support from the public that St. Ann's Hospice is financially sound and money is being contributed to establish an extension of 30 beds, which should be opened at the end of 1978. It does not aim to be a hospital but instead to provide skilled and sympathetic nursing care in a relaxed, peaceful atmosphere. It has no laboratories, no X-ray equipment, no operating theatre but it does have a high proportion of nurses to patients.

How does the nursing care in a Hospice differ from that in a General Hospital? In a hospital, staff often feel guilty that there is no active treatment for a patient, may even feel defeated. This can result in the patient being given analgesics only when pain is severe and routine care without attempting to understand the patient's needs. While in the Hospice nurses accept the fact that the patient is in the terminal stage of his illness without feeling guilty and realise that they have a very positive contribution to make in ensuring that all the symptoms are relieved, or even anticipated. The whole tempo of the Hospice is slower than in a hospital, so the nurse can devote time to understanding the needs of the patient, she does not have to work to a time-table that includes ward rounds and theatre list. Nursing care is given continually day and night.

It has been found that pain can be controlled by giving adequate analgesic drugs routinely 4 or 6 hourly. In this way one aims to keep pain out of consciousness. This routine administration of analgesic drugs controls the pain more effectively than waiting for pain to return and become severe before administering analgesic drugs. The patient also develops the confidence that pain can be controlled, with the result that the actual dose of the drug can sometimes be reduced. Not only is pain relieved but attention is paid to all symptoms whether it is nausea, vomiting, constipation, dyspnoea, or anxiety, but no attempt is made to prolong life or the process of dying by, e.g. intravenous fluids or blood transfusions. If a patient wishes to discuss his own illness or prognosis frankly staff will talk with him, but if he is not seeking information this also is respected.

About 300 patients are admitted per annum, of which 1/5th will be discharged home again after a period of nursing care. Despite the fact that a patient has been considered to be at a terminal stage of his illness, he may improve with good nursing care and relief of symptoms, stabilised on a regime of analgesic drugs, so that he can be discharged home to the care of relatives, for a further period of time. Usually there are more female patients than male patients in the Hospice, but despite this apparent predominance of female patients, statistics show that practically equal numbers of female patients and male patients are admitted in one year. The average length of stay of female patients is 42 days compared with 24 days for male patients. This difference may be attributed to either admission of female patients earlier in the terminal stage as it has been more difficult for the husband to nurse the wife at home than vice versa or to the nature of the malignancy. The dominant malignancy among men is lung cancer, while among women it is breast cancer which can be slow growing but incapacitating with bone metastases.

Criticism is sometimes made of such homes on the grounds that they will be known as a 'home for the dying' and no patient will wish to be admitted to it, also it will be impossible to staff such a home, no one will want to work there. This has not been our experience, our greatest problem is the waiting list for admission, we only manage to admit 50% of those who apply. When a bed is available it is given to the patient whose need for admission is the most urgent irrespective of when the application was received.

The nursing staff who applied to work at the Hospice did so knowing the nature of the work, and are mainly mature women, married, with families, some working full-time, others part-time. There is not a rapid turnover of staff, they come and continue to work happily in the Hospice. They derive satisfaction from the work because they see a patient on arrival, distressed, perhaps in pain or anxious but by their skill the patient becomes comfortable and relaxed, and remains comfortable until death or, in some cases, until he can be discharged home again for a further period of time.

In addition to the nursing staff there is a rota of voluntary helpers - 180, people who can be called upon to help in many ways throughout the Hospice. By having voluntary helpers there is a continual movement of people from the outside world coming in, which is of interest to the patients and helps to create a cheerful, friendly atmosphere. Relatives can visit throughout the whole day, children too and an occasional dog! With free visiting the relatives do not feel they have abandoned the patient, they may even help by feeding the patient if this is necessary.

Though Hospices are being established throughout Great Britain, on very similar lines to St. Ann's Hospice, I cannot foresee that the care of all terminal patients will eventually be undertaken at Hospices. These Hospices fill a need for patients who cannot be nursed at home and for whom there are insufficient hospital beds, but they have another very important function and that is to demonstrate how it is possible to nurse these patients comfortably, with dignity, in a relaxed atmosphere, how pain can be controlled and yet the patient remains alert. Therefore, an important aspect of the work of a Hospice is education, to train nurses and medical students in the care and management of these patients. Some of these Hospices, including St. Ann's Hospice, now have facilities for training post-graduate nurses and also undertake to demonstrate the care of these patients to medical students. Until recently little importance has been given to this aspect of patient care both in the education of medical students and of nurses. Not only nurses and medical students now seek experience at these Hospices but Medical Society Workers and theological students. The contribution that the Hospice can make is therefore not only in the actual care of the patients admitted to it but also by educating others with the knowledge and experience obtained at the Hospice. This can mean that the overall care of the terminal patient, whether at home or in hospital, will be improved.

Cancer Hostels in New Zealand

G. W. Holland

President, Cancer Society of New Zealand

ABSTRACT

With the expansion of sophisticated radiotherapy and chemotherapy, many patients have to travel long distances for therapy. Cancer hostels, financed mainly by voluntary donations and provided at minimal cost to the patient have proved very successful in overcoming this problem.

It is recommended that such hostels should be organised locally rather than nationally, and that the hostels should include facilities for counselling.

KEYWORDS

Cancer   Welfare Hostels

New Zealand, situated in the South Pacific, has a population of 3.3 million spread over two islands, with a total distance from North to South of 2000 km. The country has a high standard of living, comparable with that of Western Europe and a well developed medical service.

Treatment for the cancer patient is readily available without direct cost to the patient through the Public Hospital system, but there are also good private hospitals in most towns.

Comprehensive cancer treatment facilities are available in the six largest cities - four in the North Island and two in the South. Because of the widely scattered population, patients often have to travel considerable distances to treatment centres.

Many cancer patients requiring radiotherapy and chemotherapy are ambulant and do not require admission to hospital for treatment. However, the disease itself and the length of time required for treatment often put severe financial strains on patients, and the cost of paying hotel accommodation can only add to the worries of an already overburdened patient. For this reason most cancer centres in New Zealand, in the 1960's, considered the possibility of building hostels for those cancer patients required to travel from outlying areas, but who did not need hospital admission.

Although each centre looked at this problem independently, it is
noteworthy that the solutions have been very similar. In all cases
money has been raised by public appeal, usually with the aid of a
service organisation such as the Lions Club. No difficulty has been
found in raising sufficient money to build and furnish a hostel so
that it is debt free at the time of completion. The reputation of
the hostels has been so good that in a recent appeal for $100,000
for a hostel extension, $180,000 was raised in one night in a city of
only 80,000 people.

The emphasis in all of the hostels has been on informality, and the
construction of the buildings has usually been similar to that of a
private home. Spouses and other relatives are always allowed and
encouraged to stay in the hostel with the patient.

In all cases the hostel has been built as close as possible to the
cancer treatment centre, usually within walking distance and
sometimes within the hospital grounds.

Administration of the hostels has been kept as informal as possible
and there are virtually no rules. To promote a home atmosphere staff
do not wear uniforms and are identified only by a name badge. One of
our hostels in fact, manages without any resident staff, the patients
and their relatives doing all the cooking and light housework.

As most patients having radiotherapy can return to their homes at
weekends, rooms at the hostels are made available at weekends to
relatives of hospital inpatients. This provides low cost
accommodation for any family that is already under financial strain
through the breadwinner having cancer.

For the patients themselves, no charge is made for hostel
accommodation but many patients give donations voluntarily to cover
costs. This, together with bequests, often from previous patients,
has meant that all of our hostels have been able to break even
financially.

Adequate recreation facilities are regarded as an essential part of
the hostels and all rooms have their own radio so that the patient
can tune in to his own station. Television, games rooms, hobby
rooms and libraries are also provided.

Patient Counselling

Once the hostels were opened, it soon became apparent that they
provided an ideal environment for counselling of patients and their
relatives.

Cancer Society Welfare Officers and Medical Social Workers visit the
hostels regularly. They feel that in the relaxed and informal
atmosphere of the hostel they are able to do their work more
efficiently than in a hospital department.

A criticism of cancer hostels has been that they may foster "mutual
morbidity" and an attitude of undue pessimism by bringing closely
together patients who may be deteriorating and those who have a good
prognosis. However, we have not found this to be so. The reverse
seems to be the case. For example, a patient who is at high risk of
losing his hair from chemotherapy is often encouraged by seeing how

other patients are coping with the problem.

As a result of our experience in New Zealand the following recommendations are made for those considering similar ventures.

1.   Raising money by public appeal presents few difficulties as the project usually has widespread public sympathy and support.

2.   A home-like environment helps patients, and relatives should be encouraged to stay with the patient.

3.   Hostels should be kept reasonably small - maximum beds about 40 - to minimise administrative problems.

4.   Staff need only be minimal as patients and their relatives are usually happy to cope with cooking and light housework.

5.   Good counselling services should be provided, and the hostel is an ideal place for such counselling.

6.   Hostels should be organised on a local rather than a national basis, as requirements differ considerably in different parts of the same country.

Cancer Nursing

Charles C. Sherman, Jr.* and Josephine K. Craytor**

*University of Rochester School of Medicine and Dentistry
**University of Rochester School of Nursing
Rochester, New York, U.S.A.

ABSTRACT

In responding to an invitation to discuss cancer nursing in the United States, as seen by a physician, the authors describe several functions carried out by nurses which are particularly significant in providing cancer care: providing expert psychosocial care based on scientific knowledge, taking major responsibility in rehabilitation, teaching patients and family members, participating in screening programs, helping manage pain and anxiety, planning patient discharges, carrying out technical functions requiring specialized skills, caring for ambulatory patients in clinics and homes, teaching other professionals, staffing specialized oncology units and carrying out nursing research. In conclusion the need for increased amicable and thoughtful cooperation between physicians and nurses in the interest of improved patient care is cited.

KEY WORDS

Cancer Nursing, Nursing, Health Team, Role, Paramedical Personnel, Nurse Specialist

INTRODUCTION

In the United States today, Cancer Nursing is a growing specialty, accepted by many but still struggling to define its field. The fight for women's rights has been a major factor in the tremendous advancement in the sophistication, education and prestige in nursing generally. Developments in clinical oncology - especially in medical and pediatric oncology - have created a large demand for more sophisticated nurses to play increasingly varied roles in the care of the cancer patient. In addition to some fifty cancer centers throughout the United States, almost all of the one hundred twenty medical schools and several hundred of the larger hospitals have special cancer units in some stage of development. Cancer care is becoming more and more a function of a multidisciplinary team and nurses are earning a place on that team.

The Oncology Nursing Society, formed within the last five years in response to the great interest in the field, now has more than eleven hundred members and continues to grow. The Association of Pediatric Oncology Nurses has around two hundred members. The American Cancer Society sponsored a Second National Conference on Cancer Nursing in St. Louis in May, 1977 which drew more than two thousand

165

nurses from all over the United States and several foreign nations.(A.C.S., 1977)

A survey of the members of the Oncology Nursing Society showed that nearly half had college degrees and that six percent had either a masters or a doctoral degree. In general the educational level of this group is higher than that of the total population of professional nurses in the United States. An example of the level to which cancer nursing has developed in the United States is the case of one of my colleagues who is a university professor, an Associate Director of our Cancer Center and a member of the National Professional Education Committee and the National Advisory Committee on Nursing of the American Cancer Soceity. While the income of cancer nurses may not yet be commensurate with their educational and experience qualifications, it nevertheless represents an impressive improvement over average nurses' salaries. Forty-five percent of the ONS members surveyed were in the $15,000 range, twenty percent in the $20,000 range and two percent in the $25,000 range. The unusually high salaries commanded by this small group of nurses seem to reflect the great demand which exists for their specialized expertise (Miller and Herbst, 1978).

Functions which I see as especially important for the cancer nurse include the following:

Psychosocial Aspects of Care

There has been a tremendous increase in our understanding of the emotional and social problems of the cancer patient and of his family. Further, we are realizing more and more that often psychosocial problems must be solved before the patient will accept and respond to adequate therapy. Today's cancer nurse may have had extensive training in this area of patient care, and indeed this is the area in which many of the more highly trained cancer nurses feel they can make their most unique contributions, and in which they can carry out significant clinical investigation. Certainly the nurses spend more time with patients and families than do any other professionals, not only in the hospital setting, but in the out-patient clinic or office setting and, importantly, in the home. Understanding and dealing with the mechanisms by which patients and families cope with a continual series of problems, including those around terminal illness, requires of a nurse not only compassion but also sophisticated training and expertise.

Rehabilitation of the Cancer Patient

Therapy is provided cancer patients in the hope that they can be rehabilitated after treatment sufficiently so that they can lead normal or nearly normal lives. While a significant part of that rehabilitation begins with the management of the psychosocial concerns identified at the initial contact of the patient with the physician, the nurse or other members of the team, there are other phases of rehabilitation requiring physical and physiological approaches. Post-mastectomy patients require adequately fitted prostheses and help regarding their purchase and care. If they have had radical mastectomies they may require physiotherapy to promote proper functioning of the shoulder, and they may require counseling regarding the exercise of the arm and its protection against injury and infection. In today's world with the emphasis on the breast as a major symbol of sexual attractiveness, a mastectomy can have a devastating effect on a woman's perception of herself and on her relationship to her husband and family. The nurse can play a determining role in helping the patient back toward a normal life. Although it applies in all other situations, it is most often noted in the post-mastectomy patient, that the patient can open up and tell the nurse things that may be crucial to a successful resolution of problems, which she could never bring herself to tell the physician.

One could recite a long list of similar rehabilitative problems in patients following radical surgery of the head and neck, in patients with colostomies or
ilial conduits after urinary diversions, in patients with various amputations and
in patients with the entire gamut of rehabilitative problems following chemotherapy, radiotherapy and radical surgery. Today's cancer nurse brings special knowledge and expertise in helping the therapeutic team identify, manage and in some
cases, anticipate and prevent the development of problems during this period.

Patient Education

The nurse in cancer care can help spread the message that if we could get the
average citizen to play a greater role in his own health care, we would be doing
more to improve health than we could by doubling the number of physicians or
health facilities. People must smoke less, drink less, and eat properly. Women
should do self-examination of the breasts, seek Pap smears at appropriate
intervals. People must come to believe that cancer can be cured and that it is
important to seek and accept appropriate diagnostic and treatment measures when
they note early warning signs of cancer. If people are to accept more responsibility for their own health management they must learn more about what they can
do to prevent cancer, to take more active roles in screening opportunities and to
cooperate effectively with the health care team in early detection and to seek
and accept appropriate treatment from qualified professionals when cancer is
found. Many cancer nurses are already playing significant roles in the education
of patients and public along these lines, not only in the hospital and clinic
setting, but in the home and in the school. These nurses have learned something
of the behavioral psychology necessary for the effective teaching and motivation
of people toward health serving behavior. Indeed, in cancer screening clinics
the educational and motivational aspects of care are considered as important as
the screening examination of the breast, cervix, etc., itself.

Cancer Screening

In many screening clinics cancer nurses are performing the screening examinations
with the backup of physicians to confirm abnormal findings and to make therapeutic decisions. Nurses are trained to do all of the routine screening procedures
for cancer of the head and neck, breast, abdomen, colorectum, cervix, skin, etc.

It is not appropriate to discuss fully the problems of screening here--its
potential benefits, its defects, its costs and its priority value to a given
population in relation to others health needs. It is important to recognize that
nurses are playing an increasingly important role in this aspect of cancer care
in those parts of the world where cancer screening, particularly of breast and
cervix, is felt to be a worthwhile endeavor. Further, it should be recognized
that nurses with appropriate education and experience can play a role in the
design, conduct and evaluation of screening programs as well as in performing
the examinations.

Relief of Pain and Anxiety

The nurse spends more time in direct contact with the hospitalized patient than
does any other professional and should be uniquely able to judge the type and
degree of pain, its inter-relationship with anxiety-producing factors, including
the fear of pain, the response to medication and other comfort measures, and any
other factors which can assist in the most effective modification of narcotics
and analgesics regimens. To function in this role adequately the cancer nurse
must be compassionate and knowledgeable and must be an astute enough observer and
vocal enough advocate for the patient to be an accepted member of the multidisciplinary team.

Discharge Planning

In the past a patient was often discharged from the hospital on the spur of the moment, with little thought on the part of the physician about the patient's continuing needs at home--for medications, supplies, equipment, nursing care, social supports, on-going medical care, etc. It is particularly important for the cancer patient that careful review of his needs be made and that careful arrangements be made with the patient and family for not only the immediate but also the long-term needs. Today discharge planning is a major function of the cancer nurse in the hospital and this planning is begun as early in the hospital course as possible. A well designed plan coordinated by the cancer nurse can make a great difference not only in how the patient feels about going home, but also in how successful he and his family are in maintaining him at home.

New Technical Functions

Some new functions being carried out by nurses in special cancer clinics and physicians' offices include administering intravenous drugs and immunotherapy, obtaining medical histories and doing physical examinations as well as performing thoracenteses, lumbar punctures, bone marrow aspirations, etc. These procedures are done under physician supervision and control, and are accepted practice in only a very few medical centers where volume is great. They do, however, illustrate the possibilities for one direction in which the role of the oncology nurse can be expanded, that of physician extender. This type of expansion requires highly specialized training, and does not seem to be a direction in which many people will choose to go.

Some of the functions being taken on by cancer nurses in the United States today may cause concern on the part of other nurses and of some physicians. Many nurses will not want to become "junior doctors" and will try to restrict the expansion of nursing functions to those areas which they see as primarily related to nursing care as opposed to delegated parts of medical care. Many nurses are trying to distinguish a well-demarcated area of "health care" as being primarily the province of nursing and at the same time extend the education of some nurses so that there are sufficient nurses with advanced degrees to maintain an independent role that clearly represents nursing on the "health care team", of equal stature to the other members of the team and capable of making unique and complimentary contributions to health care. There is no question that, as individuals, many nurses have already earned advanced degrees and have the knowledge and experience to qualify as full and equal members of the "health care team." This group has at least two very important missions to perform: to give leadership to the vast numbers of nurses who cannot acquire and probably do not need the advanced education; and to delineate and demarcate the specialized body of nursing knowledge and care different from medical care. This new body of knowledge is slowly being developed through clinical nursing research and will enrich the tremendous assistance already being given by nurses in medical care.

Some physicians may feel threatened by what they see as the encroachment of nurses into the practice of medicine. Others are willing to accept well-trained cancer nurses in a variety of new roles and welcome their help on the team.

Roles of Cancer Nurses

Some of the functions being performed by cancer nurses have been discussed briefly. It seems appropriate to outline some of the roles in which they perform those functions:

Cancer hospital staffs. Obviously this is one of the most important areas for cancer nursing practice, education and research, with the appropriate staffing at all levels, as well as nurses prepared as subspecialists in such fields as pediatric oncology, radiation therapy, medical oncology, gynecology oncology, head and neck surgery, etc.

Cancer centers in university hospitals will usually require specialized and sub-specialty staff depending on the volume of cancer patients and the extent of their educational and research programs. Some of the larger community hospitals will also have sizeable specialized cancer units requiring a core of oncology nurses.

More and more frequently some of the smaller community hospitals with special programs of cancer care and research but no segregated cancer unit will find invaluable one or more trained cancer nurse specialists to coordinate the care of the cancer patients, teach staff nurses and house staff, help professional students make appropriate plans for their cancer patients and relate to the community resources necessary to help patients and family carry on management at home.

Ambulatory and Home Care

More and more cancer patients are being treated on an ambulatory basis and are managing at home. There will be an increasing demand for cancer nurses to give care and counseling to patients and families in the home either as part of "organized home care" programs, clinic outreach or home hospice programs. An increasing number of cancer units in the major hospitals will develop specialized home care programs for cancer patients requiring sophisticated nursing care.

Independent Nursing Practice

Cancer care and counseling in the home including most of the functions noted above can be given by a well-educated nurse acting independently and paid on a fee-for-service basis. A recent issue of *Cancer Nursing* describes the work of such an independent nurse practitioner who works out of the office of her physician husband. One of the limitations to the development of such practices, which could be less costly than multiple office and emergency department visits, is that most insurance companies will not yet reimburse patients for such services.

Professional Education

Many cancer nurses are now full-time faculty members in university schools of nursing. Others have joint appointments between schools of nursing, service agencies and cancer centers. Several medical schools are seeking qualified cancer nurses for joint appointments between the medical school and the adjacent school of nursing.

Research in Cancer Nursing

Most of the studies which have been done by nurses have been concerned with psychosocial aspects of patient care, with control of pain and other discomfort, with rehabilitation and with patient education. Many of these studies have been done in collaboration with professionals from other disciplines. If the special-ist in nursing oncology is to develop truly independent research or to participate as an equal partner in multidisciplinary investigations, her education will have to be at a relatively sophisticated level and will have to include experience in research techniques and evaluation. With the tremendous demand for specialists in nursing oncology to fill the many roles noted previously, research will probably be limited to a part-time activity even for those few numbers of nurse oncologists who obtain masters degrees and doctorates. Eventually, however, the numbers of nurse oncologists with advanced degrees will increase and their experience and sophistication will develop to the point where significant independent clinical investigation and perhaps even basic research will become a solid reality.

Examples of current priorities in cancer nursing reserach as selected by a large panel of cancer nurses and reported in *Cancer Nursing* follow:

1. Determine effective methods of relieving chemotherapy or radiation induced nausea and vomiting.
2. Establish discharge planning and follow-up programs which effectively mobilize patient, family and community resources.
3. Develop more effective methods of psychological support for patients and families at various stages of disease and cancer treatment.
4. Identify the unique components of cancer nursing that validate it as a specialty practice, and develop suitable educational programs in the specialty (Oberst, 1978).

Conclusion

It is apparent that interrelationships between the physician and the nurse are changing. Although there are bound to be some conflicts and differences of opinions as this process continues, willingness to compromise and to adjust to special circumstances will be necessary so that the interests of the patients come first. Unless nurses and physicians continue to work together in a cooperative friendly spirit as professionals, the patients will suffer.

American Cancer Society (1977). *Proceedings of the second national conference on cancer nursing*, A.C.S., New York.
Miller, S. and Herbst, S. (1978). Summary of O.N.S. membership survey, *Oncology Nursing Forum*, 5:22-23.
Oberst, M. (1978). Priorities in cancer nursing research. *Cancer Nursing*, 1:281-290.

Diagnosis

Ultrasound: Its Uses in Cancer Diagnosis

Barry B. Goldberg

*Director, Division of Diagnostic Ultrasound, Professor of Radiology,
Thomas Jefferson University Hospital, Philadelphia, Pennsylvania, U.S.A.*

ABSTRACT

Ultrasound has assumed an important place in the initial evaluation
of patients suspected of having cancer in various areas of the body.
Since it is a non-invasive technique, it has been used as a screening or preliminary procedure once a mass is suspected or detected
clinically. While there are limitations of its use, that is, ultrasound cannot penetrate air or dense bone, there are many organ
systems throughout the body that are amenable to visualization ultrasonically. The areas that can be examined successfully include organs
within the retroperitoneum and abdomen, as well as the chest and
mediastinum, and even such areas as the brain and eyes. Superficial
structures such as the thyroid and breast can also be evaluated in
terms of cancer detection.

Ultrasound has proven useful in cancer detection in several ways.
One important use is its ability to detect and then differentiate
the internal characteristics of a mass. A mass that is shown to be
cystic is more likely to be benign while those with major solid
components are more likely to be malignant. A second use has been
in the following of patients once cancer has been detected. This
includes the serial evaluation of masses to show their response or
lack of response to various treatments, as well as the long term evaluation of patients with known cancer to detect evidence of recurrance.
Another exciting area has been in the evaluation of ultrasound as a
potential screening test for cancer. This is still not yet proven,
but extensive work is ongoing, particularly in such areas as the
breast. If successful, it could reduce the use of x-ray mammography.
Finally, extensive research is ongoing in the development of ultrasonic tissue signature concepts, that is, the non-invasive analysis
of masses or tissues to determine if they are malignant. This has
met with some limited success in the laboratory, with applications to
clinical situations still far in the future.

INTRODUCTION

The importance of ultrasound in the detection and evaluation of masses has gained an important place in medical diagnosis. Historically, ultrasound was first used clinically after the Second World War. It's initial use was in the evaluation of midline structures of the brain followed by evaluation of the heart. No attempt was made in the 1940's to use ultrasound for the evaluation of tumors. However, by the 1950's initial work was already going on in the detection of cancer in such areas as the breast. In fact, the initial success rates in the detection of breast cancer was very encouraging, approaching 100%. This initial work, however, was carried out on large masses in an older age group. As a result, most of the solid masses were malignant. The accuracy rates in the evaluation of the internal characteristics of masses within the abdomen and retroperitoneum has been in the 90% range, similar to other non-invasive procedures. The areas that have been successfully examined ultrasonically in the evaluation of cancer are numerous. This report will discuss four major areas where ultrasound has been so used. That is (1) the detection and differentiation of a mass that is clinically suspected, (2) the serial evaluation of masses to determine their response to treatment as well as recurrance, either at the primary or distant sites, (3) cancer screening, and (4) tissue signature efforts.

I. DETECTION AND DIFFERENTIATION OF MASSES

Ultrasound since the 1950's has been used to localize masses and determine their internal characteristics. When a mass is suspected clinically by palpation, history, or through other non-invasive routine studies, such as intravenous urography, ultrasound is often performed before other more expensive and often invasive studies are ordered. It is able to detect the presence of a mass and delineate its relationship to surrounding structures. The site of origin of the mass can also be established. The internal characteristics of the detected mass can be differentiated ultrasonically. The cystic, or mixed (complex) nature of a mass is easily established.

Each organ system will be individually reviewed to indicate the usefulness of ultrasound for cancer detection.

Ophthalmologic Evaluation

Ultrasound has been used successfully over a number of years for the evaluation of tumors both within the eye and the retrobulbar region. While direct visualization will usually establish the presence of a tumor, if there is clouding or hemorrhage within the vitreous, the retinal area will be obscured. With ultrasound the detection of retinal and choroidal tumors has proven efficatious. It is the primary diagnostic approach for the detection of tumors behind detached retinas and, of course, in the retrobulbar region.

Echoencephalography

While the complete ultrasonic evaluation of the brain has been limited by its bony covering, a midline shift which is an indirect indication of tumor can be easily demonstrated. On occasion echoes can be recorded from tumors. This has been particularly true at surgery after the bone has been removed where it has been used as an aid in the localization of tumors prior to their biopsy. Ventricular dilatation can also be visualized ultrasonically.

Chest and Mediastinum

Within the chest the ultrasonic evaluation of tumors has been limited due to the aerated lung and dense bone. However, mediastinal masses that are projecting against the pleura can be evaluated. It has been used successfully to differentiate pericardial cysts from solid tumors.

Echocardiography

While echocardiography has not been used principally for the detection of tumor, certain cardiac masses can be detected. Myxomas have a characteristic pattern that is almost pathopneumonic. Pericardial effusion, often the result of tumor seeding of the pericardium, can also be detected.

Abdomen

By far the greatest use of ultrasound in cancer detection and localization has been within the abdomen and retroperitoneum. Masses that are either palpated or clinically suspected can be evaluated ultrasonically. For instance, masses within the pancreas that are cystic are usually pseudocysts while solid masses are most frequently tumors. Secondary signs or malignancy, such as the presence of dilated bile ducts due to obstruction by a tumor in the head of the pancreas can also be imaged. Tumors have been detected within the gall bladder. It has been used successfully in the detection of both primary and metastatic liver lesions. Enlarged lymph nodes have also been successfully evaluated, particularly in the para-aortic region. Ultrasound has assumed a primary role in the evaluation of renal masses, since any mass within the kidney, if it can be shown to be solid it is usually malignant, whereas if it is cystic, it is usually benign. Secondary signs of malignancy such as ascites, can also be detected.

Superficial Masses

Superficial masses have been successfully evaluated using ultrasound. Any cold thyroid nodule is examined ultrasonically in order to determine if it is cystic or has any solid components. If it is cystic aspiration is usually performed, whereas if it is solid or complex, surgery is usually the primary approach. With breast masses a similar approach has been used.

The pediatric patient has also benefited from ultrasound in the localization and detection of tumors. In the newborn, whenever a mass is palpated, ultrasound is usually one of the initial studies performed due to its non-invasive nature and lack of ionizing radiation. It easily differentiates solid, cystic, and complex masses, differentiating between such entities as multicystic kidney and Wilms' tumor.

Thus, it can be seen that ultrasound has become established as an important, often primary diagnostic procedure, in the detection, localization, and differentiation of masses. It can delineate tumors that disrupt normal organ contour or internal architecture, as well as measure the size and depth of a mass. Finally, it can delineate the internal characteristics of masses separating them into their cystic or solid components, which has a direct relationship in many instances as to whether the mass is most likely benign.

II. EVALUATION

Once a mass has been detected by ultrasound and confirmed by either arteriography, biopsy, or surgery, treatment may be initiated. When this occurs it is important not only to know the exact location of a mass but also its relationship to adjacent organs. In both of these areas ultrasound has proven useful. It is thus used extensively in radiation treatment planning to map out the ideal portal for adequate tumor treatment while sparing as much as possible exposure to normal organs. Ultrasound is also useful in obtaining total body contours. Unlike x-ray, there are no magnification factors. Once treatment is initiated, either radiation or chemotherapy, the response of the mass to treatment can be easily monitored. The volume of the mass can be easily determined. Changes in size, often a direct indication of the success or failure of treatment can be assessed ultrasonically. Secondary spread such as to lymph nodes and liver can also be determined during the course of treatment. Ultrasound has also proven effective in the long term evaluation of patients who have been treated to detect recurrance either at the primary or distant sites.

III. SCREENING APPROACHES

While ultrasound has established its usefulness for the localization, detection, and differentiation of masses, it is still under investigation as a procedure for the screening of patients with a high potential for cancer, such as can occur with some congenital abnormalities in the pediatric age group, as well as in the evaluation of non-palpable breast masses. While x-ray mammography is still the diagnostic study of choice, its effectiveness has been reduced due to public anxiety over the potential harmful effects. As a direct result, the National Cancer Institute requested research projects to evaluate the effectiveness of ultrasound for breast screening. Our group has received funds for such a project and has embarked on a two year program to evaluate the potential usefulness of ultrasound in breast screening. In our research project, approximately one thousand women will be examined each year. The ability of ultrasound to detect and differentiate masses as well as to differentiate specific breast patterns including the delineation of such structures as ducts, vessels, and hopefully, calcifications, will be evaluated. Specific ultrasound characteristics of the breast have been demonstrated including variations in general breast architecture as well as the detection of masses as small as 3 millimeters in diameter. The accuracy, however, has not yet been established.

IV.   TISSUE SIGNATURE

Extensive research is being conducted throughout the world to
determine if ultrasound can be used to non-invasively identify specific tissues. Ultrasound is transmitted, absorbed, and reflected to
varying degrees by various tissues. All of these factors, as well as
other parameters are being tested to determine if ultrasound has the
capability of specific tissue characterization. If this should prove
true, it would be of significance in cancer detection. Up to this
point, ultrasound as well as other non-invasive procedures such as
x-ray computerized tomography, do not have the ability to determine
with any specificity the type of solid tissue within organs and thus
cannot differentiate benign from malignant tissue. Preliminary
investigation of ophthalmic masses has shown some capability of
ultrasound to differentiate tumor types, however, no other clinical
work has yet supported these initial results. Laboratory studies are
showing some promise but much more research is needed.

In conclusion, ultrasound is an important primary, non-invasive,
diagnostic tool in the evaluation of cancer in various parts of the
body. It is used to localize as well as differentiate the internal
characteristics of masses. It is also used to evaluate the response
of tumors to treatment as well as to detect evidence of either
primary or secondary recurrence. Potential advances in ultrasound
cancer detection include screening, particularly in the area of the
breast, and specific tissue characterization which, if successful,
should dramatically increase our ability to detect cancer.

Flexible Bronchofiberscopy

S. Ikeda

Department of Endoscopy, National Cancer Center Hospital, Tokyo, Japan

Bronchoscopy was first introduced by Prof. Gustav Killian in 1897, then improved
by Prof. Chevalier Jackson in 1904, and since then it has been generally accepted
all over the world. On July 23, 1966 in Japan, I developed the first experimental
flexible bronchofiberscope in the world, and presented my film entitled "New
Apparatus for Bronchoscopic Cinematography and Bronchofiberscope" in the motion
picture session for the first time at the 9th International Congress on Diseases
of the Chest held in Copenhagen in August of the same year. And the first paper
was presented in the beginning of 1968, when the flexible bronchofiberscope was
completed for the practical application. Later in 1974 "the Atlas of Flexible
Bronchofiberscopy" was published in the world.

In February last year the World Conference on Bronchoscopy was held in San
Francisco with Dr. David R. Sanderson as President. Also the World Congress on
Bronchoscopy held on July 10th to 12th in Tokyo. To this World Congress on
Bronchoscopy in Tokyo, more than 650 bronchoscopists attended from about 26
countries over the world. About 90 scientific papers including two special
lectures, two symposia, panel discussions, round-table conference and free
presentations are programmed with discussions on either rigid or flexible
bronchoscope applications. At present about 5,000 to 6,000 flexible bronchofibers-
copes are used throughout the world either in diagnostic or in therapeutic purposes.

The most important subject among the purposes the bronchofiberscopy is applied for
may be the detection and diagnosis of early lung cancer. When you use the flexible
bronchofiberscope, the method in the hilar type early lung cancer is different from
that in early lung cancer in the periphery. I will, therefore, speak about the
significance of flexible bronchofiberscopy in both cases. Firstly, the flexible
bronchofiberscope, as you already know, makes it possible for us to visualize from
sub-segmental as far as to sub-sub-segmental bronchi, by inserting the scope into
any and all segmental bronchi. The bronchofiberscope, therefore, can be used to
make the locational detection of early lung cancer in hilum, and to achieve early
diagnosis by obtaining biopsy specimens directly from the lesions, since the cases
of hilar type early lung cancer are possibly found in this area. Secondly, it is
possible for you to attain the cytological diagnosis by inserting a cytology brush
or small curette through the inside channel of this flexible bronchofiberscope and
performing brushing or curettage under X-ray fluoroscopy. Even if an abnormal
shadow of 1 or 2 cm. in size is found on chest X-ray examination in mass survey,
cytological brushing or curettage should be performed correctly under X-ray

fluoroscopy so that a definitive diagnosis can be obtained even before surgical operation. Now, I would tell you the significance of flexible bronchofiberscopy in early lung cancer cases which I classify into 2 types of those in hilum and periphery.

In Japan the hilar type early lung cancer was defined as carcinoma originating in more central region up to segmental bronchi on the resected specimen and confined within the bronchial wall with N0, M0, by Ikeda Project started in 1972.

TABLE 1. The Criteria of Early Lung Cancer in Hilum

(The 1st Phase of IKEDA Project)

1. The cancer originates in the region from major to segmental bronchi.
2. In the resected lung specimen, the lesion is confined within the bronchial wall.
3. No lymph node metastasis.
4. Any histological types are allowed.

During the recent period of about 10 years, analysis of 27 cases were performed in a common method in the 3 leading institutions of National Cancer Center Hospital, Osaka City College, and National Sanatorium Kinki Central Hospital.

Fig. 1 Locations of the Cancers in 27 Cases

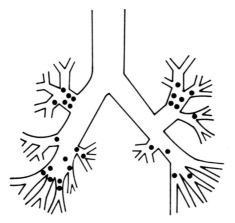

lobar bronchus   7cases
upper div. bronchus   4cases
segmental bronchus   16cases

When plotting the origins of those 27 cases on the bronchial tree diagram, there were as many as 16 cases in the segmental bronchi, 4 cases in the left upper division bronchus, and 7 cases in the lober bronchi. In all the 27 cases, the patients were male of 44 to 76 years old, 59 years old on the average, and, in their smoking history showing as a cigarette index, for which the number of daily smoking cigarettes was multiplied by the smoking years, the index of over 600 was 89% in those 27 cases. From their subjective symptoms, 3 cases were negative, 15 cases were bloody sputum, 6 cases were coughing and fever due to obstructive pneumonia, and 3 cases were only complaining coughing. In the chest X-ray findings, no findings were in 11 cases, obstructive pneumonia like shadow in 14 cases, and

Table 2
  Clinical Features in 27 Cases

Age:44 to 76 (average 59)
Sex:male 27, female 0
Smoking habit:
                          cases %
    cigarette index <600   3(11)
                    ≥600 24(89)
Symptoms:
    bloody sputum   15(56)
    cough & fever   6(22)
    cough only   3(11)
    no symptom   3(11)

Table 3
  Clinical Features in 27 cases

chest x-ray:
                              cases
    negative   11
    obstructive pneumonia   14
    segmental atelectasis   2
Sputum cytology:
    positive   22
    negative   1
    not examined   3
Bronchoscopic examination:
    localized   25
    positive biopsy   25
    not examined   2

Hostology:
    squamous cell ca   27
    others   0

segmental atelectasis in 2 cases.

The positive rate of sputum cytology was 95.6%. Bronchofiberscopy was performed
on 25 cases, and localization of tumors and histological diagnoses could be attained
in all the cases, their histological type being squamous cell carcinoma. We
classified the bronchoscopic findings of early lung cancer in hilum into polypoid
type, nodular type, and superficial infiltrating type. Particularly in the cases
of superficial infiltrating type, we studied the findings of shade of colour of
mucosa, irregularity of the surface, longitudical or transverse folds and sub-
mucosal capilaren dilatation. The data of the 25 cases in bronchoscopic findings
were 8 cases of polypoid type, 4 cases of nodular type, 9 cases of superficial
infiltrating type, and 4 cases of polypoid type accompanying superficial infiltrating type (or infiltration).

Table 4 Bronchoscopic Findings of Early Lung Cancer in Hilar Region

    1) polypoid tumor   (8)
    2) nodular tumor   (4)
    3) superficial infiltration   (9)
    4) polypoid tumor with   (4)
       superficial infiltration
                          ( ):no. of cases

The cases which a special attention should be given to were the 11 chest X-ray
negative cases. Their bronchoscopic findings, were 4 cases of granular surface, 3
cases of coarsely irregular, and 4 cases of polyp or nodular tumor. Especially in
the superficial infiltrating type, there are many cases of granular surface, which
often makes difficult to decide localization. I will report on an early case
with chest X-ray negative and sputum cytology positive I have experienced very
recently.

The patient was a 44-year-old male with a heavy smoking habit. Because of the
positive sputum cytology, bronchofiberscopy was performed to examine carefully the
orifices of all the segmental bronchi only to find out that the opening of right

Table 5

Summary in 11 cases with "occult lung cancer"

case	Symptoms	cyt. of sp.	No. of invest.	Bronchoscopy Location	Findings	Gross features
1. T.N.	bloody sp.	pos.	1	R.bas.	granular	superficial inf. type
2. E.I.	"	"	1	R.sup.	"	"
3. Z.S.	"	not done	1	LB^{1+2+3}	irregular	"
4. K.T.	"	pos.	1	"	granular	"
5. N.K.	"	not done	3	R.im	"	nodular inf. type
6. Y.K.	none	pos.	1	L.bas.	irregular	"
7. H.F.	bloody sp.	"	1	L.B*	"	"
8. I.K.	"	"	1	R.B^3	nodular	"
9. S.T.	"	"	1	R.sup.	"	"
10. K.O.	none	"	1	R.sup.	polypoid	"
11. A.U.	bloody sp.	not done	1	R.B^7	"	"

bes. : Tr.basalis', sup. : Tr. supeior, im. : Tr.intermedius

Table 6 THE CRITERIA OF EARLY LUNG CANCER IN PERIPHERY

(THE 2ND PHASE OF IKEDA PROJECT)

1. The lung cancer originates in the region from subsegmental bronchi up to the periphery.
2. The size of a tumor is less than 2cm on the resected lung specimen.
3. No infiltration to the pleura and no metastasis exists in lymph node or to any distant region.

B' bronchus had a fine granular surface with coarse irregularity in small parts, and disappearance of mucosal luster and longitudinal folds. The examination of biopsy specimen confirmed its localization, and upper lobectomy was performed. As it has become possible to obtain the findings of superficial infiltration correctly, so the localization of bronchial fouci and confirmation of resecting range have become easier to be determined.

Next, I will report about the other subject, definitive diagnosis of early lung cancer in periphery. Ikeda Project made the definition of peripheral type early lung cancer having a tumor size of under 2 cm. on the resected specimens and a very slight or no metastasis in the pleura without lymphnode or distant metastases, and its localization is as far as sub-segmental bronchi toward the periphery.

In National Cancer Center, surgical operations have been performed on 52 cases of small peripheral lung cancer of under 2 cm. during the past 9 years. The patients of these cases are 33 males and 19 females with an average year of 56. Histologically, they consist of 41 cases of adenocarcinoma, 8 cases of squamous cell carcinoma, and other 3 cases, which means naturally quite a number of adenocarcinoma cases are detected. By plotting these cases on the bronchial tree diagram, so many cases are in the periphery of upper lobes on both sides. I will report about the definitive diagnosis by flexible bronchofiberscopy.

Table 7
PERIPHERAL TYPE EARLY LUNG CANCER (52 Cases)

SEX	Cases	AGE	Cases
Male	33	31–40	2
Female	19	41–50	8
		51–60	23
		61–70	12
		71–	7

HISTOLOGICAL TYPE
Adenocarcinoma ···················· 41
Squamous Cell Carcinoma ··········· 8
Small Cell Carcinoma ············· 1
Large Cell Carcinoma ············· 1
Adeno and Squamous Cell Carcinoma.. 1

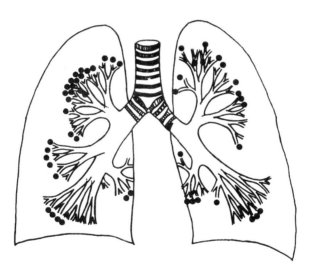

Fig.2

In the first place, such a peripheral small lesion originates in the Vth to Xth order branch bronchi in 82.7%. It is, therefore, difficult to find out the drain bronchi in the location of small lesion. The most effective method to locate such bronchi would be the selective peripheral bronchography, carefully inserting a flexible bronchial catheter into the aimed lesion and taking bronchogram to confirm the drain bronchi. Adenocarcinoma, particularly the well differentiated one,

often tends to involve several bronchi and to convert to each other in the periphery. In order to detect such drain bronchi, it is very important to take enlarged
X-ray film using 50 micron(μ) small X-ray focus. In the second place, it is
imperative to perform curettage of the drain bronchus by inserting a double hinged
curette into the bronchus through the inside channel of flexible bronchofiberscope
under X-ray fluoroscopy, since many cases of adenocarcinoma have a sharped obstruction in the drain bronchus. This fact proves the curettage more effective than
bronchial brushing. Also the double hinged curette is indispensable to hit the
bronchus complicately curved in the periphery, however, this curette must be used
most carefully under X-ray fluoroscopy. I have never had any accidents in the
double hinged curette operation in more than 10,000 examinations of 5,000 patients
owing to my careful performance.

With these methods we examined 46 cases except for 6 cases without examination, we
succeeded in definitive diagnosis in 45 cases out of 46 cases, in 6 cases of which
we performed curettage for more than twice and in 2 cases for three times, and all
resulted in positive in 2 months' period. Furthermore, the 11 cases with the tumor
under 1 cm. were all positive in these methods. To obtain such good results, it
is by all means necessary to perform energetic bronchofiberscopic curettage under
X-ray fluoroscopy after confirming the location of the drain bronchus by correct
and selective peripheral bronchogram.

Table 8 DEFINITIVE DIAGNOSIS OF PERIPHERAL CANCER

		Less than 2 cm. (Resected Cases) (1969 --- 1977)		
Total Number	Bronchoscopic Curettage Case Under X-ray T.V.	Definitive Diagnosis on Curettage		
		(+)		(−)
52 Cases	46 Cases	45 Cases		1 Case

Flexible bronchofiberscopy is the most effective weapon not only in visualization
and biopsy of the hilar lesion but also in curettage of the small peripheral lesion,
and I should say that it is impossible to diagnose early lung cancer without the
flexible bronchofiberscope.

Value of Mammography

Philip Strax

Medical Director, Guttman Institute,
200 Madison Avenue, New York, NY 10016, U.S.A.
Assoc. Clin. Prof., Preventive and Community Medicine
New York Medical College, New York, NY 10019, U.S.A.
Director of Radiology, LaGuardia Hospital, Forest Hills, NY 11373, U.S.A.

ABSTRACT

Clinical examination with inspection and palpation for detection of breast cancer has been found increasingly inadequate in recent years. It is becoming evident that breast cancer is present for a substantial period of time in a non-palpable stage. It is also apparent that detection and treatment of the disease in this occult stage leads to increased survival and improved cure rate. Mammography is the only practical means available today to detect and localize the lesion before it can be felt.

Mammography is of great value under the following conditions:

a. In the presence of a questionable mass on palpation, mammography can help clarify the issue.
b. When a palpable lesion is present which appears benign but requires surgery, another lesion which is not palpable may be present in the same breast and be detectable only on mammography. The latter lesion may be a cancer.
c. The breast opposite to the one with a palpable lesion may harbor a non-palpable cancer.
d. The greatest value of mammography may lie in screening for breast cancer. In all studies to date, up to 45% of cancers are negative to palpation and detected on mammography alone. These are in a particularly early stage with a high degree of curability.

The radiation dose used has been reduced by use of film-screen combinations to under 5% of 1 rad to the mid breast, at the same time that quality has been greatly improved. Such minute doses are considered negligible in light of the great potential benefit.

Mammography is widely accepted as a valuable modality in the detection and diagnosis of breast cancer. It is becoming increasingly apparent that breast cancer may exist for a substantial period of time before it becomes clinically obvious by palpation. During this time, it may be detectable by mammography. Such detection may be possible when the immunocompetence of the host is intact and when removal of the growth results in a high rate of curability.

Keywords: MAMMOGRAPHY / NON-PALPABLE CANCER / LOW-DOSE RADIATION / XEROMAMMOGRAPHY / RISK VS. BENEFIT

MAMMOGRAPHY: WHY SHOULD WE DO IT, HOW SOULD WE DO IT, AND IS IT SAFE?

Introduction

Mammography is not new. It is an old technique. The first recorded use, on amputated breasts, was described by the German pathologist Salomon (1913). He characterized the irregular mass density and microcalcifications. We still consider these important signs of malignancy on a mammogram. The procedure has had a varied career since that time. It was taken up by various radiologists in various countries with various modifications but never found general acceptance. In particular, LeBorgne (1953) in Uruguay, Gros (1963) in Strasbourg, and Gershon-Cohen (1963) in the U.S.A. continued to promote the modality. It was not until 1960 when Egan (1964) in the U.S.A. developed his technique of using industrial-type fine grain film with low kilo-voltage and high milliampere-seconds that mammography began to receive greater attention. All this time, mammograms were difficult to produce with acceptable quality, probably because films were too grainy and details were often obscured. Even the Egan technique required considerable close scrutiny, much experience, and even much intuition. Because of the technical difficulties in performing mammography and the problems of interpretation, xeromammography - also an old technique - was revived and perfected by Wolfe (1972) as an improved method of mammography. Finally, it was the support of the United States Public Health Service and the development of teaching centers for mammography that stimulated increased interest in this procedure. The big push came with the reports from the Health Insurance Plan study that the use of mammography combined with palpation, under mass screening conditions, was leading to the saving of lives from breast cancer.

Today, mammography is in widespread use all over the world wherever breast cancer is a dread disease. And, whenever a procedure achieves fame in medicine, opponents and detractors begin to appear to emphasize weakness or dangers. Since mammography uses x-radiation, concern has been expressed over its safety. Now we are in a new era in mammography. Most investigators agree that it is indeed very useful and probably life-saving but some question whether the harm of radiation exceeds the good.

Why Should We Do Mammography?

The female breast is readily accessible to inspection and palpation. Why then do we need mammography (Strax, 1975)?

The time-honored method of clinical examination with inspection and palpation for detection of breast cancer has been found increasingly inadequate in recent years. It is becoming more and more evident that breast cancer is present for a substantial period of time in a non-palpable stage, when the fingers of a woman herself or those of the most proficient breast clinician cannot feel the growth. It is also becoming apparent that detection and treatment of breast cancer in this occult stage leads to long survival and increased cure rate. Mammography is the only practical means for detecting the lesion before it can be felt.

We need mammography because:

1. The breast is normally a multi-nodular structure which practically always is made up of varying-sized small or large "lumps." The dominant mass that suggests pathology may not be clearly evident to inspection or palpation. This is particularly true of an early cancer. The mammogram is our most useful modality that very often - not always - gives the physician that extra

assurance that he may be dealing with a malignant - or benign - process. It is often the added bit of suspicion that leads to prompt exploration.

2. In the face of a definite lesion on clinical examination that is about to be explored, the mammogram can yield additional information about the rest of the breast or the opposite breast. A cancer may be lurking elsewhere in either breast which is completely non-palpable and that "other" lesion may be the cancer, not the mass leading to exploration.

3. One of the most cogent reasons for mammography, particularly in the symptomatic woman, who feels a vague mass, severe localized pain or nipple discharge, is the varied expertise of physicians in breast clinical examination. The average woman who sees her primary-care physician with a breast that is a problem to her often presents an even greater problem to her physician who does not have the experience of the breast expert. A mammogram under such conditions can be life-saving in avoiding delay, especially under screening conditions.

4. It has been known for many years that a breast cancer may not be palpable by even the most expert hands and yet be in the early stages of a deadly disease. The breast cancer screening activities, using mammography in addition to clinical examination, that have been going on for about fifteen years, have turned up hundreds of such lesions. It is these non-palpable cancers, which have a high degree of no nodal involvement and are accompanied by a substantially increased survival, and often reduction in mortality, that have brought the importance of the x-ray examination of the breast to the fore.

How Should We Do Mammography?

Mammography. Mammography, which uses low-kilovoltage, and therefore low penetrating x-rays, produces a two-dimensional gross anatomical view of the breast. Breast structure, normal and abnormal, is visualized. These images are correlated with the pathologist's findings and criteria are set up for differential diagnosis of breast lesions. It should be remembered that mammography is an anatomical display with potential for accurate localization of a lesion. It offers the possibility of accurate comparison with the pathologist's study (Strax and Pomeranz, 1968).

Mammography delineates details of normal breast structure with its varying amounts of glandular tissue, ductal structures and stroma of fibrous tissue and fat. Detectable within this framework are:

- Benign masses, such as fibroadenomata, cysts and lipomata, usually with regular margins and often with homogeneous calcifications;
- Cancers, displayed as: (1) masses, usually with irregular margins; (2) irregular calcifications, usually grouped and with varying densities; and (3) areas of trabecular distortions.

Mammography can detect non-palpable cancer when it is still localized and probably curable in three ways:

- By finding a dense mass which is too small in proportion to the size of the breast to be felt;
- By detecting the microcalcifications of intraductal carcinoma, often non-invasive, before a mass has developed;
- By detecting the trabecular distortion of a cancer before the fibroblastic response has developed which makes it palpable.

The value of film mammography has been enhanced in recent years by improved radiographic equipment especially designed for this purpose. Such improvements include molybdenum anode tubes and compression which increase the contrast of breast soft tissues with improved accuracy of interpretation.

The importance of mammography versus clinical examination varies with the type of breast, the stage of the cancer, and the type of patient. Thus, in the small glandular breast, the large cancer mass, and in the premenopausal woman, clinical examination is more efficient. In the large fatty breast, as in the older woman, in the small cancer mass, or the cancer without a mass, the x-ray examination may be more informative.

An important principle in breast cancer therapy needs to be emphasized here. Because neither palpation nor mammography is 100 percent in accuracy, if a cancer is suspected on palpation, a negative mammogram should never be allowed to delay exploration of a breast. Similarly, a clinician whi is faced with negative clinical findings, but with a positive mammographic report, should seriously consider exploration. The two modalities are truly complementary. They should never be considered competitive.

Xeromammography. Xeromammography is merely a variation of mammography in which the same x-rays are used to produce the image. A charged selenium plate is used instead of film and the end result is a mammographic image on paper with considerable edge enhancement. There is difference of opinion amongst radiologists about which display medium is superior, some preferring one and some the other. Most experienced mammographers think the microcalcifications may be more easily detected on the Xerox plate but that masses are more easily detected on the improved film mammography.

When xeromammography was first introduced, it produced better detail and lower radiation dose than was possible with the Egan fine-grain film techniques. The present film-screen combinations, such as are used at the Guttman Institute in New York City and in other centers in the U.S.A., are producing high-quality films with considerable reduction in dosage over xeromammography so that many radiologists prefer the new film techniques.

Radiation Dosage

Recent years have seen a dramatic improvement both in the quality of mammography and in the radiation dose used. The most widely-used technique, purporting to produce the highest quality, in the 1960's was that of Egan, involving a slow industrial Kodak type M film, a tungsten tube, close Coning, no compression with low kilovoltage and high milliampere-seconds. This technique produced high quality mammograms with radiation doses ranging from 8 R to 12 R to the skin per examination. In the last few years, under the leadership of British radiologists like Price, Sellwood and Nathan (1975) and Ostrum, Becker and Isard (1973) in the U.S.A., the use of faster film-screen combinations in vacuum cassettes has seen a remarkable improvement in contrast and resolution of the mammographic image plus a reduction in radiation levels of .2 R to .3 R to the skin. The latest measurements by Miller and others (1977) in the Northeastern Physics Center in the U.S.A. indicate that such skin radiation, with low kilovoltages used plus the molybdenum-anode tubes and compression techniques, is delivering doses to the mid breast of .02 rads to .03 rads for a right-angle pair of films. These techniques are readily available and are being used by an increasingly number of radiologists. Revision of techniques in xeromammography with the introduction of the negative mode and increase of kilovoltage has resulted in reduction of radiation, though not to the low levels available by the newer film-screen techniques.

Table 1 is a list of varying radiation dosage in various mammographic techniques. Notice that the dose has dropped from 8-12 R to the skin, per exposure in the Egan technique - which was used essentially in the Health Insurance Plan study - to .2-.3 R to the skin, per exposure in techniques presently in use at the Guttman Institute.

TABLE 1   Film-Screen Combinations and Dosages for their Operation

Film-Screen Combination, Compared with Other Methods	Radiation Dosage (R)	
So-called Egan technique (type M-tungsten, no screen)	8 -12 +	
Xeromammography		or
Tungsten tube	2 -3	1-2 with
Molybdenum tube	3 -4	minimal filtration
Senographic-type machine (molybdenum)		
Kodak SO-146, no screen	5 -6	
AGFA Osray M, no screen	2 -3	
DuPont Lo-dose (screen no. 1)	1 -1.5	
DuPont Lo-dose (screen no. 2)	0.8-0.9	or little
Kodak Min-R (rare earth screen)	0.8-0.9	less, to
AGFA rare earth screen	0.8-0.9	0.6-0.7
GM special alpha rare earth screen	0.3	
Kodak 105 mm RFC 874 with Min-R screen	0.3	
105 mm with United States Radium special screen	0.2	
DuPont 105 mm SF 2 with Min-R screen	0.3	

Wilkinson and others (1978) with Xerg (Xonics) techniques in the U.S.A. have produced high-quality mammograms with markedly reduced radiation to levels even lower than the best of the film-screen techniques. This process holds great promise for the development of mammography techniques with radiation dosage so low as to be negligible in comparison with the potential benefit to the x-ray study of the breast.

RADIATION RISK VS. BENEFIT

The problem of radiation risk from mammography revolves around two facts:

1. The breast is sensitive to x-radiation. Previous studies on women subjected to substantial doses of radiation, such as with the Atomic Bomb, fluoroscopies in the course of tuberculosis treatment or radiation treatment for breast abscess, have indicated increased incidence of the disease in those exposed. Such breast cancer initiation had a latent period of about 10 years and varied in proportion to dose. Although no evidence exists for absence of a theshold dose, it has been considered prudent that such a dose be postulated and that a linear radiation effect be assumed down to the smallest quantity of radiation. A figure of "1 rad to the body of the breast given to a million women would produce 6 cancers per year for a lifetime of the woman after a latent period of 6 - 10 years" has been offered by Dr. Arthur Upton, noted radiobiologist and at present, Director of the National Cancer Institute, as a fair statement of radiation risk from mammography.

2. Risk, however, is directly proportional to dose. The state of the art in mammography has changed radically in the years since the H.I.P. study. In that study, doses of 7-8 R to the skin were given per examination. New film-screen techniques, as used at Guttman Institute and other places, now deliver .2-.3 R to the skin per exposure or, as we have noted above, doses of about .02-.03 rads for a complete examination of the breast, instead of 1 rad in the formula mentioned above means that if all 40 million at risk for breast cancer in the U.S.A. were to receive a breast examination, including mammography, every year for the 30 years that even the youngest member would be exposed, the following would happen. The usual present annual incidence of 96,000 breast cancers would be found with 34,000 deaths expected from the disease per year. With screening (using mammography plus palpation) we would reduce the death rate by at least one-third or save 12,000 lives. The cost from the radiation would be 6 cases of breast cancer per year or 180 cases in the 30 years of lifetime, after a 10-year latent period, and one-third of these would probably be saved. In other words, at least 12,000 women would be salvaged at a cost of, at most, 120 lives over 30 years. In short, such dosage is negligible by all radiological standards and should permit more liberal interpretation of risk vs. benefit.

We must always remember that the symptomatic woman with a dominant mass, localized persistent pain or nipple discharge has the real possibility of harboring a cancer which may be non-palpable. All diagnostic means, including mammography - with the best techniques - must be used for elucidation of the problem. The question of radiation dose does not apply at all to the symptomatic woman.

CONCLUSION

The radiation dose used in mammography has been reduced by the use of film-screen combinations to under 5% of 1 rad to the mid breast at the same time that quality has been greatly improved. Such minute doses are considered negligible in light of the great potential benefit.

It can be said categorically today that mammography is turning out to be the best single modality for detecting curable breast cancer.

REFERENCES

Egan, R.L. (1964). Mammography. Chas. C. Thomas, Springfield, IL.

Gershon-Cohen, J., and Berger, S.M. (1963). Mastography. Radiol. Clin. North Am., 1:115.

Gros, C.M. (1963). Les Maladies du Sein. Masson et Cie., Paris, France.

LeBorgne, R.A. (1953) The Breast in Roentgen Diagnosis. Impresora Uruguaya, Montevideo, S.A.

Miller, D.W., and others. (1977). Radiation absorbed dose in mammography. Presented at Annual Meeting of American Association of Physicists in Medicine, Cincinnati, OH.

Ostrum, B.J., Becker, W., and Isard, H.J. (1973). Low dose mammography. Radiology, 190:323.

Price, J.L., and Nathan, B.L. (1975). Radiological aspects of the West London Screening Program for Breast Neoplasms. Proc. R. Soc. Med., 68:438.

Salomon, A. (1913). Beitrage zur Pathologie und Klinik des Mammakarzinoms. Arch. Klin. Chir., 101:573.

Strax, P., and Pomeranz, M.M. (1968). Non-malignant variations in mammography Am. J. Roentgenol., 102:941.

Strax, P. (1975). Breast cancer diagnosis: mammography, thermography and xero-
    graphy; a commentary. J. Reprod. Med., 4:265.
Wilkinson, E., Jacobson, G., and Muntz, E.P. (1978). Preliminary clinical mammo-
    graphy study using electron radiography. In: H.E. Nieburgs, ed., Prevention
    and Detection of Cancer, Part II, Detection, Vol. 2. Marcel Dekker, Inc.,
    New York. (in press).
Wolfe, J.N. (1972). Xeroradiography of the Breast. Chas. C. Thomas, Spring-
    field, IL.

Infra-red Thermography of Breast Cancers. An 8-year Experience. (Diagnosis, Detection, Prognosis, Follow-up)

R. Amalric,* D. Giraud,* C. Altschuler,* J. M. Spitalier,**
H. Brandone,** Y. Ayme,** J. M. Paoli,*** J. F. Pollet,*** and
R. Burmeister***

*Department of Radiology
**Department of Surgery
***Pluridisciplinary Laboratory
Cancer Institute, Marseilles, France, POB 156 F 13273 Cedex 02

SUMMARY

This paper is a very short summary of our experience of the reliability and the place of infra-red thermography (IRT) in mammary oncology. This experience is based on 30,000 different women, 3,682 palpable breast tumors, 2,226 consecutive breast cancers (BC) confirmed with full physical, radiological and microscopic studies, and on 779 operable breast cancers followed over 3 years (373 of these ones over 5 years).

Amid the means of medical examinations of breast diseases, IRT takes an original part. IRT does not produce static anatomical images, but it brings physio-pathological thermal pictures at 16 frames per second. IRT is still not appreciated by many physicians, specially because of its false indication rate in mass screening of breast cancer. Among asymptomatic people IRT taken by itself in isolation has a limited value. In order to achieve its proper use, it is necessary to practice it on a large scale within a multi-disciplinary oncology team. Concerning high risk or symptomatic women, IRT gives valuable data of energizing behaviour of BC.

Key words: Infra-red thermography, diagnosis, detection, prognosis, breast cancer.

INTRODUCTION

IRT represents a <u>non-invasive method</u> at clinician disposal. In the <u>strategy against BC</u> (7) <u>IRT has an original place in diagnosis, detection, prognosis and follow-up.</u>

193

IRT picks up at distance electromagnetic infra-red emission from the tegument by high speed cameras with quantic detectors and translates the received energy into black-white and colour images in an instant manner.

A thermographic pioneer R.N.LAWSON (5) demonstrated in 1956 that BC is a heat producing tumor. Blood warms up at the cancer fire. M.GAUTHERIE (4) has measured BC thermogenesis and found a range of values between 0.015 and 0.075 watt/cm^3 . The rate of cancer growth (3) is directly proportional to this specific thermogenic power.

A continuous thermal exchange chain must be present from cancer to camera, which implies that :
* the cancer must emit sufficient thermal message.
* the thermal messa-ge must be transmitted towards the tegument (reasonable depth of cancer, conducting intermediate tissues without excess of fat, convecting veins draining towards superficial levels).
* the thermal message must be reemitted outwards by the tegument in the form of infra-red ra-diations (ulcerations, crusts, phaneres, sudation, ointments may considerably decrease skin surfa-ce emissivity).
* the thermal message must be picked up by the high speed camera which processes it and converts into a visual image through controlled manipulations of position, sensitivity, definition, speed and isotherms (by specialized technician under supervision of physicist).

For a good interpretation of mammary thermograms, by a professional thermographer physician, two steps are necessary: first of all analysis of objective parameters (tab. 1), then synthesis with classification into categories of increasing dia-gnostic weight (tab. 2).

table 1   INFRA-RED THERMOGRAPHY SIGNS

PARAMETERS	SUSPICION	MALIGNANCY
HYPERVASCULARIZATION	ASYMETRIC	ANARCHIC
HOT SPOT	2.5°C.	>2.5°C.
WHOLE BREAST HYPERTHERMIA	2 °C.	>2 °C.
EDGE SIGN	LOCALIZED	EXTENDED

table 2   INFRA-RED THERMOGRAPHY GRADING

TH 5	MALIGNANT TYPE THERMOGRAM WITH SEVERAL SIGNS OF MALIGNANCY (OR ONLY ONE SIGN OF MALIGNANCY WITH SEVERAL SIGNS OF SUSPICION).
TH 4	MALIGNANT TYPE THERMOGRAM WITH ONLY ONE SIGN OF MALIGNANCY (OR SEVERAL SIGNS OF SUSPICION).
TH 3	SUSPICIOUS OR DOUBTFUL THERMOGRAM WITH ONE SIGN OF SUSPICION.
TH 2	BENIGN TYPE THERMOGRAM (WITH SYMETRIC HYPER-VASCULARIZATION).
TH 1	NORMAL THERMOGRAM WITHOUT ANY VASCULAR MANIFES-TATION.

Equipped with such device, working on well defined parameters and strictly classified data, the oncologist has a new way to approach the behaviour of BC.

I   DIAGNOSIS

Since June 1970, the clinical experience of our medical community has been supported by mammary IRT of 30,000 different symptomatic patients with 3,682 consecutive palpable breast tumors, which have been confirmed microscopically later on (tab. 3).

table 3   IRT GRADING OF 3,682 PALPABLE BREAST TUMORS

IRT GRADING	BENIGN TUMORS		MALIGNANT TUMORS		
TH 5	30	0.02	855	0.38	885
TH 4	131	0.09	722	0.33	853
TH 3	320	0.22	441	0.20	761
TH 2	626	0.43	184	0.08	810
TH 1	349	0.24	24	0.01	373
	1,456	1.00	2,226	1.00	3,682

IRT OF BENIGN TUMORS was true-negative (TH1 + TH2) in 67 %, suspicious (TH3) in 22% and falsely-positive in 11 % of cases.

IRT OF BREAST CANCERS was true-positive (TH4 + TH5) in 71 %, suspicious (TH3) in 20 % and falsely-negative in 9 % of cases. IRT was abnormal in 91 % of cases of malignancy.

Cancer probability in cases of palpable breast tumor, according to our infra-red thermography grading, is the following (tab. 4).

table 4   IRT CANCER PROBABILITY OF PALPABLE BREAST TUMOR

	CANCER	NO CANCER
TH 5	0.95	0.05
TH 4	0.78	0.22
TH 3	0.48	0.52
TH 2	0.16	0.84
TH 1	0.04	0.96

The significant thermographic level of high cancer probability is indeed 2.5ºC. gradient (between TH3 and TH4).

THE CAPITAL QUESTION OF FALSE-NEGATIVES

The rate of IRT false-negatives depends on the size of the BC (tab. 5) and varies from 2 to 30 % .

table 5   RATES OF IRT FALSE-NEGATIVES (IUAC T CATEGORIES 1969)

	T0	T1	T2	T3	T4	
TH1 + TH2	3	51	132	18	4	208
TOT	28	170	1,204	590	234	2,226
%	0.11	0.30	0.11	0.03	0.02	0.09

The figure of 30 % false-negatives in small size BC (palpable mammary carcinoma s T1 category) is indeed considerable. Is IRT useless for BC detection ? It is necessary to compare it with the false-negatives of clinical and radiological examinations for the same cancers (tab. 6).

table 6   FALSE-NEGATIVES OF 200 SMALL SIZE BREAST CANCERS
            (30 TO + 170 T1 , IUAC 1969)

CLINICAL EXAMINATION	80 / 200	=	0.40
RADIOLOGICAL EXAMINATION	50 / 200	=	0.25
INFRA-RED THERMOGRAPHY	56 / 200	=	0.28

It is obvious that any isolated mehod is not infallible not even radiography which makes 25 % of errors by default in small size cancers in spite of a strict methodology.

Infra-red thermography should not be used alone.
Fortunately the errors are not always made in the same direction as the methods used are based on different principles.
Each one is able to rectify the other's errors: about two
times out of three. IRT must enter a combined non-invasive
diagnosis with clinical, radiological, microscopic examinations.
At this price the errors before histologic control are reduced
to about 1 % of existing carcinomas.

In positive diagnosis of palpable breast tumors IRT
gives 11 % of false-positives and 9 % of false-negatives
(between 2 and 30 % according to the diameter of the cancer).

II   DETECTION

IRT may misknow a palpable breast cancer, but paradoxically it is able to see a certain number of unpalpable
carcinomas...

With the help of IRT we have identified 30 unpalpable infiltrating BC. Two thirds of these patients had a palpable cancer on the opposite breast, which had been or were
about to be treated. The only true screening that we do is
" the other breast expected cancer screening" among women whose
high risk has been proved by the first side. Now we detect during the three years following the first treatment 7 % of carcinomas on the second side, which are unpalpable in 18 % of
cases.

We have performed 40 exploratory wedge resections in
strictly normal breasts (clinically) on account of thermographic and/or radiologic alarm. In an unexpected manner IRT
produces fewer false-negatives (4/30= 0.13) than radiology
(18/30= 0.60). However radiological significant images of
the wedge resections sites in operative research remain absolutely necessary for histological swabs.

IRT often gives the first alarm of unpalpable BC,
nine times out of ten and one out of twice alone (tab. 7).
Sometimes radiography shows abnormal opacities after several
months or years. Before disregarding a single thermal alarm
we must keep an eye on these patients (clinically and radio-

logically) for many years, above all among high risk women.

table 7   NATURE OF THE FIRST ALARM OF UNPALPABLE BREAST CANCER

INFRA-RED THERMOGRAPHY ALONE	15 / 30 = 0.50
INFRA-RED THERMOGRAPHY AND RADIOLOGY	12 / 30 = 0.40
RADIOLOGY ALONE	3 / 30 = 0.10

On the other hand we have identified 37 carcinomas in 575 mammary benign dysplasias (6 %) : 11 of these carcinomas (30 % ...) after initial single IRT alarm.

Among 744 well women with abnormal IRT A.STARK (UK) has found 12 % of breast carcinomas, and during the following 7 years: 7 % more. In a retrospective study concerning 1,245 women with abnormal thermograms M.GAUTHERIE (4) has collected, from 1 to 12 years: 40 % of breast cancers...

IRT is the highest risk marker we have to date, according to W.B.HOBBINS.

The apparent three different birth dates of breast carcinomas can be separated by long intervals, sometimes several years: often the thermal birth is the first, the radiologic is the second and the clinical is the last.

Don't be careless: yesterday's false-positive might become tomorrow's true-positive !

III   PROGNOSIS

We owe to the English School the first clinical verification of the value of the IRT prognosis (6). Sometimes a false-negative is not only an error but also good news.

Our experience is supported by 779 3-year cases and 373 5-year cases of consecutive operable breast cancers, with initial IRT and followed after curative treatment.

Generally speaking, over 3°C. gradient we register a loss of about 20 % of survivors (tab. 7).

table 7   3 AND 5 YEAR SURVIVAL RATES

	3 YEARS	5 YEARS
TH4 + TH5 ($\geq$3°C.)	407/552= 0.74	179/281= 0.64
TH1 + TH2 + TH3 ($<$3°C.)	207/227= 0.91	74/ 92= 0.80

Being parallel to some elements of prognosis (histological local grading and axillar staging, for instance) IRT has
however an personal anticiped meaning at equal stage (tab. 8).
It is able to foresee some unexpected failures and unhoped-for
successes.

table 8   3 AND 5 YEAR SURVIVAL RATES OF STAGES II (IUAC)

	3 YEARS	5 YEARS
TH4 + TH5 ($\geqslant$3°C.)	0.80	0.65
TH1 + TH2 + TH3 ($<$3°C.)	0.97	0.96

Under 3°C. gradient we only register 1 % of additives
failures between 3 and 5 years: for " cold" stage II cancers the
time slows down.

THE CAPITAL QUESTION OF FAST GROWING UNAPPARENT CANCERS

IRT squares with a fast growing cancer (anatomicaly
operable):
* for a hot spot at least of 5°C.
* for a hot spot of 4°C. at least, with abnormal hot surface
  exceeding two quadrants.

Thermograms of this type bring a very poor prognosis
(tab. 9).

table 9   SURVIVAL RATES WITH OR WITHOUT FAST GROWING TYPE IRT

	3 YEARS	5 YEARS
FAST GROWING TYPE IRT	53/112= 0.47	13/ 52= 0.25
NO FAST GROWING TYPE IRT	577/667= 0.86	241/321= 0.75

The great merit of the thermo-prognosis is that it
provides the clinician with an objective non-invasive test helping him before any invasive investigation in the selection,at
an equal stage, of two groups:
* high failure risk patients (for additive medical treatment,
  for instance).
* low failure risk patients (for curative treatments with conservative hope, for instance).

IRT shows us how dangerous are the " warm microcancers".
It is high time to consider the thermal stage of the carcinomas
of the breast.

IV   FOLLOW-UP

Following curative treatments IRT must be performed, every year for instance, after radiotherapy or surgery for detecting local recurrencies and metastatic disease as well as new neoplasms of the other breast. After the first normalized post-therapeutic thermogram, **any new hot spot** has a very high diagnostic relief.

Following curative radiotherapy of operable BC IRT shows a **thermal tide** withdrawing slowly (18 months and over), with 70 % cooled down at 3 years. Failures correlate with persistance of abnormal patterns or **flare-up** after improvement. After conservative treatments IRT has played a great part in early detection of 11 % evolutions and 2 % of recurrences.

IRT will also help in assessoring the effects of chemotherapy and endocrine management of advanced cancers with local visible manifestations. IRT provides precociously objective data of initial therapeutic response, before any perceptible effect by physical examination. IRT is the first spy satellite in oncology.

DISCUSSION

We are particularly aware of the value and interest of infra-red thermography in clinical research on the behaviour of breast cancers. It seems to us that the concept of energy production by mammary carcinomas brings in a new dimension to the whole conception of malignant disease. Facing those who disregard infra red thermography our experience shows that more work, more care and more imagination are still required for the future of oncology.

REFERENCES :   Vol. 3, No 1-2, 1978.
1 ACTA THERMOGRAPHICA? Editor Pr Pistolesi Dept Radio. Verona(I).
2 AMALRIC and al. Acta Therm. Vol. 1, No 2, 1976.
3 FOURNIER D.V. and al. Méditerranée Médicale, 111, 89-99, 1975.
4 GAUTHERIE M. and al. Biomedecine, 22, 328-336, 1975.
5 LAWSON R.N. Canada Med. As. J., 75, 309, 1956.
6 LLOYD WILLIAMS K. Medical Thermography, Karger Ed., 1969.
7 SPITALIER J.M. and al. Acta Therm. Vol 1, No 3, 1976.

****

Automated Cytology Using a Quantitative Staining Method Combined with a TV-based Image Analysis Computer

E. M. van Ingen*, L. Leyte-Veldstra**, I. Al**, G. Wielenga* and J. S. Ploem**

*Laboratory of Pathology, Erasmus University, Rotterdam, The Netherlands
**Leiden University Medical Center, Department of Histochemistry and
Cytochemistry, Leiden, The Netherlands

ABSTRACT

One of the aims of the research of our group is the development of an automated
system for prescreening and for quantitative evaluation of cervical cytology preparations. As an approach towards this goal a relatively large number of slides
obtained from patients of different clinics has been analyzed by semi-automated cytofluorometry for the presence of cells with a strongly increased DNA content
(> 5C). Such cells were found in 95% of the preparations of patients with at least
a severe dysplasia and were absent in 91% of the negative preparations. Strongly
increased DNA content was therefore chosen as a parameter to detect suspect cells.
For the automated procedure LEYTAS (Leyden Television Analysis System) was
developed. The system permits rapid detection of nuclei with a strongly increased
DNA content and effective rejection of detected artifacts such as overlapping
cells, leukocytes, dirt etcetera. A second screening criterium based on increased
nuclear contrast has also been tested with LEYTAS. Data obtained from a limited
number of preparations are presented to demonstrate the principle of these methods.

INTRODUCTION

At present several screening methods for cancer are being applied such as cytology,
imaging techniques (X-ray, ultrasound, infrared), serum markers, cytochemical markers and radioactive tracers. Cytologic screening for precancerous and cancerous
lesions of the female genital tract has proven to be most valuable (Berlin, 1976).
Automated screening could be of great assistance since application of objective
criteria can eventually lead to more objective and standardized diagnostics.
Furthermore rapid performance is possible of a constant quality provided that the
present instrumentation for automated cytology can be optimized. Also a need exits
for a better classification of precancerous lesions of the uterine cervix reflecting their biologic behaviour regarding disappearance, persistance or progression
(Koss, 1978; Reagan, 1953). Quantitative evaluation of cytology specimens of which
detailed information can be obtained about a large number of cell types, can be
expected to contribute to the improvement of visual diagnostic work. This is important because, although visual diagnosis enables the interpretation of a large
number of observations, it still shows a considerable inter-observer variation
(Langley, 1973). Testing of a large number of objective criteria, obtained with
rapid automated cytology may perhaps reveal facts that will correlate with the
biological behaviour of cervical neoplasms. In a limited number of applications
quantitative cytological methods have revealed differences between cell types that

could not be detected by visual means (Bartels, 1978; Durie, 1978).

Technical Approaches
The approaches that have been followed in cytology automation can be categorized
as follows:
Dynamic systems (Flow systems). In flow systems cells are suspended in a liquid
stream and pass rapidly (up to 5000 cells per second) one or more detector systems.
Multiple parameters can be recorded such as light absorption, light scatter,
fluorescence or electrical resistance. These systems are low resolution systems,
having a measuring field larger than the objects of interest. Although more time-
consuming, sorting of cells, in different batches is possible, on the basis of various preset sort criteria. Flow systems, that provide more detailed morphological
information are being developed (Cambier, 1979).

Static systems (Slide-based systems). In static systems conventional slides are
analized by means of optical scanning methods at moderate to high resolution in
order to extract a large number of parameters per cell. Data acquisition is
achieved by using fast scanning stages, scanning mirror systems or television scanning. The two dimensional data matrix can be analyzed by means of pattern recognition methods. Static systems, of which an example will be described in this paper,
permit analysis both at low and high resolution.
In general low resolution methods are used for screening and high resolution methods for cell classification. A combination is used in dual resolution systems, in
which relevant objects are selected rapidly at low resolution and are subsequently
analyzed at a higher resolution (Bacus, 1974; Tanaka, 1977; Zahniser, 1979).
Early attempts in the detection of malignant cells in cervical and sputum cytology
specimens were made using a microfluorometric scanning method (Mellors, 1952).
Further developments led a.o. to the CYTOANALYZER (Tolles, 1961) and the CYDAC
(CYtophotometric and DAta Conversion) system which was applied to the problem of
morphological analysis, recognition and classification of normal and abnormal chro-
mosomes (Mendelsohn, 1964). Recently, systems like TICAS (Wied, 1970), LARC (Megla,
1973), CYBEST (Tanaka, 1977), LEYTAS (Al, 1979; Ploem, 1979) and BioPEPR (Zahniser,
1979) became available for automated quantitative cytology.

Cytochemistry. Besides technical developments for automated cytology, the development of specific cytochemical staining methods contributed to quantitative evaluation of certain cell constituents. Especially the quantitative staining of DNA has
been of great importance, as a large number of investigators has demonstrated the
presence of (cell) nuclei with an increased DNA content in many premalignant and
and malignant lesions of the cervix uteri (Atkin, 1964; Böhm, 1973; Hrushovetz,1969
1970; Nishiya, 1977; Ploem-Zaayer, in press; Sandritter, 1976; Sprenger, 1977).
For application in prescreening, this type of cell would have to be present in all
or nearly all preparations from patients with a malignant or a premalignant lesion
and absent in negative preparations. Some authors were not able to find cells with
an increased DNA content in positive preparations (severe dysplasia, carcinoma in
situ or invasive carcinoma). This could be due to the limited number of measured
cells, as a result of the rather time consuming measuring procedure with a non-
automated microscope. In flow measurements nuclei with an increased DNA content
are often indistinguishable from groups of cells, or groups of leukocytes or may
be hidden in the background noise. Cells with a high DNA content may also occur
in some normal cervical smears or with inflammatory conditions (Kiefer, 1976). In
our relatively large number of specimens, cells with a high DNA content occur in
less than 10% of the negative smears as will be shown in the following study.

The Approach of the Leiden Group
In a introductory study the usefulness of DNA content as a prescreening parameter
has been tested. Entire cervical smears were screened for nuclei with a visually
estimated high DNA content, using a rapid semi-automated microfluorometer. To cor-

relate the DNA measurements with the morphology of the preparations, a morphological classification as well as DNA fluorometry would have to be possible in the same
smear. A new bicolor staining for DNA and protein was used to meet these requirements (Cornelisse, 1976; Tanke, 1979). In addition to a fluorescent image, this
staining method also gives a good absorption image of the nucleus permitting analysis of chromatin patterns. The fluorescence of nuclei with a visually expected
high DNA content (based on size and/or intensity) was selectively measured. In this
paper the results of the selective fluorometry method on 864 cervical smears in
relation to the histological and/or cytological diagnosis of the patient and to
the morphological diagnosis of the same maesured smear will be given.
There after two studies have been carried out using LEYTAS. In the first study with
LEYTAS the DNA parameter was tested for its use in an automated image analysis system, directed to the automated detection of cells with an increased DNA content.
The use of a quantitative DNA staining permits a relatively simple procedure of
detecting such cells, since the DNA content is directly proportional to the product
of fluorescence intensity and size of the nucleus. The results are described by
Al and co-workers and will be summarized in this paper.
The second study with LEYTAS was carried out to test the use of high "internal nuclear"-contrast as a prescreening parameter. The contrast method makes use of the
more sophisticated possibilities of the TAS and was developed by Meyer (1979) in
close collaboration with our group. A preliminary test on 90 cases will be described in this paper.

SPECIMEN COLLECTION AND SLIDE PREPARATION

Cervical samples of patients with a suspect smear on an earlier occasion, were
taken by general practitioners (from all parts of the Netherlands) and by gynaecolo-
gists from clinics of the universities of Rotterdam, Utrecht and Leiden. Control
samples were taken from a group of women visiting the clinic for pill control or
during mass screening programs. Part of the material has been taken under colposcopic control by the same gynaecologist. The cervical cells were collected from
the ecto- and endocervical regions, using a cotton tipped applicator. Immediately
afterwards the applicator was immersed in a preservative solution of 24% ethanol
in phosphate buffered saline (0.15 M NaCl, pH 7.2) and sent by mail to the laboratory where it arrived 1-4 days later.
Slides were prepared as described by Tanke and co-workers (1979). This method includes syringing of the cell suspension to minimize cell clumping. As a diploid
standard for DNA-measurements, human lymphocytes were added to the suspension.
Cells were deposited on glass slides with centrifuge techniques and stained using
a bicolor fluorescent staining method (AFS, Acriflavine-Feulgen-SITS).
The acriflavine-Feulgen procedure was used for quantitative staining of DNA, including an acid-ethanol wash for the removal of non-covalently bound dye (Van Ingen,
1979); proteins were stained with SITS (Stilbeneisothiocyanato-disulfonic acid).
The entire staining procedure and subsequent dehydration were performed automatically in an adapted Shandon staining machine. Stained slides were mounted in
Fluormount (Gurr, Germany) and stored in the dark at 4°C. Routine PAP smears were
prepared according to conventional laboratory procedures. Prior to measurements,
the AFS-stained slides were judged for quality of cell material, fixation and
staining. Only slides with a good technical quality have been included in the series.

CYTOFLUOROMETRY

Method
Analysis of the DNA content of cells was performed using a semi-automated procedure
with a specially adapted microfluorometer (MPV II, Leitz, Germany) allowing rela-

tively rapid visual screening of the entire slide as well as quantitative fluorescence intensity measurements on single cells.
Added human lymphocytes were measured as a 2C (diploid) reference value. Nuclei with an expected high DNA content (based on fluorescence intensity and/or size) were visually selected and measured. The obtained value was stored in a computer. A DNA value of more than 5C was chosen as a preliminary threshold to differentiate the negative cases from the positives, i.e. moderate dysplasia and more sever lesions. In this way an overlap with normally dividing cells (2C-4C) would be avoided. The results of the measurements were compared with the histological diagnosis if available or with the cytological diagnosis of a Papanicolaou stained cervical smear taken at the same time or at an earlier occasion. The measured data were also compared with the morphological diagnosis of the same measured AFS-stained preparations. This diagnosis was assessed without knowledge of the cytological or histological diagnosis based on Pap-stained slides.

Results
Selective DNA measurements were performed on 864 cervical suspension preparations. The results are given in table 1. In the left column the most probable diagnosis is given of the cervix from which the cell suspension was taken. The number of histologically diagnosed cases is indicated between brackets.

TABLE 1   DNA values of acriflavine-Feulgen stained nuclei in cervical suspension preparations measured by cytofluorometry

Histological/Cytological Diagnosis	Number of cases in which cells were found with DNA content as indicated			Total
	≤5C	>5C ≤7C	>7C	
negative	290	18	9	317
mild dysplasia	38 (2)*	23 (4)	21 (1)	82
moderate/severe dysplasia, atypical reserve cell hyperplasia	17 (5)	34 (17)	126 (51)	177
carcinoma in situ	7 (4)	37 (26)	203 (155)	247
invasive carcinoma	0	6 (6)	35 (33)	41
				864

* The numbers of histologically verified cases are indicated between brackets.

The results are divided into three classes. The first class gives preparations in which no nuclei were found with a DNA content of more than 5C. The second class consists of preparations in which nuclei were found between 5C and 7C and the third class depicts those preparations that contain at least one nucleus with a DNA content of more than 7C.
Nuclei with a DNA content of >5C are detected in 9% (27/317) of the negative cases (false positives). These cases usually contained very few nuclei with a high DNA content. Cases classified as at least moderate/severe dysplasia mostly showed DNA values of >5C, many cases even above 7C. No high DNA content has been found in 5% (24/465) of these cases (false negatives). Of these 24 preparations 20 were also negative on morphological examination. The mild dysplasia group demonstrated variable results. No nuclei with a high DNA content were found in 38/82 preparations, 29 of these preparations were also morphologically negative.

PRESCREENING USING LEYTAS

Methods
Automated detection of suspicious cells on the basis of DNA content or nuclear contrast is based on television scanning of microscopic images with simultaneous analysis by the Texture Analysing System (TAS, Leitz, Germany) as described by Serra
(1973). The TAS can be described briefly as an image analysis computer, permitting
processing of selected cells by special purpose hardware, as well as by software
using a PDP 11 minicomputer connected to the TAS. The system is equipped with an
autofocus system and stage movement, filter selection and selection of magnification are computer controlled. TAS instructions were programmed using an interpreter
language especially developed for this purpose.

1. Automated detection of cells with an increased DNA content. For the trials described in this paper a computer program was run to search a sufficient number of
microscopic fields (200 sq. microns each) for the occurrence of suspect events.
Detection was based on fluorescence intensity and nuclear size. Suspect objects
were displayed on a TV monitor. Operator intervention took place to distinguish
visually between artifacts (cell clumps, stained acrylcotton, debris) and cells.
After searching 1000 fields, the results were compared with a total diagnosis obtained as described previously. When less than 4 suspect cells were in positive
preparations found the program continued to analyse the entire slide.

2. Automated detection of cells with an increased nuclear contrast. For this trial
1000 microscopical fields (250 sq. microns each) have been analysed by the program
Detection was based on the presence of large density differences within an individual nucleus. For the rest the same procedure as described above was used.

Results
In a first blind study 42 cervical cytology slides were tested for the presence
of nuclei with a DNA content of more than 7C (table 2). This trial consisted of
13 negative slides and 29 positive slides (moderate dysplasia and more severe lesions). One false positive slide was found. The false negative case was reanalyzed,
using another slide. This resulted in the finding of several suspicious cells.
The second trial was carried out on 21 slides, 12 positive cases and 9 negative
cases (table 2). One negative slide was classified as "suspect". All positive cases were confirmed.

TABLE 2   Results of two studies using the "DNA parameter"

Histological/Cytological diagnosis	Number of cases in which cells are found automatically by LEYTAS with DNA content as indicated					
	Trial I	>7C		Trial II	>5C	
	−	+	total	−	+	total
negative (−)	12	1	13	8	1	9
positive (+)	1	28	29	0	12	12

In a study testing nuclear contrast, 90 preparations were analysed for the presence of single cells with an increased nuclear contrast (table 3). In the 3
false positive cases only one cell was detected. No single sell was detected in
the false negative case after analysis of 15000 objects.

TABLE 3   Results of a study using the "contrast method"

Histological/Cytological	no cells detected	cells detected	total
negative	29	3	32
positive	1	57	58
total			90

DISCUSSION

In the first introductory study using the semi-automated method for a relatively large clinical trial, the entire cervical smear was visually searched for nuclei with a high DNA content (>5C), with subsequent measurement of fluorescence intensity. Nuclei with a high DNA content were not present in 24/465 (5%) cases classified as moderate/severe dysplasia, carcinoma in situ or invasive carcinoma. As the case diagnosis consisted of a histological diagnosis, or a cytological diagnosis of a Papanicolaou stained smear, taken at an earlier occasion than the AFS stained preparation, sampling errors may have played a role when no atypical cells were observed in the suspension preparation. Only 4/24 preparations without a high DNA content cell, contained atypical cells. These cases might be considered as "true errors" or "machine errors" to be compared with visual screening errors made in conventional cytology. But even if we take together the false negative rate consisting of sampling and machine errors (5%), this rate compares well with visual screening errors made in conventional cytology, which are estimated at about 5% (Patten, 1976; Soost, 1976; Tanaka, 1977; Wied, 1976). Cells with a high DNA content (>5C) were found in 27 of the 317 preparations from normal cervices or benign lesions (9% false positives). Other authors (Böhm, 1973) reported on the occurrence of cells with a high DNA content in some negative cases, which is in accordance with our own observations. The mild dysplasia group is considered seperately with variable measurement results (nuclei with a high DNA content were present in 44/82 cases). Evaluation of these results, await cytological follow-up data.
The use of LEYTAS for the automated detection of nuclei with an increased DNA content shows promising results. A total false negative rate of less than 3% was achieved with 41 cervical cytology specimens. The false positive rate for the 7C and 5C threshold were 7% and 11% respectively. A large number of samples is being tested at present.
Also the detection of nuclei with an increased internal nuclear contrast shows good results. Testing 90 specimens a false negative rate of 2% and a false positive rate of 9% were obtained. Combination of the screening for nuclei with an increased DNA content and/or an increased nuclear contrast, together with sophisticated automated procedures for the discrimination between artifacts and real cells or nuclei, may lead to a reliable and fast automated prescreening procedure. In the future, other cellular features such as nuclear size, cytoplasmic size, nuclear and cytoplasmic shape and especially chromatin pattern and chromatin distribution are now studied with LEYTAS for possible correlation with the cytological diagnosis "suspect smear".
Two approaches will then be followed. The first is the development of a fully automated procedure for prescreening of cervical slides in a period of approximately 6 minutes per slide.
A second procedure will include interaction with the cytotechnologist. Suspicious events or fields will be stored in a computer memory and will be displayed on a TV monitor after the entire slide has been searched. This should be effective in establishing the more precise diagnosis of positive cervical cytology slides in a short time.

ACKNOWLEDGEMENTS

The authors wish to thank Dr. J. van Meir, Dr. J.C. Hage, Mrs. J. Laar,
Mrs. G. Kroessen, Mrs. T. Burgerhout, Mrs. A. Frangenheim and Mrs. L. Rooks for
their skilful work in obtaining the specimens, and Mrs. J. van der Voorn and
Mrs. I. Reit for their help in preparing this manuscript.

REFERENCES

Atkin, N. B. (1964). The deoxyribonucleic acid content of malignant cells in cer-
    vical smears. Acta Cytol., 8, 68-72.
Al, I., and J. S. Ploem (1979). Detection of suspicious cells and rejection of
    artefacts in cervical cytology using LEYTAS. J. Histochem. Cytochem., 27,
    629-634.
Bacus, J. (1974). Design and performance of an automated leukocyte classifier.
    In Proc. Second International joint conference on pattern recognition,
    Copenhagen.
Berlin, N. I. (1976). The need for automated cytology: Goals of the program of the
    National Cancer Institute. In G. L. Wied, G. F. Bahr and P. H. Bartels (Eds.),
    The automation of uterine cancer cytology, Chicago. pp. 1-5.
Bartels, P. H., C. Yin-Pao, B. G. M. Durie, G. B. Olson, L. Vaught, and
    S. E. Salmon (1978). Discrimination between human T and B lymphocytes and mono-
    cytes by computer analysis of digitized data from scanning microphotometry. II.
    Discrimination and automated classification. Acta Cytol., 22, 530-537.
Böhm, N., E. Sprenger, and W. Sandritter (1973). Absorbance and fluorescence cyto-
    photometry of nuclear feulgen DNA. A comparative study. In A. A. Thaer and
    M. Sernetz (Eds.), Fluorescence techniques in cell biology. Springer Verlag
    Berlin, Heidelberg, New York. pp. 67-77.
Cambier, J. L., D. B. Kay, and L. L. Wheeless (1979). A multidimensional slit-scan
    flow system. J. Histochem. Cytochem., 27, 321-324.
Cornelisse, C. J., and J. S. Ploem (1976). A new type of two-color fluorescence
    staining for cytology specimens. J. Histochem. Cytochem., 24, 72-81
Durie, B. G. M., L. Vaught, Y. P. Chen, G. B. Olson, S. E. Salmon, and P.H. Bartels
    (1978). Discrimination between human T and B lymphocytes and monocytes by com-
    puter analysis of digitized data from scanning microphotometry. I. Chromatin
    distribution pattern. Blood, 51, 579-589.
Hrushovetz, S. B. (1969). Two-wavelength Feulgen cytophotometry of cells exfoliated
    from uterine cervix. Acta Cytol., 13, 583-594.
Hrushovetz, S. B., and S. C. Lauchlan (1970). Comparative DNA content of cells in
    the intermediate and parabasal layers of cervical intraepithelial neoplasia
    studied by two-wavelength Feulgen cytophotometry. Acta Cytol., 14, 68-77.
Ingen, E. M. van, H. J. Tanke, and J. S. Ploem (1979). Model studies on the acri-
    flavine-Feulgen reaction. J. Histochem. Cytochem., 27, 80-83.
Kiefer, C., and W. Sandritter (1976). DNA and the cell cycle. Beitr. Path. BD.,
    158, 332-362.
Koss, L. G. (1978) Dysplasia, a real concept or a misnomer. Obst. and Gynec., 51,
    332-362.
Langley, F. A., and A. C. Krompton (1973). Epithelial abnormalities of the cervix
    uteri. Springer Verlag, Berlin, Heidelberg.
Megla, G. K. (1973). The LARC automatic white bloodcell analyzer. Acta Cytol., 17,
    3-14.
Mellors, R. C., A. Glassman, and G. N. Papanicolaou (1952). A microfluorometric
    scanning method for the detection of cancer cells in smears of exfoliated
    cells. Cancer, 5, 458-468.
Mendelsohn, M. L., W. A. Kolman, and R. C. Bostrom (1964) Initial approaches to
    the computer analysis of cytophotometric fields. Ann. N. Y. Acad. Sci., 115,

998-1009

Meyer, F. (1979). Interactive image transformations for an automatic screening of cervical smears. J. Histochem. Cytochem., 27, 128-135.

Nishiya, I., T. Kikuchi, S. Moriya, and I. Sawamura (1977). Cytophotometric study of premalignant and malignant cells of the cervix in an approach towards automated cytology. Acta Cytol., 21, 271-275.

Patten, S. F. (1976). Sensitivity and specificity of routine diagnostic cytology. In G. L. Wied, G.F. Bahr, and P. H. Bartels (Eds.), The automation of uterine cancer cytology, Chicago. pp. 406-419.

Ploem-Zaaijer, J. J., M. E. Beyer-Boon, L. Leyte-Veldstra, and J. S. Ploem. In N. J. Pressmann and J. L. Wied (Eds.), The automation of cancer cytology and and cell image analysis. In press.

Ploem, J. S., N. Verwoerd, J. Bonnet, and G. Koper (1979). An automated microscope for quantitative cytology combining television image analysis and stage scanning microphotometry. J. Histochem. Cytochem., 27, 136-143.

Reagan, J. W., I. L. Seidemand, and Y. Saracusa (1953). The cellular morphology of carcinoma in situ and dysplasia or atypical hyperplasia of the uterine cervix. Cancer, 6, 224-235.

Sandritter, W. B., and N. Böhm (1976). Ploidy of normal and malignant cells. In G. L. Wied, G. F. Bahr and P. H. Bartels (Eds.), The automation of uterine cancer cytology. Chicago. pp. 289-304.

Serra, J. (1973). Theoretical bases of the Leitz-Texture-Analysis System. Leitz Sci. Techn. Inf. Suppl., 1, 125-136.

Sprenger, E., W. Sandritter, H. Naujoks, M. Hilgarth, D. Wagner, and M. Vogt-Schaden (1977). Routine use of flow-through photometric prescreening in the detection of cervical carcinoma. Acta Cytol., 21, 435-440.

Soost, H. J. (1976). Clinical application of automated prescreening methods. In K. Goerttler and C. J. Herman (Eds.), Technologies for automation in cervical cancer, Heidelberg. pp. 2-14.

Tanaka, N., H. Ikeda, T. Ueno, S. Watanabe, Y. Imasato, and R. Kashida (1977). Fundamental study on automatic cyto-screening for uterine cancer. III. New system of automated apparatus (CYBEST) utilizing the pattern recognition method. Acta Cytol., 22, 85-88.

Tanke, H. J., E. M. van Ingen, and J. S. Ploem (1979). Acriflavine-Feulgen Stilbene (AFS) staining: A procedure for automated cervical cytology with a television based system (LEYTAS). J. Histochem. Cytochem., 27, 84-86.

Tolles, W. E., W. J. Horvath, and R. C. Bostrom (1961). A study of the quantitative characteristics of exfoliated cells from the female genital tract. I. Measurement methods and results. Cancer, 14, 437-454.

Tolles, W. E., W. J. Horvath, and R. C. Bostrom (1961). A study of the quantitative characteristics of exfoliated cells from the female genital tract. II. Suitability of quantitatibe cytological measurements for automated prescreening. Cancer, 14, 455-468.

Wied, G. L., G. F. Bahr, and P. H. Bartels (1970). Automatic analysis of cell images by ticas. In G. L. Wied and G. F. Bahr (Eds.), Automated cellidentification and cellsorting. Academic Press, New York, London. pp. 195-360.

Wied, G. L., G. F. Bahr, and P. H. Bartels (1976). Defining the problems of automating uterine cancer cytology. In G. L. Wied, G. F. Bahr and P. H. Bartels (Eds.), The automation of uterine cancer cytology. Chicago. p. 6.

Zahniser, D. J., P. S. Oud, M. C. T. Raaymakers, G. P. Vooys, and R. T. van der Walle (1979). BioPEPR: A system for the automatic prescreening of cervical smears. J. Histochem. Cytochem., 27, 635-641.

Psychological Impact of Cancer

The Oncologist and the Psychologist

Melvin J. Krant

Professor of Medicine and Director of Cancer Programs,
University of Massachusetts Medical Center, Worcester,
Massachusetts, U.S.A.

ABSTRACT

There are at least three areas where the study of psychological behaviors of people relate to the cancer problem. Firstly is the elusive question of whether previous life experiences, and manners of psychological adaptation, may be instrumental in the development of cancer. If there is a relationship between cancer and the psyche, what is it's relevance as compared to other oncogenic forces, such as chemicals, viruses, and altered immunological processes? Secondly, once cancer develops, do psychological forces bear on the rapidity of spread of the cancer, and on the patient's response to treatment. Thirdly, can the psychological needs of cancer patients and their families be elucidated in a way that allows for effective interventions that can alter a sense of suffering?

The literature of the past 100 years is rich in implications that the psychological history of an individual bears a definite relationship to the development of cancer. Carefully done perspective studies, however, are minimal but the needs for such observation is crucial. Likewise, there is some evidence that short or long survival in cancer is related to psychological adaptation, and this raises the question of whether more intense psychological support for patients and their families might not alter responses to therapeutic maneuvers and change the progress of the cancer.

Several groups in the United States are attempting to define the helplessness so often found in cancer patients, and to provide a sense of power to the patient to help in the fight against cancer, and the response to treatment. The use of hypnosis, meditation, and auto-reflection are part of such attempts.

Beyond changing therapeutic responses and cancer progress, is the issue of human suffering experienced by patients and families, relative to their psychological makeup and their communication styles. When understood, certain interventions are possible in order to relieve some of the mental anguish associated with cancer.

Psychological Causality, Supportive Therapy, Helplessness, Self Esteem.

We are each of us persons in our bodies – an embodied self – and events occuring in the objective world of our physical form register in, and are interpreted by, this self and recorded as either pleasure, insignificance, or hurt. It is this

211

registration that is central to the concept of suffering in cancer. While the
body, as materialistic form, is relatively easy to grasp intellectually, the self,
the ego, or psyche, or soul, or spirit, or personhood, or whatever terminology
one wishes to apply to that concept that is over and beyond the physical body,
is harder to grasp ideationally and operationally. For the oncologist, as
medical scientist and practitioner, cancer in the body can be described, and
set against normality and other pathological conditions by a set of determinants
and observations that are recordable in precise physical form. These physical
forms, be they measurable and evaluable in pathological, biochemical, endocrono-
logical, radiological or immunological terms, have distinct, and therefore
attractive characteristics that allow for discussion, debate, accusation, and
best of all, standardization. Scientific language accomodates these characteristics, and they are then said to be free of cultural, racial, emotional, or
other humanistic biases. Normative characteristics of the psyche, or ego, or
spirit, are much harder to elucidate across languages, across cultures, across
races, across religions – yet for each unique person, these normative properties
are the base for understanding pain, hurt, and suffering. When cancer appears
in the body, a human response occurs, and this response is the heart of suffering.
It is the responsibility of the psychologist, or medical psychiatrist, or
medically-oriented minister, or any student of the human proposition to elucidate
the nature of that suffering.

There have been three lines of study relating cancer and the human psyche. The
first line has dealt with etiology and epidemiology. The question asked is,
"Does there exist psychological characteristics that can be recognized and
recorded that influence the emergence of cancer?" A number of studies, in
different medical settings, in different countries, and using different investi-
gational instruments, have indicated that such, indeed, is the case. Two major
hypothesis have emerged, namely, life events leading to feelings of isolation
and estrangement, and secondly, a repression of the ability to express emotions.
Neither theory postulates that the psyche is solely related to the emergence of
cancer, but instead speculates that the psyche participants in carcinogenesis as
one of multi-causal factors. I believe that other discussants will examine this
line of endeavor further.

A second avenue of investigation has dealt with the question of whether the
progress of cancer, once established, is related to personality characteristics;
that is, do people with a short, rapidly spreading, course of cancer have certain
psychological traits that distinguish them from individuals with slow, indolent
courses? A further question relates to therapeutic responsiveness; namely, is
response to a therapeutic maneuver, such as ablative endocrine surgery, or chemotherapy, at all inter-related to certain psychological characteristics?

The third line of endeavor is of another order, in which survival outcome, as a
numerical figure of weeks, or months, is less crucial than is an understanding of
the nature of suffering, and how relief might be brought about for the individuals
caught in the web of hurt that deviously develops when cancer is diagnosed. We
might call this approach existential, in that it attempts to recognize and
ameliorate life problems. It is here, in this dimension, that the oncologist
treating the cancer, and the psychologist, treating non-physical suffering, may
interact to the best advantage of every one – the patient, the family, and the
medical staff itself.

There are many potential psychological paradigms that we might discuss. For the
sake of reasonable brevity, let me examine three human existential elements that
apply to the interacting trilogy of patient, family, and medical staff. These
three themes are helplessness, self-esteem, and mortality but should not be seen

as independent entities, for they are quite related, one to the other. Helplessness is an extremely painful feeling, for it is the revelation that one can do nothing to prevent an inexorable fate from doing what it will. Revealed helplessness usually breeds great anxiety; people will go to great lengths to avoid this feeling of being out of personal control of their destiny. Cancer patients, in my experience, will not spontaneously talk about their helpless feelings to the physician; they are more apt to keep the feeling as a personal secret. However, if questioned, they will talk freely of their helplessness to do anything themselves about their illness. They frequently feel that they must place themselves completely in the hands of the physician, and trust his judgment. Cancer patients will compare themselves to patients with heart disease, or diabetes, and will point out that in these latter disorders, people can do something about it, while cancer is beyond a person's personal power to intervene. Thus a cancer patient often feels that he must place himself completely in the physician's hand, and this act requires extensive trust. Where that trust does not fully exist, a person may feel forced to give himself over to a physician, but with great misgivings. Such situations cause extreme anxiety. Many cancer patients, and their families have had some exposure to the surgical, chemotherapeutic, and radiotherapeutic treatments available to them, and thus find themselves in an unenviable position of needing the physician's power, but uncomfortable in the potential consequences of accepting his advise. Patients may challenge a physician's authority, or act out by skipping appointments, postponing therapies, or behaving badly with family members, or with members of the medical team. Helping a patient, a family member, a physician or a nurse to understand the genesis of behaviors can avoid, or eliminate, considerable anguish.

Helplessness also breeds both over-dependence as well as guilt. The overly dependent patient, who is constantly seeking medical reassurance, or refusing to do anything without the physician's approval, can cause great consternation in the medical system, as well as in the family. The patient may resort to the psychological defense of denial to prevent excessive anxiety of his helplessness from overwhelming him - many a physician, and many a family member have been awed, and made uncomfortable, with the excessive degree of denial that the helpless patient may exhibit. Again, assisting the family and the medical staff to understand the nature of this reaction, and other behaviors, such as excessive clinging, can relieve the tension created between the patient and others in his environment.

When an individual exhibits his helplessness, and seeks our help in dealing with overwhelming fate, guilt may be generated if we cannot provide him with adequate assistance. Such guilty feelings on the part of the physician, or the family, can result in excessive medical tests and treatments, or in flight. Physicians do abandon patients, not infrequently, with the comment of "there is nothing more I can do for you". Patients, especially those with advancing diseases, often feel this abandonment, and their despair is worsened. A psychologically minded staff member can assist in an understanding of the dynamics involved in such behaviors and by helping the medical staff verbalize and get in touch with their feelings, prevent flagrant abandonment from occuring. In this situation, the psychologist helps the physician to relate authentically to the patient, the family, and other members of the medical staff.

Families frequently feel helpless and guilty when faced with a loved one whose disease is progressing. Helping the family to examine their own feelings, and providing assurances that they are playing a vital part in the care of the patient, can assuage guilt considerably. We have seen many families refuse to visit relatives in the hospital, or even at home, when they are made uncomfortable by the helpless feelings they experience, especially in the presence of an uncomfortable, or demanding patient. Helping family members to verbalize their

helplessness, and providing reenforcing feelings of control, is also critical.
Physicians frequently seek patient compliance and capitulation, and often are
not aware that they do so to overcome their (the physician's) own feelings of
inadequacy to deal with the responsibility of being in charge of a cancer
patient's life.

Self-esteem is a vital aspect of each human life. To feel esteemed is to feel
worthy, to be felt worthy and deserving of attention. Self-esteem, while an
abstraction, is rooted in day-by-day life, in the doing of those roles, tasks,
and pleasures that constitutes authenticity. Working, self-caring, participating
in life projects are all elements of self-esteem. Cancer patients frequently
fear becoming burdens - becoming that kind of person who can no longer carry out
roles, activities, behaviors, that have given them their station in life. Such
a role might be cooking, gardening, working - any specific task that defines an
individual. Self-esteem is secured by feeling in control, and by feeling the
opposite of helpless, namely, that something is being done that is sensed to
be a correct action for whatever the problem may be. Self-esteem is related to
doing pleasurable things, and in finding pleasure in things. Self-esteem is
related to feeling partnership, to sensing respect, to feeling listened to, to
having an influence.

Sickness cuts sharply into a person's self-esteem, especially if one feels
confused, misunderstood, bereft of playing out one's roles, totally dependent but
unallied to the people upon whom one is dependent. When there is an erosion of
self-esteem, patients may act belligerantly to save face, may become deeply
moody and depressed, become clinging, or act as if they have no real purpose
in life. Physicians frequently do not comprehend the personal injury that both
disease and treatment may produce, and frequently misinterpret a patient's
behavior as an attack upon themselves. Patients may oftentimes be labelled as
"bad", or "difficult" patients, without an awareness of the narcissistic injury
that they are undergoing. The psychologist can be of great help in clarifying
such matters, and helping the patient, the family, and the oncologist both
understand, and ameliorate the suffering or the hostile reactions of all parties.

Cancer invaribly symbolizes death. Even though many patients may undergo curative
therapeutic procedures, for years they live in the shadow of potential recurrence. It is hard to bring closure to the illness and its existence. For
those people who are not cured, or who have a recurrence, death and suffering
loom large. People come into their doctor's office, informed of cancer through
stories and personal observations of friends and relatives. They have watched
or participated in the dying of others, and have seen pain, withering, and
personal terror. They have often watched dying as an event of horror and helplessness. Patients frequently worry that they will inflict terrible pains on
loved ones who must watch them die.

To make confrontation with death is overwhelming for some, bearable for others,
and for a few, almost pleasurable. Again, many psychological styles can be
employed to cope with that confrontation, and some of these defenses may be
difficult for the family and the physician to deal with. Some patients use
denial of their status almost excessively, and their family members become angry
at such patients who can't "face up" to what is happening. Physicians may
scornfully look down at patients who refuse to acknowledge that they are dying,
but continue "begging" for treatments. Just as frequently, physicians abandon
patients who are dying, or at any rate, many patients feel that they are being
abandoned. When a physician has not realistically appraised the realty of his
treatment options, or has invested too heavily in physical treatments as his
way of relating to his patients, then indeed the failure of a treatment to be
successful may well result in the physician's pulling away from the patient as

the latter enters into a dying pathway. Switching into a mode of palliating and
comforting may be a problem for the physician, especially the oncologic specialist, who has invested his physicianhood into a specific treatment mode, rather
than into personal relationship with a patient. Excessive treatment, or
excessive control of the patient's destiny, may result in an excess of perceived
suffering as dying occurs.

Most patients and families need to integrate dying and losing into their lives
gradually. Too rapid a movement in this direction can result in hopelessness
and despair. The physician's role, be he oncologist or psychologist, is to
support this gradual integration by valuing the patient's defenses and styles,
and by helping the family members accept the gradual, yet perceptable, changes
that occur to the patient. Helping in the communication systems between family
members and patients and medical staff can serve a dramatic requirement for
appropriate easing into death. Helping a patient, or a family member, ack-
nowedge their fears (whatever they may be), their depressions, their sense of
helplessness is a vital role for the psychologist. Helping to open lines of
communication, and thus allowing a patient and family to talk together, and thus
feel together in regard to the dying experience, frequently improves the sense
of togetherness and support for the patient and his loved one. Understanding
the dependency needs of family members of the patient may help the family
member avoid excessive demands "to do something", that is frequently the mark of
excessive anxiety in someone who needs the patient to stay alive for some
unfinished business, and thus prevents an easeful dying.

The psychologist thus has many roles and functions in assisting the patient,
family member and medical staff in meeting the many emotional, communicative and
role-relating needs that are disrupted by cancer. The psychologist's role is
less than "curer" of cancer - but more the helper in resolving problems brought
to all, the patient, the family members, and the medical staff, by the illness.
The psychologist can assist people with ongoing life, as well as with an easeful
dying that occurs in an appropriate manner that minimizes hostility and dysphoria
and leaves all concerned with the feeling that the best that could have been done
was done!

Impacto Psicologico del Cancer
Decodificacion del Impacto Psicologico del Cancer en el Staff Terapeutico

Lily S. de Bleger

Las Heras 1750, 24° F. Buenos Aires, Argentina

Para comenzar, explicitaré los modelos científicos a que recurro en el desarrollo del tema, ya que creo facilitar con ello la comprensión del mismo.

En primer lugar, partiendo del esquema de la lingüística, recordemos que, en toda relación humana, la comunicación se da a través de señales, signos y símbolos, verbales y preverbales. Participan de ella, por lo menos, dos individuos llamados 'emisor' -el que envía, transmite, comunica un mensaje-, y 'receptor' -el que escucha recibe y adjudica un significado, o sea responde al significante del emisor. Este vínculo caracteriza el diálogo entre dos personas. Aquí lo aplicaré específicamente a la relación interpersonal médico-paciente, médico-médico y paciente-familia, entendiendo por familia a la esposa, hijos o persona más allegada al grupo familiar primario.

Las relaciones interpersonales son, en general, sumamente complejas: sobre todo si nos proponemos decodificar la riqueza contenida en el mundo interno de los seres humanos que las dinamizan. Cuando el vínculo se amplía, involucrando a varias personas, esta complejidad, naturalmente, aumenta.

Estas características sin duda definen también a la relación médico-paciente que nos ocupa; ésta adquiere notas particularmente llamativas toda vez que juegan en ella elementos como la salud, la enfermedad, las respectivas personalidades del profesional y del enfermo, las de sus familiares y los miembros de la comunidad que puedan tener alguna implicancia en ella.

La vastedad de este tema es visible. Es mi intención recortarlo y encuadrarlo para posibilitar así el abordaje de los puntos que configuran el objeto de este trabajo. Me referiré entonces al cáncer y concretamente orientaré el presente desarrollo hacia las significaciones psicológicas de esta enfermedad en lo que atañe al quehacer médico dentro del cual, obviamente, me incluyo. Es mi deseo transmitir mis propias experiencias y reflexiones sobre el tema, como así también las de otros colegas enfrentados a esta difícil tarea; y traigo como propuesta desde este panel, analizar el significado y valor del rol del psicólogo y de la ciencia psicológica en el campo que nos atañe.

Considero justo aquí señalar el mérito de este Congreso que en su notable afán por poner al día a los profesionales del área en los adelantos de la oncología, dio cabida a la ciencia psicológica tomándola como otra perspectiva de abordaje. Este panel, coordinado por el Dr. José Schavelzon, -un pionero en la problemática psicosomática en este campo-, es muestra indiscutible de ello.

Durante toda mi trayectoria profesional, y desde mi juventud -época en que era gi-
necóloga-, me preocupó siempre develar el 'misterio' de la medicina psicosomática.
Eso marcó de alguna manera el camino que me llevó a convertirme en psicoanalista.

La ciencia psicológica plantea una nueva dimensión de investigación tan importante
como las de otras especialidades tales como la química, la biología, etc., y el enfoque psicosomático se refiere en particular al ser humano enfermo como a una tota-
lidad gestáltica que se comporta como tal en la salud y en la enfermedad. Este es
el encuadre con el cual, en medicina psicosomática, se enfrenta la tarea del diagnóstico, pronóstico y tratamiento.

Como dicen Menninger y sus seguidores, los procesos psicológicos son funciones del
coordinador central del organismo, es decir, el más elevado centro integrador del
sistema nervioso central, como sucede también con otros procesos vitales. La diferencia estriba en que a los hechos psíquicos se los percibe subjetivamente y como
tal deben ser estudiados con técnicas propias, técnicas psicológicas, que difieren
de los métodos empleados por las otras ciencias. Es así que nuestro campo posee, como las ciencias biológicas, su metodología de observación y experimentación que es-
taría representada por la entrevista psicológica, los tests y lo que llamamos la e-
valuación global biopsicosocial.

En el enfoque conductista de Watson, la conducta se describe en términos de motiva-
ciones y fines. Comparto sólo parcialmente este concepto ya que pienso que tanto mo-
tivaciones como fines son, a su vez, emergentes de un condicionamiento psicosocial,
al cual debe sumarse la herencia del sujeto y su historia personal intra e interpsí-
quica.

Todo ser humano es engendrado por una madre que le da la vida y un padre que ayuda
y participa de ese proceso: a partir de esta constelación primigesta crece, sufre,
aprende y, si tiene suerte, llega a la adultez. Según esto diría que nuestras conductas, en la medida que somos entes y emergentes de un entorno psicosocial son, en
última instancia, pautas específicas y singulares de nuestras relaciones interpersonales e intrapsíquicas. Esto constituye un esbozo general que nos abarca también a
nosotros, médicos y psicólogos, tanto como a nuestros pacientes.

Prefiero, por más enriquecedor, el enfoque de los estructuralistas y gestaltistas,
que aunque pertenecientes a dos campos teóricos diferentes, tienen puntos de coinci-
dencia interdisciplinaria. Toda estructura conductual, ya sea en la vida cotidiana,
como en situaciones propias de las crisis vitales (niñez, latencia, pubertad, adultez, desprendimiento, vejez previa madurez, etc.) como en las crisis de salud y enfermedad, es una forma de respuesta a diferentes estímulos. Es así que cada ser humano tiene su repertorio de estructuras privilegiadas de comportamiento que constituyen su personalidad. Es decir, que se puede caracterizar la personalidad a través
de codificar las pautas defensivas que se hallan privilegiadas, tomando los modelos
de personalidad de Ruesch, que en nuestro medio el Dr. David Liberman ha trabajado
y enriquecido con el aporte psicoanalítico.[1]

1 Personalmente me ha sido muy útil este enfoque para entender una entrevista, ya
sea hospitalaria o en consultorio privado; también es de utilidad en entrevistas de
preparación psicológica para una intervención quirúrgica de urgencia y lo he emplea-
do asimismo en trabajos de investigación en esterilidad, cuando actuaba en la sec-
ción psicosomática de ginecología que dirigía el Dr. G. di Paola en el Hospital de
Clínicas de Buenos Aires. El Dr. di Paola trabajaba en colaboración con un psicoanalista, el Dr. Teodoro Schlossberg, cuyos estudios psicofisiológicos realizados en
U.S.A. con el Dr. Cannon, abrieron rumbos y muchos colegas argentinos les debemos
gratitud por brindarnos sus experiencias con generosidad.

Tanto la conducta normal como la patológica (enfermedad, síntoma) obedecen a una po-
licausalidad que Freud sistematizó con el nombre de Series Complementarias. En e-
llas intervienen:

      1a. Serie: factor HERENCIA más VIVENCIAS INTRAUTERINAS: da la CONSTITUCION

      2a. Serie: CONSTITUCION más EXPERIENCIAS INFANTILES: da la DISPOSICION

      3a. Serie: DISPOSICION más CONFLICTO DESENCADENANTE: dan la ENFERMEDAD.

Detallaré ahora los distintos tipos de personalidad universalmente normal que, al
descompensarse ante las crisis vitales, rompen ese delicado equilibrio llamado 'salud'. Empezaré por enumerar las estructuras con mayor grado de organización, es decir, que en el devenir de la vida han llegado a desarrollar e instrumentar conductas y defensas que, desde la perspectiva genética de Freud, pertenecerían a la etapa fálica secundaria.

PERSONALIDAD HISTERICA

Son personas que establecen un buen contacto afectivo, rápido y fluído, pero todas
sus manifestaciones tienen un sello de teatralidad, gran desarrollo y utilización
de la fantasía que en algunos casos llega a la fabulación. Aprenden todo con gestos y palabras en términos simbólicos, pero no lo integran con hechos reales. Hay
un predominio en el empleo de modificaciones somáticas (lenguaje corporal) como medio de expresión simbólica. El sistema nervioso autónomo juega en la expresión de a-
fectos y conflictos: es decir, la musculatura lisa es usada como si fuera estriada.

Se caracterizan por un desarrollo infantil favorable, pero entre los tres y cinco a-
ños se produce una fuerte represión a nivel de la sexualidad, los órganos genitales
y las partes del cuerpo ligadas a la función sexual, mecanismo este que subsiste en
forma disociada del resto de la personalidad.

PERSONALIDAD FOBICA

Han alcanzado un buen nivel de integración. Sienten variadas inhibiciones, los contactos interpersonales están interferidos por la angustia ante lo que se llama el
'objeto fobígeno'. Necesitan a veces ir acompañados, como por ejemplo en la agorafo-
bia. La discriminación entre lo agradable y lo desagradable está regido por la angustia. Pueden tener puntos ciegos para ciertos peligros reales e hipersensibilidad
a peligros internos proyectados en el mundo exterior. Esto es condicionado por represión de fobias infantiles a la castración y al abandono. La valorización de personas y hechos está monopolizada por la angustia y su control. Viven muchas situaciones de rivalidad llegando a enfrentar trances de riesgo con actitudes contrafóbi-
cas.

Los padres son vividos, el del mismo sexo tentador y el del sexo opuesto como objeto fobígeno, castrador.

PERSONALIDAD LOGICA Y OBSESIVA

Son personas ordenadas, limpias, escrupulosas y puntuales en quienes el control es
su preocupación fundamental. Este control puede ser mantenido en ellos a través de
rituales y ceremoniales, con predominio de la formalidad, pero que los aísla de los
contactos afectivos.

La enfermedad es sentida por ellos como una perturbación del orden y de la limpieza
de sus funciones corporales.

PERSONALIDAD PARANOICA

Son personas que, por su estructura predominante, se constituyen en agudos observa-

dores del otro, a expensas de escotomas en su propia personalidad. La problemática
se da más en el área mental y cuando se enferman, son pacientes desconfiados que
no se entregan al médico y hacen generalmente malos post-operatorios

PERSONALIDAD DEPRESIVA

Fijada en una etapa más regresiva, la oral sádica secundaria. A esta etapa están fi-
jadas también las ciclotimias y las psicosis maníaco-depresivas. Son personas cuya
objetividad está regulada por la autoestima. Tienen ideales exigentes, pero, al no
satisfacerlos, caen en colapsos depresivos. Su ideal del Yo está regido por una óp-
tica infantil. Tienen prejuicios, rigidez en las normas, una tendencia a la culpa.
y una autoestima precaria porque su superyó es muy sádico. Necesitan pertenecer a
un grupo porque su capacidad de independencia es interferida por una permanente necesidad de afecto; el otro es un reflejo de la propia conciencia, es decir, las
personas son vividas como parte de ellos o ellos como parte del otro. Por eso hay
cierta sumisión y la adaptación sexual se rige por la adhesión y siempre tienen miedo de que se los abandone. Pueden adaptarse a actividades en que dependen o si se
sienten formando parte de un grupo.

PERSONALIDAD HIPERACTIVA

Es la persona de acción. Se expresa fundamentalmente por medio del comportamiento
en el mundo externo. Sus tensiones, conflictos y enfermedades también se exteriori-
zan en esta área (actuación psicopática, delincuencia, prostitución,etc.)

PERSONALIDAD HIPOCONDRIACA

Su relación con las personas es a través de la queja, la autoobservación y la preocupación. Manejan al grupo familiar a través de somatizaciones para atraer la atención del otro. Las ecuaciones simbólicas son de origen más primario que en la his-
teria de conversión. No relaciona sus trastornos con conflictos, porque la problemática de sus conflictos es más regresiva.

PERSONALIDAD INFANTIL

Estas personalidades merecen un estudio especial porque en ellas las manifestaciones psicológicas se expresan casi exclusivamente con el lenguaje del cuerpo, y así
hay que saber diferenciarlas de la personalidad histérica. Tienen un real déficit
de formación simbólica, del mundo fantasmático o imaginario como dirían los france-
ses.

Toda conducta del área de la mente o mundo interior casi está ausente, de manera
tal que en vez de percibir sensaciones o sentimientos a través de señales o símbolos, los expresan casi directamente con el cuerpo. Por ejemplo, no sienten rabia,
angustia, pero lo derivan en otro lenguaje quejándose de un dolor de estómago o mejor dicho, del sistema del plexo solar. No sienten la tristeza y el vacío existen-
cial lo llenan comiendo y engordando.

Su dependencia los hace poco diferenciados. Dependen intensamente de su grupo primario (padre, madre, hermanos) y posteriormente cuando se desprenden por ejemplo
casándose, que es lo más frecuente, son nuevos dependientes del marido o hijo (grupo secundario), sin desprenderse de su grupo primario. Son mujeres u hombres con u-
na fuerte parte del yo inmersa y no diferenciada del entorno social, porque no sa-
ben decodificar; es lo que muchas escuelas han llamado la parte no diferenciada o
primitiva de la personalidad.

José Bleger ha estudiado a fondo este tipo de personalidad en su obra 'Simbiosis y
ambiguedad'. Para ello ha creado una tercera posición o estructura gliscocárica,

siguiendo a la escuela inglesa que describe sólo dos posiciones o estructuras: la esquizoparanoide y la depresiva; cada una de ellas tiene su propio repertorio de re- laciones objetales, tipo de ansiedades y defensas inherentes. En la primera, las de- fensas más frecuentes son la omnipotencia, bloqueo afectivo, negación, disociación o clivaje y represión primaria. En la segunda, se darían defensas semejantes con la diferencia de que la omnipotencia y la negación son menos intensas y hay mayor capa- cidad de insight al dolor y la discriminación.

Concepción Unicista

Al hablar de Medicina Psicosomática incurrimos ya en un error hipocrático, porque va implícita en este concepto una decodificación confusionante: el ser humano es u- no solo, ente biopsicosocial que expresa sus conflictos normales y patológicos como puede, en tres áreas: mente, cuerpo y mundo externo, alternativa y dialécticamente. También podría decirse 'situacionalmente', o sea que, en momentos cruciales de la vida todos nosotros, médicos, nuestros pacientes y los que nos rodean, no podemos escapar a este contínuo fluctuar de las defensas para seguir viviendo.

Para esclarecer esta importante cuestión, propongo el concepto unicista ya estudia- do por Griessinger y desarrollado posteriormente por Menninger y su escuela en Chi- cago. En nuestro medio trabajó sobre este punto el maestro por excelencia del psico- análisis en Argentina, Dr. Enrique Pichón Riviere. El concepto sería el de la enfer- medad única donde en sucesivos momentos se privilegia un área determinada, en este caso el cuerpo. Quedarían de este modo englobados los conceptos dinámicos con los de constitución (tomando la tipología clásica de Kretchmer o los perfiles psicológi- cos de Florence Dumbar), junto a los de constelación que se van configurando en el decurso de los cinco primeros años de vida, y que se reactivan con el devenir del crecimiento en la latencia, la pubertad, la primera y segunda adultez, la madurez y la vejez.

La enfermedad displásica evoca en sí viejos resabios mágico animísticos ligados a la muerte; y aunque los médicos abocados al quehacer oncológico sabemos que los ex- traordinarios adelantos en esta rama de la medicina van a la par de otras especiali- dades, el cáncer sin embargo, representa un temor arraigado ancestralmente y que nos acompaña como una fantasía fantasmática de terror, dolor, invalidez, dependencia, deterioro físico y psíquico y finalmente de muerte. Funciona, en última instancia, como un temor universal.

Si partimos del concepto unicista, el ente humano es un magma vivencial indiscrimi- nado, un conjunto de procesos defensivos con un yo incipiente, que avanza en el des- arrollo para llegar a diferenciar -después de un largo aprendizaje- dónde están los conflictos, si en la mente o en el cuerpo o en ambos. La discriminación es lo que permite constituir el cuerpo y la mente con una existencia recíproca.

Pero esa misma discriminación se puede tornar clivaje, disociación o aislamiento y es así como entramos en el dominio de los procesos psicosomáticos patológicos en el campo de acción del médico, del especialista de cada área. Es en este mismo campo donde se verifica la necesidad de la presencia concreta de la ciencia psicológica, a cargo del psicólogo, como un especialista más en la vida cotidiana normal o pato- lógica de un staff terapéutico.

Quiero en este momento adelantar mi primer sugerencia, haciendo resaltar -visto el avance científico y tecnológico interdisciplinario de nuestro tiempo-, la necesi- dad de la presencia de los psicólogos en el staff terapéutico con la finalidad pri- mordial de llevar nuestra experiencia al campo médico y recoger de él valores seme- jantes.

En ciertas áreas de la medicina, y en buena hora como freno a la pseudología iatro-
génica, bajo el dominio del pensamiento rector de la Patología Celular, se dice
que toda enfermedad tiene, como punto de partida, una perturbación a nivel celular,
demostrable por métodos experimentales concretos, materiales, visibles, registra-
bles y confrontables. Esto es cierto si el problema es enfocado desde una vertiente
parcial y no integradora como es la de mi postulación.

Está demostrado que la perturbación inicial reside en la modificación de la actividad normal de células, tejidos y órganos. Es decir, sería de carácter funcional.
Esta perturbación produce sufrimiento celular y reacción tardía o, secundariamente,
enfermedad celular con cambios protoplasmáticos definidos y cada vez más irreversi-
bles.

Está demostrado también que estas lesiones celulares secundarias aparecen siempre
como expresión de cansancio, de desgaste, de agotamiento de la capacidad de rendi-
miento; y este cansancio es, a su vez, consecuencia de expoliación protoplasmática,
que se produce, por ejemplo por una prolongada privación de nutrición (como sucede
en la isquemia). Y por qué la privación mencionada? Por fallas, ya de exceso o de
defecto, en la actividad que rige el equilibrio funcional de los órganos efectores:
esto es, el sistema nervioso central y la organización endócrina.

Se comprueba igualmente que la perturbación funcional se inicia siempre en el sistema nervioso, ya que es él quien pone al individuo en contacto con el medio ambiente, a través de la faceta 'promundo', y es justamente en este medio ambiente
donde se encuentran los estímulos que hacen impacto contínuo sobre los receptores
sensoriales y, por su intermedio, sobre la corteza cerebral. Ponen así en marcha
las secuencias de alteraciones funcionales, que, por medio de la fracción 'vital'
del sistema nervioso, culminarán en lesiones celulares.

En resumen, esto significa que los estímulos del ambiente, si actúan sobre el sistema nervioso en magnitud y tiempo suficientes, son capaces de provocar fenómenos
vegetativos por exceso de estimulación, inhibición funcional o desviación de la actividad específica de los protoplasmas. Provocarían así, entonces, enfermedades de
naturaleza celular definida.Este tipo de estudio se debe, en su mayoría, a Menninger y su escuela.

Pienso entonces que lo que acabo de enunciar deberá ser replanteado a nivel de nuestro quehacer y que ello incidirá sin duda en la necesidad de trabajar solamente en
grupos interdisciplinarios que incluyan al psicólogo. El psicólogo es quien ha a-
prendido en su preparación profesional específica, cuál es la mejor manera de decodificar lo que está ocurriendo detrás del staff terapéutico que aborda un enfermo
de cáncer.

La inclusión de un psicólogo puede cuestionarse como factor disociante ya que nuestro quehacer propio es diferente al del médico de cualquier otra especialidad. A
qué se debe esta desigualdad? Es simple: nuestros supuestos básicos son diferentes
y lo son también nuestras técnicas de abordaje de la problemática del paciente.

El psicólogo usa la entrevista, como he dicho, preferentemente, ya que confluyen
en él la función profesional y la de investigador; su técnica es, así, el punto de
interacción entre las ciencias y las necesidades prácticas.

En las entrevistas, sean con el staff médico o con el paciente (solo o con su familia), el psicólogo logra la aplicación de conocimientos técnicos y al mismo tiempo
posibilita colocar la vida diaria del ser humano a nivel de la elaboración científica.

Aportaciones de las diversas escuelas a la teoría de la entrevista.

Confluyen en la teoría de la entrevista, conocimientos provenientes de diferentes escuelas psicológicas. Reseñaré a continuación, brevemente, las más importantes.

El Psicoanálisis ha aportado el conocimiento de la dimensión inconciente de la conducta, como así también de la transferencia y la contratransferencia, la resistencia, la represión, la proyección e introyección.

La Gestalt trajo la comprensión de la entrevista como un todo, en el cual el entrevistador (el psicólogo) es uno de los elementos integrantes: considera el comportamiento humano como una parte del todo.

La Topología ha conducido a plantear y reconocer el campo psicológico, con sus leyes, tanto como el enfoque situacional.

El Conductismo por su parte, ha resaltado la importancia de la observación del comportamiento total.

Todos estos aportes han contribuido, de alguna manera, a que hoy podamos realizar la entrevista en condiciones metodológicas más estrictas, transformándola en un instrumento científico en el cual 'el arte de la entrevista' se ha visto, naturalmente, reducido, en función de una mayor sistematización de las variables. Esta sistematización es la que posibilita mayor rigor en su aplicación y obviamente, en sus resultados. El estudio científico de la entrevista (la investigación del ser humano enfermo) ha reducido hoy su proporción de arte e incrementado su operancia y manejo a nivel de técnica científica. Por eso, los psicólogos nos encontramos en condiciones de mostrar a los colegas médicos la técnica de la entrevista sin tener que dejarlos librados a un don o virtud innata o a un talento artístico imponderable.

Estos últimos conceptos forman parte de un artículo de José Bleger sobre la entrevista psicológica, que editara el Departamento de Psicología de la Universidad Nacional de Buenos Aires[2].

La técnica de grupos operativos aplicada al staff terapéutico.

En la medida que consideremos a los seres humanos como entes singulares, aún cuando su formación en términos de rigor científico pueda ser similar, con todo, el Dr. X no será igual al Dr. Y. He aquí lo difícil: hemos aprendido a ser excelentes especialistas en las diferentes ramas de la ciencia médica, pero en la medida que en nuestro quehacer profesional entran a operar nuestros sistemas de valores, nuestras propias ideas acerca de la vida y la muerte, esto se traslucirá en nuestra diaria tarea.

Si tomáramos por ejemplo un staff terapéutico interdisciplinario ideal, con una formación científica bastante homogénea, el comportamiento de cada integrante de ese equipo tendrá sin embargo aspectos singulares, que provienen del propio acervo que en un profesional competente, ha decantado el curso de su vida. Este hecho incide, sin ninguna duda, cuando se plantea una discusión científica en un grupo de colegas de la misma o diferente especialidad como muchos en los que me ha tocado actuar, ya como profesional psicóloga o como coordinadora. En estos casos, la tarea ha sido enriquecedora para todos ya que lo psicológico representaba sólo un nivel

---

[2]Bleger, quien fuera mi maestro, tenía incorporada la metodología como parte de su personalidad altamente científica y rigurosa. Yo, en cambio, más pragmática, sigo pensando que si bien es cierto que no podemos operar dentro del caos, sin embargo en todo quehacer médico hay algo de arte, de humanismo y de imponderables personales.

de integración más.

La metodología de los 'grupos operativos' o 'grupos de entrenamiento' promueve situaciones en las que los procesos grupales pueden ser claramente observados y estudiados. La tarea del coordinador debe ser adjudicada en primera instancia al psicólogo, aunque cuando haya transcurrido ya un tiempo de trabajo en el grupo, los roles podrán alternarse.

Lo operativo de la tarea será que el grupo llegue a deducir por sí mismo experiencias significativas y que las condiciones sea tales que permitan aprender de esas experiencias. El grupo o staff terapéutico en general opera en medio del uso conciente del método experimental, bajo condiciones que deben revestir el suficiente grado de motivación como para permitirle pensar lo más objetivamente posible en los problemas subjetivos y singulares.

Dónde residiría el miedo? Creo que en la circunstancia de que muchos profesionales confunden grupo operativo con grupo terapéutico, y, como tal, les intimida por ejemplo el temario: la relación médico-paciente, las dificultades de obtención de datos en una anamnesis, la comprensión del material, el compromiso afectivo en el binomio médico-paciente: todo esto influye en algunos miembros en forma positiva, les hace sentir que se enriquecen, los distiende, sienten el diálogo en el grupo como un receptor de sus ansiedades y una desalienización de la tarea; mientras que en otros provoca una retracción que deberá ser respetada, ya que implica una disociación de su personalidad médica, que quizá no pueden superar en ese momento. No es fácil resolver una disociación organicista. Otro sería el caso si al estudiante de medicina se le familiarizase desde el principio con el acontecer psicológico igual que con el orgánico. De otro modo, se hace difícil medir las ansiedades que la problemática psicológica despierta en cada uno de nosotros.

Manejo de grupos operativos

En las discusiones de los grupos operativos se trata inicialmente la relación médico-paciente. Cada uno comienza identificándose con alguna de las dos partes y, por ejemplo, si corresponde al paciente alguien dirá: por qué no le preguntaste tal cosa?, no ves que te lo señaló muy claro y esperaba que lo ayudaras?. En otro caso, la identificación será del grupo con el médico y entonces, por ejemplo frente a un paciente muy invasor que lleva enquistado un duelo con situaciones hipocondríacas de queja y reproches, se le señalará al colega que se ha dejado invadir, tratando de no herir su susceptibilidad profesional.

Se torna a veces difícil evitar el alto nivel de dramatización que alcanza el grupo y aunque el psicólogo pueda devolver en forma de explicaciones teóricas o señalamientos, pienso con todo que el aprendizaje decanta en su continuidad, en la medida que los integrantes participan de un aprendizaje activo y empiezan a instrumentar y decodificar los mismos con su repertorio de respuestas maduras, lo que predomina en sus propias estructuras de personalidad, cualquiera sean. Me refiero básicamente a las estructuras defensivas o de comportamiento de los niveles maduros que se deben instrumentar en el quehacer médico cotidiano.

Los integrantes del staff terapéutico deben funcionar en condiciones normales, armónicas, creando así un campo dinámico que se refuerza y potencia paulatinamente. Por ejemplo: si un médico, por circunstancias afectivas personales se halla con su capacidad de conflictos interferida, bloqueada, y por ello no asumida en su área de trabajo, esta parte -excluída de su quehacer profesional y ahora de su personalidad-, entraría a funcionar para decodificar, cuando él observa y participa del grupo, el área de conflicto de los otros colegas, siempre claro está, que esos conflictos no sea de naturaleza semejante.

La instrumentación de la dramatización ayuda al médico que presenta sus dificultades a vivenciar el conflicto no percibido, en la medida que se deja ayudar por la
parte observadora y discriminadora de los otros, que colaboran en la exterioriza-
ción del conflicto.

El grupo exterioriza las tres ansiedades básicas: confusional, paranoide y depresiva, a través de aquellos miembros del staff que tienen más facilidad para la
dramatización, mayor espontaneidad o menos dificultades para zafarse de estereoti-
pos formales o fijos.

Puede ocurrir también que aparezcan defensas como la disociación y aún negaciones
masivas: se deberían a una regresión en el grupo, por haberse tocado ideologías o
modalidades médicas muy estereotipadas, que es difícil desarraigar y cuyo cuestio
namiento genera ansiedad. He aquí el momento importante de la acción del psicólogo que tenderá a esclarecer el por qué de la situación planteada: esta acción técnica ayudará sin duda a detectar la presencia del conflicto, la inherencia del mismo a la naturaleza humana y también al quehacer médico.

Si el equipo es de médicos de distintas especialidades, el área de personalidad
del profesional que no se halla comprometida en su tarea cotidiana, aporta a los
colegas sugerencias muy valiosas y permite que, el que en cada momento expone, pueda decodificar y reincorporar con poca rivalidad sus partes disociadas; mientras
que tratándose de un grupo de colegas de idéntico campo de trabajo, estas observa-
ciones resonarían quizá más agresivas.

El paciente

El paciente es alguien que depende de nosotros, que nos entrega su enfermedad lle-
no de temor y de expectativas; con la decisión por tomar acerca de una intervención quirúrgica que cambiará las características de su vida quizá para siempre.
Frente a él, es necesario que el staff terapéutico refuerce su identidad profesional. Ello implica no sólo el afianzamiento de sus conocimientos científicos, sino,
y principalmente, la mayor comprensión posible de los problemas que alienan al grupo en su quehacer. Aquello que no puede concientizar, por tratarse de un aspecto
disociado, su área de conflicto, que no le permitirá buenas proyecciones y reintro-
yecciones si no le son proporcionadas las condiciones para hacerlo.

Esto constituye el por qué de la necesidad de orientar la labor del staff terapéutico en forma de grupos operativos, donde los psicólogos crean el contexto apropia-
do para desarrollar armónicamente la actividad profesional específica.

Esta forma de trabajo permitirá además que en el grupo emerjan los mecanismos defensivos de sus miembros, incluído el coordinador psicólogo. Así, el equipo cono-
cerá experiencialmente cómo cada uno ha elaborado el monto de ansiedad que provoca
en todos el quehacer médico: la permanente confrontación con la muerte, la locura,
las enfermedades incurables como el cáncer, la diabetes, los problemas renales con-
génitos, etc.

Este modelo, dirigido a una elaboración desalienizante, operará inlcuso en las vi-
das privadas de los profesionales médicos, en las de sus familiares y en las de
los pacientes. Cuando he tenido la oportunidad de recurrir a un colega para ser
tratada, esto es, como paciente, algunas veces al salir del consultorio he pensa-
do 'pobres pacientes...' y no precisamente refiriéndome a la enfermedad que los a-
queja. He observado como puede maltratarse innecesariamente al enfermo, dejando
fuera, conciente o inconcientemente, lo psicológico.

En muchos casos, el paciente acude posteriormente a pedir ayuda psicológica, cuando en realidad debió recibir este tipo de asistencia desde el comienzo de la inves-

tigación médica, es decir, a partir del diagnóstico, la verificación, la intervención quirúrgica o un equivalente sucedáneo tipo cobalto o quimioterapia.

No soy ajena a que las condiciones en que a veces se debe ejercer la profesión
son precarias y no me pasa desapercibido tampoco que las carencias de material de
investigación, de personal auxiliar y de medios en general representan un factor
que, obviamente, tensiona al profesional médico que se siente también él inmerso
en esa precariedad.

En estos casos, que no son pocos, el profesional trabaja en situación de stress
subliminal y, naturalmente, sus pacientes sufren parte importante de las consecuencias de ese stress.

Propongo desde aquí que hagamos todos una corta reflexión sobre lo que acabo de
exponer y quizá podamos entonces retomar nuestra tarea en mejores condiciones.
Cuando el equipo terapéutico de cualquier rama de la oncología ha sometido su quehacer profesional y su identidad a este tipo de experiencia, ello ha redundado en
una actuación más sincronizada del staff y con aperturas humanas enriquecidas que
se han vertido en la forma de enfoque de cada paciente. El paciente, reitero, es
un ente singular que pasa a depender de nosotros, de nuestros gestos, de cómo lo
tratamos, de cómo le hablamos y de qué le decimos. Recordemos que nuestro quehacer contiene una gran dosis de sadismo metabolizada en nuestra identidad profesional y que debemos cuidarnos de ser innecesariamente crueles.

Trabajar con la muerte agazapada en un paciente descompensado, con una familia
desestructurada por la incertidumbre y el miedo, puede conducirnos a dos modalidades extremas, caricaturescas, de nuestra forma de comunicación: o nos protegemos
poniendo una exagerada distancia, y entonces el binomio médico-paciente es un fantasma deshumanizado donde los dos pueden llegar a no conocerse, o nos lanzamos a
un excesivo acercamiento. De parte del paciente se expresa la alternativa de 'distancia' en forma de olvido de las prescripciones médicas y aún de la apariencia
física del profesional tratante. El médico, por su lado, salva la amnesia que res-
pecta a este paciente recurriendo a su ficha.

Lo distinto es cuando se da una corriente empática, donde el enfermo consulta sobre algo estructurado y concreto: aquí el médico puede optar por dejarlo hablar o
iniciar él el interrogatorio.

Para nuestra especialidad, a mi juicio, lo más correcto sería un modelo de entrevista de características mixtas donde en cada caso, y según las circunstancias la
misma se desarrolle en forma abierta, pautada o semilibre.

Todos los dinamismos giran alrededor de la ansiedad de ambas partes: médico y paciente. El paciente, por el solo hecho de venir a pedir ayuda se encuentra ansio-
so y están perturbados sus mecanismos defensivos. Suele hablar mucho o quedar to-
talmente paralizado. De la habilidad del médico dependerá que pueda percibir como
vive el paciente esa situación, que es nueva para él, donde teme que el médico le
confirme sus temores, es decir, le hable de aspectos enfermos de su personalidad
que puedan focalizarse en un síndrome canceroso en cualquiera de sus localizacio-
nes.

Generalmente, cuando el paciente acude al especialista es porque ya pasó por la
consulta con su médico particular, quien trata de enviarlo a un oncólogo conocido,
con quien puede ligarlo o no una relación amistosa. Suelen suscitarse, a esta altu-
ra, extrañas y esotéricas relaciones entre los dos profesionales: hay colegas especialistas que están envueltos en un halo de narcisismo y autismo que los lleva
a actuar en forma muy impersonal y con un pobre contacto con los colegas que les
derivan pacientes. Nuevamente juega aquí la ansiedad del médico que se hace muy

difícil de decodificar. Y surge a nuestro desarrollo entonces la necesidad de la presencia del psicólogo en el staff que aborda el tema oncológico.

Vale la pena diferenciar entre lo que aquí llamo 'presencia del psicólogo en el e-quipo' con la habitual consulta al servicio de psicopatología que suele haber en hospitales o clínicas. Esta alternativa no es el camino, a mi entender, ya que no todos los colegas del quehacer psicológico nos hallamos en condiciones de manejar situaciones con algo contenido ansiógeno, donde interviene el fantasma de la muer-te real, elemento no siempre bien tolerado por todos los psicólogos y psicoanalis-tas.

Todos los profesionales de la ciencia psicológica manejamos fantasías sobre la muerte, como así también un fantástico mundo de ansiedades, temores, serias cri-sis de identidad y graves desestructuraciones de la personalidad de nuestros enfer-mos. Pero la muerte real es otra cosa: es un hecho vivencial palpado concretamen-te en el quehacer cotidiano. Aseguraría que todo médico se ha enfrentado alguna vez con el hecho de la muerte de su paciente. Nosotros, en cambio, nos encontramos con una problemática de distinta índole: frente a un intento de suicidio, por ejem-plo, por lo general rápidamente tomamos nuestros recaudos, internamos al paciente compartiendo así la responsabilidad.

Sostengo que significa más grave impacto el deceso provocado por una enfermedad de origen prevalentemente orgánico, que la muerte por suicidio. En el primer caso, nos enfrentamos seguramente con un paciente que pide ayuda; como tal, no quiere mo-rir ni tampoco sufrir; se aferra a la vida y el sentimiento del médico es la impo-tencia para evitarle ese trance. Probablemente lo que ocurre es que es más directa la identificación con este tipo de dolor que remueve las propias ansiedades frente a la muerte, al sufrimiento, a la futilidad de nuestro quehacer y a las limitacio-nes de la medicina, a pesar de los enormes avances científicos y tecnológicos de que, con justicia, nos enorgullecemos.

En el caso del suicidio, si el profesional sabe que tomó las medidas para tratar de evitarlo, reconocerá que el paciente ha hecho una opción; opción que podrá o no coincidir con su ideología de vida pero que debe aceptar como lo que es: la de-cisión del otro, ya que la vida no significa para él lo mismo que para su médico.

A modo de acotación al tema 'entrevista', quiero señalar que cuando llega el pa-ciente con su familia el médico no debería aceptar de entrada el criterio fami-liar acerca de quién es el enfermo, sino que haría mejor en actuar considerando al grupo familiar como enfermo y a todos sus miembros implicados en la enfermedad. De este modo el interjuego de roles y la dinámica propia del grupo familiar, son ele-mentos que le servirán de orientación para observar cómo el que para la familia es 'el enfermo', puede serlo en realidad pero puede también tratarse por ejemplo, del cónyuge que proyecta en él sus ansiedades hipocondríacas. Este tipo de manejo po-dría interferir el claro pensar del médico acerca del diagnóstico.

No olvidemos que la culpa es un fenómeno que siempre deberá ser tenido en cuenta por el staff para poder valorarlo adecuadamente y manejarlo. En muchos casos se ha visto como, quien hace las veces de 'acompañante' puede ser el que se siente más culpable o incluso quien desea reparar en ese familiar a una hermana, un hijo, etc., tratándose de que sus conflictos con el supuesto enfermo, le dan la oportuni-dad de actuar adecuadamente con él y frente al staff terapéutico.

El médico tendrá en cuenta también y evaluará las preguntas pertinentes que duran-te la entrevista le sean formuladas: lo que infiera a través de ellas deberá ser convalidado más tarde por medio de pruebas auxiliares. Tratará asimismo de detec-

tar el grado de ansiedad frente a lo desconocido que el paciente está debiendo so-
portar y cómo lo hace: el entrevistador mismo, el consultorio, la enfermedad en sí
y los miedos que la entrevista reactiva, son elementos cuyo manejo más o menos a-
daptado dará idea de la fortaleza del yo del paciente.

Casi todos los individuos que sospechan que están enfermos de gravedad incurren
en mecanismos regresivos para sobrellevar el impacto: aparecen la negación, las
conductas evitativas y fóbicas y las defensas paranoides cuando niega lo que el
médico le dice acerca de su verdad. Esto lo llevará a él y a sus familiares a recurrir a la magia y a la omnipotencia, a nuevas consultas que reforzarán sus mecanismos de negación.

En mi postulación final sugiero no flaquear, seguir investigando y no quedar de
brazos cruzados lo cual configura el otro extremo de la omnipotencia: la Nada,
que es muerte asumida en forma inconciente.

--ooOoo--

BIBLIOGRAFIA

Alexander F. y Szasz . El enfoque psicosomático en medicina y en psiquiatría.
    Editorial Paidós, Buenos Aires.
Baranger M. y W. y colab. Mecanismos hipocondríacos 'normales' en el desarrollo
    femenino. Rev.Urug.Psico-Anál., Vol. VI, N° 1, Año 1964.
Baranger M. y W. y colab. Problemas del campo psicoanalítico. Editorial Kargie-
    man, Buenos Aires.
Baranger W. Posición y objeto en la obra de Melanie Klein. Editorial Kargieman,
    Buenos Aires.
Blessler B. Per Nyhus and Fin Mag nussen: pregnancy fantaseis in psychosomatic
    illness en simpton formation: a clinical study. Psychosomatic Medicine, May-
    June, 1958. Vol. XX, N° 3.
Bleger J. Simbiosis y ambiguedad. Editorial Paidós, Buenos Aires, 1972.
Bleger L. Cuerpo y mente en la gestación. (Trabajo para optar a miembro titular
    de la Asociación Psicoanalítica Argentina, 1965).
Bleger L. La presencia del hijo en la pareja estéril. (Trabajo para optar a miem-
    bro titular de la Asociación Psicoanalítica Argentina, 1966. Análisis aplica-
    do a dos obras teatrales: "Yerma", de Federico García Lorca y "Quién le teme
    a Virginia Woolf?", de Edward Albee.).
Bleger L. Estudio correlativo somatopsíquico de la pareja estéril. Presentado al
    Congreso Latinoamericano de Psicoanálisis, 1964.
Bleger J. y Bleger L. Algunas correlaciones entre Freud, Melanie Klein y Fairbairn.
    Rev.Psico-Anál., T. XIV, N° 1 y 2. Buenos Aires, 1962.
Klein M. El psicoanálisis de niños. Versión directa del inglés por Enrique Pichón
    Riviere. Editorial El Ateneo, Buenos Aires, 1948.
Fenichel O. Teoría psicoanalítica de las neurosis. Editorial Nova, Buenos Aires,
    1957.
Liberman D. La comunicación en terapéutica psicoanalítica. Eudeba, 1962.
Liberman D. Linguística, interacción comunicativa y proceso psicoanalítico. Tomo
    I. Editorial Galerna.
Mahler M. On human symbiosis and the vicissitudes of individuation. Edit. Interna-
    tional Universities Press, Inc. New York, 1968.
Pasqualini R.K. Stress. Vol. I. Editorial Ateneo, 1952.
Pichon Riviere E. Conceptos básicos en medicina psicosomática. Prensa médica ar-
    gentina, vol. 35, N° 36. Buenos Aires, 1948.
Rothenberg S. Depressions in psychosomatic desorders. Psychosomatic Medicine, Vol
    XVI, N° 3. May-June, 1954.
Ruesch J. Disturbed Communication. Norton C. New York, 1957.
Segal H. Notas sobre la formación de símbolos. Int.J.Psycho-anal., vol. 38, 1952.

The Psychology of Cancer Patients and Cancer Doctors: Shock of Recognition

Arthur S. Levine

*Pediatric Oncology Branch, National Cancer Institute, Building 10, Room 3B-12,
National Institutes of Health, Bethesda, Maryland 20014*

Psychologic and social management of the patient with cancer (and the family
of such a patient) is often complex and anxiety-provoking, as any doctor can
testify who has witnessed the contrived support of the patient who "doesn't
know the truth," the endless demands on the medical staff's time in pursuit
of seemingly trivial matters, the frenzied flight from one physician to another
seeking a cure, the withdrawal, anger, depression, and/or paradoxic euphoria
of the dying patient, and the driven energy of a patient seeking support for
a questionable malpractice suit. As important as the patient's reaction to
cancer may be, the reaction of the physician to his patient is equally complex
and important. The almost uniform but transient depression of oncology fellows
during their second and third month of fellowship is familiar, but the enduring
degree to which anxiety-provoking factors in the doctor-patient relation may
cripple a physician's effectiveness is often not appreciated. The oncologist
may adjust to his practice in a way which causes discomfort to his patients
and himself, but the generalist often arranges not to "spend a lot of time
with cancer patients," thus avoiding possible discomfort. What is the price
paid by the cancer patient for such arrangements?

If one is to speak to these critical matters in a helpful way, it is necessary
to explore questions which are as much philosophic as technical. One must
inquire about the structure of man's psyche and the society of which he is
a part, the techniques man uses to deal with stress, and specifically, the
response he makes to the fear of dying. Death is what the word cancer means
to most people, and what it means to most physicians as well.

Few of us are sufficiently transcendent to consider that personality (indeed
what we call culture) represents an inevitable reaction to the shock of man's
recognition that while he is capable of conceptualizing the infinite, he nonetheless remains ultimately doomed to death. Becker refers to this paradox as
the condition of individuality within finitude, and writes that,

> "Man is literally split in two: he has an awareness of his own splendid
> uniqueness in that he sticks out of nature with a towering majesty, and
> yet he goes back into the ground a few feet in order blindly and dumbly
> to rot and disappear forever. It is a terrifying dilemma to be in and
> to have to live with ... to live a whole lifetime with the fate of death
> haunting one's dreams and even the most sun-filled days." (Becker, 1973).

The fear of death reflects our instinct for self-preservation; yet, this anxiety must be decisively repressed as a condition for normal daily functioning. The complex psychologic mechanisms involved in this self-protecting repression often are maintained in paradoxic and energy-demanding ways. Thus, human actions, particularly when they occur in situations of great stress, may appear bizzarre unless they are examined in the context of a ubiquitous human fear of death.

> "Men are so necessarily mad that not to be mad would amount to another
> form of madness. Necessarily because the existential dualism makes an
> impossible situation, an excruciating dilemma ...everything that man
> does...is an attempt to deny and overcome his grotesque fate. He literally
> drives himself into a blind obliviousness with...personal preoccupations
> so far removed from the reality of his situation that they are forms
> of madness-agreed madness, shared madness, disguised and dignified madness,
> but madness all the same." (Becker, 1973).

The physician dealing with a patient who has a potentially fatal disease cannot usually be considered, and should not consider himself, to be an objective observer in this setting. One may speculate that physicians in particular sense the finite quality of life, and more than most, experience the fear of death. The manipulative, controlling, potent posture is a common one among physicians - it is, after all, the student with an "A" and not a "C" in organic chemistry who has the best chance of medical school acceptance. Paradoxically, it is this same individual who may be least equipped emotionally to deal with the dying patient and the frustration attendant upon the physician's inability to manipulate the situation.

Nearly every physician has a large element of the hero in his self-concept, and this quality, so important to getting him into and through the rigors of medical school, becomes a handicap at certain points in the doctor-patient relation (Artiss, 1973), for it makes him peculiarly susceptible to the patient's praise and flattery - offered by the patient in an attempt to persuade the physician to enter a subtle contract: the good and flattering patient will be rewarded with a cure. It is easy for the physician to come to expect a "larger-than-life" performance from himself. The patient says, "Between you and me and God, we'll make it, won't we, Doctor?" The doctor nods his head or makes some other reassuringly agreeable response and he has thus made a contract as far as the patient is concerned. The doctor learns later to rue those few seconds when he was caught off guard, because in effect he has promised something he cannot deliver. The dependency implicit in this relation between doctor and patient appears to be at the very crux of medical practice - always seeming to be in the best interest of the patient, but the worst interest of the doctor, if the latter fails to appreciate his situation and permits himself to believe, even for an instant, that he is in fact, "larger-than-life."

In considering the patient's and the doctor's fear of death and their relation to one another, we must introduce still more complexities. The child of five has begun to conceptualize death but his mechanisms for dealing with the anxiety of dying differ remarkably from the child of ten who has probably learned the adult's pattern of repression (Evans, 1968). One might further consider the dependency relation of a pediatric patient to his parents and the parents' relation with each other, the relation of the family members to their community, and the relation of one or more physicians to the family, to each other, and to society. There obtain almost infinite combinations of repression, anxiety, dependency, and delusions of invulnerability. It is no wonder that, particularly in oncology, there are factors in the doctor-patient relation that frequently provoke crises in management.

With the dependency relation of doctor and patient, and the denial of death
common to both as the setting, we might now proceed to describe certain phenomena
which recur with sufficient frequency that they should always be anticipated.
As is true elsewhere in medical practice, anticipation and prevention are
usually more useful than treatment when one considers the psychologic management
of the patient with cancer.

PSYCHOLOGIC STAGES OF DEATH

Kubler-Ross has described five stages in a patient's response to terminal
illness (Kubler-Ross, 1960). These are, in sequence: denial, anger, bargaining,
depression, and acceptance. Depending on the patient and the rapidity of
the terminal illness, these stages may be of variable duration and the sequence
may be incomplete. Further, certain elements of each stage may appear intermittently throughout the clinical course. Thus, some patients may employ denial
as a mechanism throughout the major portion of their illness or denial may
only comprise a brief episode followed by a prolonged stage of anger or depression.
Bargaining is usually evanescent, but may occur at several points, and it
is not uncommon to see anger manifested intermittently throughout the course
of the disease. Acceptance of the imminence of death is usually a relatively
brief phenomenon shortly before death, associated with a gradual voluntary
separation of the patient from his friends and relatives. The patient's family
usually progresses through a similar pattern of stages in its adjustment to
the patient's illness.

Kübler-Ross has described the activities of a program designed to provide
supportive psychologic care for cancer patients and their families. She has
pointed out the initial reluctance of professionals to accept the role of
such a unit in patient care, their overt and covert hostility, and even frank
anger when patients, learning of the unit from other patients, requested consultation. Such reactions are not surprising in view of the often desperate need
of the hospital staff to deny themselves the reality of dying patients and
by extension, the reality of their own mortality, usually by becoming deeply
involved in the technical aspects of case management. Even the clergy, who
accepted the need for Kübler-Ross' program, have often avoided dealing with
the patients' true concerns by using prayer or biblical readings as their
major method of communication with the patient.

SOCIAL DEATH

The phenomenon of social death may be an area of extreme difficulty (Sudnow,
1967). The fact that families and communities must undertake a series of
rituals when one member dies is frequently overlooked. Many physicians are
unaware of the possibility of profound social reaction to the diagnosis of
cancer, professing ignorance of the fact that cancer is frequently seen as
a punishment for misdeeds. Not being aware of these social phenomena, they
may have serious altercations with members of the patient's family as misunderstand-
ings are compounded, the doctor repeating "medical facts" and the family pleading
with him for social solutions. Often, family members avidly receive the words,
"Everything is being done that can be done. You were very smart to come to
this hospital so quickly." Once given this statement, the family can report
to the community that superb doctors at a fine hospital are doing everything
possible: The family is surely absolved of wrong-doing or neglect. It is
only when the doctor permits hemself to be seduced by such a statement that
the words pose a danger.

GUILT

There is no more extreme instance of guilt than that commonly displayed by
the parents of a dying child. To the extent that procreation represents a
parent's bridge to eternity, death in his child awakens the parent's own fear
of death to a degree that the death of any other loved one cannot. Becker
paraphrases Aristotle, "Luck is when the guy next to you gets hit with an
arrow," and indeed, no human is transcendent enough to avoid a sense of good
fortune at having been spared when death strikes nearby. This "luck" may
even be conceived by a parent. Yet the inevitable consequence of such good
fortune, given our cultural frame of reference, is overwhelming guilt. An
additional, though probably lesser source of guilt is the accumulation of
real or imagined wrongs perpetrated on the patient by his relatives. One
common method for diminishing the anxiety produced by guilt is the use of
a scapegoat. All the power of the intellect and profound attention to detail
is brought to bear on the selection of a scapegoat, since to be effective
in reducing anxiety, the scapegoat must be made part of a rational, credible
system. It is for this reason that the physician must exercise extreme caution
in his discussion with a family of the causes of the malignancy, or questions
concerning previous management by other physicians. Given the parents' natural
guilt and their tendency to relieve the anxiety associated with guilt by identification of a scapegoat, even the vaguest suggestion will fall on fertile ground.
In all probability, a scapegoat will always be identified, but the physician
must be careful not to be drawn into the logic system created by the family.
The consequences of becoming involved in questions of management by previous
physicians, exposure to insecticide sprays or diagnostic x-ray, etc., are
obvious. Less apparent is the subtle trap which can be set when a busy physician
innocently agrees that the onset of malignancy could have had a relationship
to some trivial viral infection, only to discover later that a sibling or
neighbor, who may have "given the infection" to the patient, has been blamed
by the parent.

When a family identifies a doctor as its scapegoat, the anxiety provoked in
both doctor and patient is profound. One of the most common mechanisms for
handling anxiety is to transfer responsibility for one's fate to a leadership
or authority figure. The extent of this transference is often not apparent
until the leader gives evidence of his fallibility (LeBon, 1960, and Bion,
1961). In the case of a patient with malignancy, the family looks to the
physician as a key source of psychologic support. Any suggestion that he
is less than excellent results in profound anxiety, yet the family, to relieve
its guilt, is constantly searching for just such a scapegoat. The potential
for a misstep under such circumstances is very great indeed.

Once a scapegoat has been identified, the mechanism is usually amplified.
To be effective in diminishing the family's guilt, the scapegoat must be believable.
Thus the family, to sustain its own belief, must convince others of its validity.
Like new religious converts therefore, they set out as evangelists to convince
nurses, doctors, other families, any who will listen, of their belief in the
chosen scapegoat. In its extreme form, this process can have a devastating
effect, not only on the medical staff, but on the well-being of other patients
and families as well. Often, the most effective way of insuring that the
scapegoat is not a member of the medical staff is for the family to be continuously
assured that "Everything is being done that can be done," and especially to
provide consistent information to patient and family from all staff members.

TRUTH

The physician of an older generation often remained aloof, not explaining disease or treatment to patient or relatives, and writing in Latin to emphasize the sacred mystery. This role may have evolved because it is an effective device to alleviate patient anxiety (ultimately the fear of death) by transferring personal responsibility for one's fate to a leadership figure: "It's his responsibility now." The naturalness and ubiquity of this enduring role in society can be appreciated by a study of primitive cultures. In contemporary society, however, the patient's apparent sophistication may make the divestiture of personal autonomy all the more subtle and complex. Truth, while it may not entirely avert suspicion and pretense, is clearly the minimum requirement for dealing with such a situation (Glaser, 1965).

A great deal has been written about the question of whether to tell a patient the truth about terminal illness. However, we often fail to recognize that patients (and relatives) hear only what they want to hear or are ready to hear. In effect, people have protective mechanisms which prevent the acceptance of knowledge they are not ready to accept, even when told these truths directly (Weinstein, 1955).

On the other hand, a patient cannot be brought into a large medical center or community hospital, receive the constant attention of a large number of physicians, nurses, and technicians and undergo numerous tests and treatments day after day without knowing something indeed very serious is wrong. "Not knowing" what it is that is wrong may be far more anxiety-provoking than the harshest reality. In most circumstances the truth, tactfully told, is the best approach; one must then remain sensitive to evidence that the patient has not "heard" what was said. In such circumstances, the truth should not be labored, but time allowed to pass and the subjuect discussed later, always watching for clues that the patient or relative is now ready to hear more.

When patients and relatives are past their initial denial, the physician must be prepared to deal with their anger. Anger, always a defense against anxiety, is an almost constant concommitant to serious illness, and in relatives, especially the parents of a dying child, anger resulting from strong feelings of guilt must be managed skillfully. The threat of guilt and anger in the family often makes us less than eager to deal with them in a truthful manner but it is in this very situation that we must demand of ourselves utter honesty.

Before the age of three to five, death has been thought to have little or no meaning to children, since they do not speak of it in conventional terms. The subject is best avoided, unless we are prepared to deal with the child in symbolic language or in another investigative fashion. From five to ten years of age, it is probable that adult concepts of death are being formulated, the human paradox is being faced, and adult patterns of dealing with the issue are being developed. The seriousness of their illness is generally apparent to such children from their parents' reaction. Depending on the child, the parents, and the institution, the fear of death may or may not arise in discussion. The description by Evans provides a useful guide to techniques which may be employed with young children (Evans, 1968). After the age of ten, however, the adult pattern of dealing with the fear of death has probably been established and truth is undoubtedly the most efficient approach; defensive delusions of invulnerability are probably not so strongly developed as in the adult.

HOPE AND ABANDONMENT

Hope cannot be given nor destroyed by the physician; it comes (or fails to
come) from within the person himself. A judicious and honest statement of
the facts will be incorporated by patient and relatives into the matrix of
their ego defenses in a surprisingly appropriate fashion. Just as the physician
should not force the patient to abondon denial before he is ready, so too
the physician need not dwell on formulating a reason for hope, since he has
no special skill or endowment in this regard. Honest and simplicity suffice.

It is often tempting to abandon the patient with intractible disease or an
"intractible" emotional state. Yet cancer patients and their relatives are
exquisitely sensitive to abandonment. Even in a situation where both patient
and relatives are in the stage of "acceptance," attention must be paid to
unspoken needs. Regrettably, abandonment usually occurs when the anger of
a patient and relatives literally forces the staff to stay out of the room
and avoid contact except for the required minimum. It is this avoidance which
is interpreted as abandonment, even in the presence of technically excellent
care. Probably nothing done by a staff can have a more destructive impact
on a patient and family than abandonment. Yet the staff, confident that their
technical duty is being done and failing to appreciate the anxiety-anger-guilt
reaction as being inherently biologic, console one another in stunned bewilderment
over the perceived ingratitude of patient and family alike.

No element of the doctor-patient relation justifies abandonment, although
a particular doctor-patient relation may not be viable (after thorough exploration)
and infrequently, there may be a need for referral.

Just as the paralytic who has lost spincter control may be viewed by the staff
as troublesome but not malicious because the problem is understood, so too
the attitude of the staff to the anxious, angry, and ultimately silent patient
and relatives will inevitably be conditioned by the extent to which the staff
views the trouble caused by the family as beyond their control, i.e., - a
universal and ultimately irrepressible response to the fear of death.

THE DOCTOR'S BEHAVIOR

The experience of death among his patients weakens the physician's defensive
armoring against this issue in his own life, and he is thrown into conflict
(Artiss, 1973). On the one hand, he longs for the peace of mind that he possessed
before he began to confront death, but on the other hand, he is driven by
his own scientific curiosity and heroic tendencies to explore this conventionally
unknown territory. He may find such existentialist authors as Camus quite
helpful in this regard, expecially in that writer's awareness of the "absurd" -
the gap between human needs and the unreasonably unresponsive world (Camus,
1955).

The physician's attempt to confront the "absurd" is commonly represented by
the question, "What should I say to the dying patient?" In fact, there is
often nothing to say. As death approaches, a patient may psychologically
come to accept its imminence. One consequence of this acceptance is a dramatic
change in the patient's pattern of communication - having no future, he is
not interested in discussing anything that bears implications for the future.
He is left with virtually nothing to talk about, and conversations become
stilted or meaningless. Unprepared for this phenomenon, and heavily oriented
by virtue of his training to provide patients with hopeful words about the
future, the physician may experience a sense of helpless, almost foolish embarrass-
ment.

But the physician's presence, without words, may now be as helpful to his
patients as were talking and listening early on.

Seeing existences terminate all around him, the young oncologist usually becomes
quite reflective about his own. As he becomes increasingly aware of his personal
responsibility and recognizes that his seniors do not have more answers than
he has, the young physician is singularly confronted with himself. His patients'
discussion of how fully they have lived their lives has an effect upon him
and he is directed toward an ontologic form of existential anxiety that results
from his being finally confronted with his own question, "Am I fulfilling
my potentialities?"

The existentialist anxiety is a liberating one for the physician charged with
the care of a dying patient, for it forces him to enter the human equation
with his patients as he confronts the basic issues of his own life:

> "Man does not really begin to live until he has begun to take his own
> mortality seriously." (Kaufmann, 1956)

Artiss, K. L., and Levine, A. S. (1973). Doctor-patient relation in severe
    illness: A seminar for oncology fellows. New Engl. J. Med., 288.
    1210-1214.

Becker, E. (1973). The Denial of Death. The Free Press, New York.

Bion, W. R. (1961). Experiences in Groups and Other Pages . Basic Books,
    New York. pp. 105-113.

Camus, A. (1955). The Myth of Sisyphus, and Other Essays. Vintage
    O'Brien, J. (Trans), New York. pp. 3-68.

Evans, A. E. (1968). If a child must die... New Engl. J. Med. 278. 138-142.

Existentialism from Dostoievsky to Sartre. (1956). In. W. A. Kauffmann (Ed.).
    Meridian World, Cleveland. pp. 221, 307-311.

Glaser, B. G., and Strauss, A. L. (1965). Awareness of Dying. Aldine,
    Chicago, pp. 29-63, 64-115.

Kübler-Ross, E. (1969). On Death and Dying. Macmillan, New York.

LeBon, G. (1960). The Crowd: A Study of the Popular Mind. The Viking
    Press, New YOrk. pp. 23-100, 117-140.

Sudnow, D. (1967). Passing On: The Social Organization of Dying. Prentice-Hall,
    Englewood Cliffs, N.J. pp. 63-107, 181-193.

Weinstein, E. A., and Kuhn, R. L. (1955). Denial of Illness. Symbolic and
    Physiological Aspects. Charles C. Thomas, Springfield, Illinois.
    pp. 3-9, 10-22, 23-37, 122-129.

Modifications of Therapeutic Procedure for Psychological Reasons in Breast Cancer

J. A. Urban

Attending Surgeon, Memorial Sloan Kettering Cancer Center,
New York, N.Y.
Associate Clinical Professor of Surgery, Cornell University Medical School

ABSTRACT

The female patient who undergoes mastectomy for breast cancer is exposed to two stressful, emotional problems: 1) she must cope with the knowledge that she has a potentially fatal disease and must overcome the fear of cancer recurrence and death; 2) she must adapt to the loss of her breast, which is a source of femininity and self esteem. The initial response of most patients to the possible diagnosis of breast cancer is one of fear and anxiety at the prospect of losing her breast. In most cases, this initial anxiety is ultimately replaced by an overriding concern regarding the possibility of recurrence and death from disease.

Both problems must be faced resolutely by the patient and her surgeon. Recently, there has been a tendency to downgrade the adequacy of primary surgical therapy and to perform more conservative and, oftentimes, inadequate surgical treatment, in order to preserve the breast, and thus, prevent the onset of emotional and social problems resulting from the loss of the patient's breast. Unfortunately, these more conservative procedures have not proven to be as effective in controlling disease as more adequate primary surgical therapy. Several studies in which conservative surgery has been compared with radical mastectomy are cited, and show improved longterm survival rates at 10 years in the patients treated by the more adequate primary surgery. The use of adjuvant multi chemotherapy and adjuvant x-ray therapy should be applied to patients after adequate primary surgical treatment has been performed, and should not be used as a crutch for inadequate primary treatment. Because of the chronicity of breast cancer, 5 year follow up data, or less, is inadequate to evaluate the effectiveness of a primary therapeutic measure. Such evaluation must be based upon the follow up of at least 10 years at the minimum.

Both dominant emotional problems can be managed best through the initial application of adequate primary surgical therapy to afford the patient the optimum chance for long term control of breast cancer - followed at a suitable time interval by the implantation of a prosthesis to restore a more satisfactory appearance in patients who desire this.

The female patient who undergoes mastectomy for breast cancer is exposed to two stressful, emotional problems. She must live with the knowledge that she had a potentially fatal disease, and must overcome the fear of cancer recurrence and consequent pain, suffering and death. Also, she must adapt to the loss of her breast, which is a source of femininity, self esteem and attraction to others. These problems are difficult and not infrequently, patients fail to make the necessary psychological adjustments and develop severe emotional and social problems. Often, the initial response of the patient to the possible diagnosis of breast cancer is one of fear and disappointment at the prospect of losing her breast. In most cases, when this possibility has been confirmed through biopsy and primary treatment, this initial fear is largely replaced by an overriding concern regarding the possibility of recurrence of cancer and subsequent suffering and death from this disease. Both problems must be faced resolutely and directly by the patient, her family, her surgeon, and associated therapists.

Ours is a breast oriented society, in which preservation and enhancement of the breast is being emphasized with increasing enthusiasm regardless of other, more pertinent, consequences. The psychological trauma of removal of the breast for the treatment of breast cancer is being stressed, while the need for adequate surgical treatment of this disease is being minimized. Well meaning enthusiasts for conservative surgery, aided and abetted by the female Lib Movement are preserving the breasts while losing the patients. Currently, there is an increasing awareness of the breast cancer problem in the general public. This has resulted in the detection of "minimal" breast cancer in an increasing proportion of patients. This development presents a tremendous potential for improved salvage of breast cancer patients, which may easily be negated by the current trend toward conservative , inadequate primary surgical treatment. Since the advent of the Cronin prosthesis,(ref in 1964, and subsequent modifications of this prosthetic device which have occurred since, it is feasible and practical to reconstruct the breast following adequate primary surgical treatment for breast cancer with facility and satisfactory cosmetic results. We believe that the thoroughness of the primary surgical procedure should not be diminished in a misguided effort to help the patient cope with the emotional stress secondary to the loss of her breast. Rather, both dominant emotional problems can be handled best through the application of adequate primary surgical therapy, which will realistically support the patient in coping with her fear of recurrence of disease and subsequent death, followed at a suitable time interval in those patients who desire reconstructive surgery, by the implantation of a suitable prosthetic device. This plan of action most effectively helps the patient to cope with the two main emotional problems which arise following the detection and treatment of breast cancer.

Maguire (ref. 14) recently summarized the psychiatric problems which arise from the presence of breast cancer. He found that 20% of patients developed marked anxiety, before undergoing surgery for a breast tumor. This is no different in patients who were ultimately found to have carcinoma, or in those who were found to have benign disease, or in patients who underwent biopsy in the out-patient department. 56% of his patients developed emotional problems following mastectomy - the degree of this distress was directly related to the preoperative level of distress and worry. 45% of his patients complained of a lack of opportunity to discuss their emotional problems while in the hospital with anyone in a position to help. These worries were intensified when the need for adjuvant chemotherapy or x-ray therapy presented. Most patients considered this added therapy an indication of a poor prognosis. Torrie, (ref. 21) found that 83% of his patients developed a sense of depression during the year following mastectomy for breast cancer. This depression was compounded by the inability to discuss their emotional problems with anyone capable of helping them. During this early phase, following mastectomy, patients were helped tremendously by loving, supporting husbands and family. Following mastectomy, 32% of Maguire's patients still had marked anxiety and depression.

Almost half of his patients experienced sexual difficulties, and 60% had difficulty in carrying on their normal work. A third of the patients lost interest in social activities. A year following mastectomy, the degree of anxiety had diminished, but still persisted, particularly in those who had had x-ray therapy or adjuvant chemotherapy.

Maguire presented several positive approaches to aid the breast cancer patient. These patients should be supported with information regarding good prognosis, particularly, when lesions have been detected early, and have been treated adequately. With more advanced lesions, truthful answers, plus support may lead to initial shock, but eventually lead to a better adjustment in most patients, rather than an inconsistent approach of initial enthusiasm, not finally borne out. The support of a loving husband and family is most crucial in the recovery of most women. Provision of adequate prosthesis to provide satisfactory appearance is most important. The rehabilitation team, oftentimes, is of great help in supporting the patients and diminishing social and psychological problems. The personnel involved in this rehabilitation team must be well trained and flexible in their approach to patients. Most important, it has become possible recently to replace the mastectomized breast with an attractive well tolerated prosthesis inserted beneath the operative area, and presenting an adequate substitute for the lost breast. Reconstructive surgery represents the most positive and helpful aid in the psychological support of the mastectomized patient. However, this should be done only following adequate cancer surgery, depending upon the stage of disease found in the individual patient. Thoroughness of the primary surgical treatment of breast cancer must be given precedence over the maintenance or replacement of the breast. When feasible, however, the operative procedure can be tailored to facilitate satisfactory plastic reconstruction several months following primary therapy - provided that this does not jeopardize the prognosis of the patient. The quality of life following mastectomy requires a cooperative, supportive role by the patient's family, her husband, her surgeon, and at times the psychotherapist, and, with increasing frequency, the plastic surgeon.

We have recently experienced an explosion in developments of several methods for coping with the patient's disappointment and fear of losing her breast. Several beneficial developments have occurred - Reach to REcovery, Rehabilitation Programs, etc. (ref. 7). However, other trends have led to neglect of the overriding fear of most patients - that of losing her life to recurrent breast cancer. With increasing frequency, many patients are being treated inadequately in order to preserve the breast, or to facilitate immediate reconstructive measures. While this may please the patient in a short term manner, it ultimately places her future in jeopardy, and should nt be countenanced. Current use of unorthodox, inadequate primary surgical procedures supplemented by radiation therapy or chemotherapy, are experimental procedures at best, and are not proven to be as effective as more thorough, adequate surgical procedures supplemented by similar adjuvant therapies in any long term statistical studies. Subcutnaeous mastectomy with immediate insertion of a prosthetic device should not be accepted as a proven therapy for any stage of breast cancer. Although adjuvant chemotherapy may prolong life and delay the appearance of recurrent disease, it should not be used as a substitute for adquate primary surgical therapy, since there is no evidence that this will affect the long term salvage of the patient with breast cancer (ref. 2, 3).

The multicentric nature of breast cancer is an established fact, as shown by the pioneer work of Gallager, Martin and others (ref. 8,9). 47% of their infiltrating cancers were found to be accompanied by separate foci of infiltrating cancer, presenting elsewhere in the breast parenchyma. The great majority of breasts containing carcinoma were found to have multicentric areas of in situ carcinoma elsewhere in the breast. On this basis, the minimal effective treatment for breast cancer of any extent should include a total mastectomy. Involvement of the regional nodes

increases in extent and frequency as the size and the degree of anaplasia of the
primary tumor progresses. With smaller infiltrating cancers under 1 cm. in diameter, approximately 15 to 18% of patients will have axillary node involvement, but
usually of a minimal extent. In these situations, the presence of nodal involvement usually is not apparent clinically. However, when minimal involvement - micro-
metastases (ref. 12) are found, in the lower axillary nodes and an adequate axillary
dissection has been performed, along with total mastectomy, the great majority of
these patients are salvaged longtermwise - over 90% 10 year survival in our own experience.

The individual patient should receive the most adequate and suitable primary surgical therapy appropriate for her clinical, pathologic stage of disease (ref. 23).
At a subsequent time following adequate healing and after the development of adequate blood supply to the mastectomized site, the patient then may undergo reconstructive surgery with the insertion of a suitable prosthesis. This approach covers
the emotional problems of the average female patient undergoing treatment for breast
cancer most adequately. It gives her the best opportunity for long term survival,
free of recurrent disease, and, she can anticipate later reconstruction of her
breast with satisfactory appearance, a sense of self esteem, and confidence in her
dealings with others (ref. 19). The fact that a very small minority of patients,
who originally expressed the desire for breast reconstruction, following mastectomy,
ultimately proceed with this operation, indicates the overwhelming effect on the
patient of her fear of cancer recurrence and death from spread of cancer. The ideal
situation is found in patients who undergo early diagnosis, during which a "minimal"
cancer is found. This stage of disease can be handles adequately by a Patey type
modified radical mastectomy, in which the pectoralis major muscle is preserved
(ref. 11). This facilitates later reconstruction procedures with insertion of a
prosthetic device. As cancer therapists, we must always remember that our ultimate
goal in treating patients with breast cancer is to cure the patient of her disease.
We have come a long way in approaching this ideal situation through the development
of Cancer Screening Clinics, the use of modern laboratory aids - particularly
mammography, combined with frequent, carefully physical examination of the breast.
All of these contribute to the early diagnosis of this disease in its localized
stage, when it is confined to the breast and most amenable to current therapy.
Modern plastic reconstruction procedures should be carried out only after adequate
control of the breast cancer has been accomplished. We can only support the patient
honestly when we have made our best effort at controlling her disease, and yet, afford
the patient an opportunity for later satisfactory reconstructive surgery.

The use of subcutaneous mastectomy in order to facilitate immediate reconstruction
should not be accepted as a proven method for the treatment of breast cancer. Incomplete partial removal of the breast parenchyma usually occurs, since acceptance
of the prosthesis depends upon adequate tissue coverage, and unimpaired blood supply.
In most instances, only about 85% of the breast parenchyma is removed during this procedure. When attempts are made to perform an adequate mastectomy, with immediate
insertion of a prosthesis, the incidence of slough and rejection of the prosthesis
becomes unacceptable. This is an experimental approach and has not been prove to
be effective for the long term control of breast cancer. It should not be used as
a proven method of primary treatment for curable breast cancer. Reliance upon the
use of adjuvant multi chemotherapy to control residual breast cancer following
partial mastectomy represents wishful thinking. There is no evidence that breast
cancer can be destroyed permanently by the multichemotherapy which is currently in
use. All the clinical trials in which adjuvant multichemotherapy has been applied
to patients with operable breast cancer following surgery, demonstrate that this
therapy does result in delay in the progression of disease. However, to date,
there is no evidence that long term salvage will be affected by this approach. The
potentiality for iatrogenic carcinogenesis through exposure of the patient to toxic
radio mimmetic drugs, or exposure of the breast to aggressive x-ray therapy over

the long term, (ref. 13, 15) must be considered. These procedures must be applied
to the individual patient, as an adjuvant, to proven effective surgical therapy,
and only on a relative benefit versus risk basis.

Statements have been made to the effect that patients will be encouraged to come
to their physicians earlier, if they can be treated by less than a total mastectomy.
The intimation being that the patient can have her cake and eat it. This, unfortunately, is not true and is mesleading, when one reviews the poor, long term results of partial mastectomy (ref. 10,20, 24). The appeal of preservation of the
breast, while treating the patient with less than a total mastectomy is without
basis, as demonstrated in the data presented in favor of this approach by the pro-
ponents of conservative surgery. If one could assure the patient a similar salvage
rate with less than the total mastectomy, women would be justified in demanding this
type of therapy. Careful evaluation of current clinical data lends no credence to
the claims of these conservative surgeons. Crile (ref. 4, 5) treated a small number
of patients with partial mastectomy alone, and although his patient material was
excellent, he obtained a 10 year survival rate of only 34%. Mustakallio and Rissanen, in Finland, (ref. 17, 18) compared a series of patients with clinical stage 1
cancers, treated by partial mastectomy with radiation therapy to the remaining
breast and regional nodes, with a group treated by radical mastectomy with radiation
therapy to the regional nodes. Although they found no significant difference in
survival at 5 years, there was a definite diminution in 10 year survival rate in the
patients treated by the more conservative approach. This was most obvious in patients with larger tumors, measuring 2 to 5 cm. in diameter. Less difference was
noted in the small lesions, although in both categories, patients treated by the
radical mastectomy showed a superior 10 year survival rate. Atkins and Hayward
(ref. 1) in Guys Hospital in London conducted a truly randomized study in which
patients were categorized according to the clinical stage of their disease into
stage 1 and stage 11 groups. Alternate patients were then treated by "extended
tylectomy" with x-ray therapy to the remaining breast and regional nodes, or, by
radical mastectomy with x-ray therapy to the regional nodes. Again, no significant
difference in survival rate was noted at 5 years, but there was a tremendous difference in 10 year survival rate, particularly in the stage 11 cases, in which the
survival rate of patients treated by the conservative approach was only 22%, as compared with 67% for the more thorough surgical procedure. The difference at 10 years
in stage 1 patients, was less dramatic, but still in favor of the more adequate
surgical procedure.

Currently, all conceivable types and varieties of conservative surgery, plus x-ray
therapy, immunotherapy, and multichemotherapy are being applied to patients with
curable breast cancers. Some patients with minimal lesions which can be treated
most adequately by total mastectomy with low axillary dissection alone, are being
treated by segmental resection of the breast followed by extensive radiation therapy
to the remaining breast and regional nodes, and long term multichemotherapy. This
type of therapy may preserve the breast, but it is more exhausting, more time consuming, more expensive, and often yields a less attractive cosmetic result. Others
are being treated by injection of toxic chemicals into the breast, followed by
partial mastectomy with insertion of a prosthesis into the breast, and subsequent
systemic multichemotherapy and immunotherapy. These approaches are completely in
the experimental stage and yet, are being presented as proven methods of treatment
on the basis of 1 to 2 year follow up data. In order to prove the worth of a therapeutic procedure, the clinical material must be well documented, and long term
survival data must be available - with at least 10 year survival rates. Many papers
are being presented on the basis of 5 year follow up. This is completely inadequate
to evaluate the effectiveness of a therapeutic method for managing breast cancer,
because of the chronicity of this disease. In addition, these more unorthodox procedures, which include radiation exposure of the breast and long term exposure of
the patient to toxic chemicals, expose the patient to the iatrogenic carcinogenic
potentials of these methods of treatment. The possibility of subsequent development

of malignant tumors - leukemia, lymphoma, etc., is of real concern. The attempt
to treat breast cancer solely by partial mastectomy has proven unsatisfactory, and
has been abandoned by almost all individuals who have attempted it.

A great deal of effort is being expended in an attempt to develop an efficient systemic means of therapy for the control of breast cancer. Adjuvant multichemotherapy
is being applied to large groups of patients with stage 11 disease, who are being
studied in control groups (ref. 2, 3). All evidence at present does demonstrate
that such therapy can delay the appearance of recurrent disease. However, at present,
there is no evidence that increased long term survival rate will accrue from this
approach. Multi chemotherapy does not represent an alternative for adequate primary
surgical therapy. Instead, it should be used as an adjuvant following adequate primary
surgical treatment. It has its best place in patients with extensive local disease
with a high risk of occult systemic disease and ppor prognosis for long term salvage
on a historical basis. Every effort should be made at the time of initial surgical
treatment to remove all disease present in the breast and regional nodes. This
approach may be altered when preoperative survey of the patient demonstrates evidence
of systemic disease - however, in the absence of such evidence, appropriate primary
therapy should be applied to each individual patient on the basis of local extent of
disease present. We cannot honestly support our patients in their fear of recurrence
and ultimate death from breast cancer, unless we do our best to control this disease
through a combined approach, consisting of thorough, adequate primary surgical treatment combined with adjuvant radiation therapy and adjuvant multichemotherapy and/or
immunotherapy - when indicated. Further developments in the field of these systemic
modalities are being evaluated and further innovations and new trials in this direction
should have first priority in the field of breast cancer.

Satisfactory reconstruction of the breast with an excellent cosmetic result can be
obtained through the use of currently available prosthetic devices, implanted in the
operative field following adequate cancer operations for breast cancer. The pop-
ularity of the Patey type of modified radical mastectomy, in which the pectoralis
major muscle is preserved, is well founded. When applied to early, operable breast
cancers, and performed with meticulous technique with thorough axillary dissection,
this procedure is as effective as the radical mastectomy procedure, and provides an
improved base for further reconstructive surgery. This trend from the radical
mastectomy to the modified procedure is a valid one, and is effective when applied
to patients with "minimal" cancers, and when performed in a thorough manner (ref.27).
However, much harm will result unless this procedure is performed with meticulous,
thorough technique. We have seen too many patients in whom a "modified mastectomy",
has been performed in which only 3 to 5 axillary nodes have been removed, and in
whom, despite the institution of such therapy in patients with minimal disease, has
ultimately resulted in recurrence and death of the patient. Although the modified
mastectomy does offer an improved base for future reconstructive surgery, at times,
other more extensive procedures are indicated for the individual patient (ref. 22,
23). Patients with a high risk of internal mammary disease, particularly when they
are young, with comparatively localized disease in the breast, with primary tumors
lying in the parasternal region of the breast, have been shown to have the best 10
year survival rate, following surgical excision of these involved nodes (ref.25, 26).
In some cases, particularly when the tumor is adherent to the pectoral muscle, radical mastectomy has a definite advantage over the modified approach. At the Memorial Hospital in New York City we have applied a selective plan of adequate surgery
to patients with breast cancer in which the scope of the operative procedure is
correlated with the clinical pathologic extent of disease in the individual patient.
Three distinct operative procedures have been utilized: total mastectomy with axillary
dissection, radical mastectomy and the extended radical mastectomy - the primary aim
being complete removal of all disease in the breast and regional nodes in each patient. A 10 year survival rate of 61% with a local recurrence rate of 7.7% has been
attained in a group of 565 patients with 40% proven axillary nodal involvement

treated by us between 1955 and 1964 (ref. 25).

Most recently, two new approaches have been developed in the reconstruction of the
breast. These should be most helpful in coping with reoncstruction of the more
extensive, more deforming operative procedures. The use of a pedical graft made
from the omentum (ref.6), which is swung up through the upper anterior abdominal
wall and spread through a tunnel into the subcutaneous tissue over the chest wall,
does afford improved circulation, smooths out and fills in the deformity resulting
from radical and extended radical mastectomy procedures. This additional blood
supply also provides a much better base for later implantation of a prosthetic
device. The manufacturers of artificial prostheses are now capable of fabricating
custom models, for concealing operative defects and replacing the normal tissues,
which were sacrificed in order to adequately remove the breast cancer. While these
two devlopments are in the formative stages, it is possible to perform all types
of adequate cancer surgery for the appropriate patient, giving her the best chance
for long term freedom of disease while still providing the patient with the option
of later undergoing satisfactory reconstructive surgery.

At present, the psychological impact of loss of the breast following surgical
therapy for breast cancer can be managed best by deferring reconstructive procedures until adequate healing and good blood supply has been restored following an
adequate cancer operation. Removal of the cancer must take precedence and must
be the first consideration in the management of each patient. Many patients who
fear the loss of their breast and its psychological and social consequences will
accept this plan of therapy. Strangely enough, the great majority of these patients,
who originally expressed extreme interest in undergoing later plastic reconstruction
ultimately do not wish to undergo reconstructive surgery, and do adapt to their
situation in a positive manner following primary breast cancer surgery.

Our ultimate role as cancer therapists should be the cure of the patient from her
cancer. If we can facilitate later reconstructive measures without jeopardizing
the patient's prognosis, by preserving additional normal tissues in the operative
field, this may be done. However, all efforts should be made to remove the cancer
completely from the breast and its primary regional lymph nodes. We must depend
upon our current limited methods of primary therapy as the mainstay in the management of the patient with breast cancer. Until an effective, reliable, systemic therap
is developed, we should not diminish the adequacy of the primary surgical treatment for breast cancer.

1. Atkins, H., Hayward, J.L., Klugman, D.J., Waite, A.B. (1972). Treatment of early
    breast cancer-report after 10 years of clinical trial. Brit.Med. J., 2, 423-
    429.
2. Bonadonna, et al. (1976). Combination chemotherapy as an adjuvant treatment in
    operable breast cancer. N. Eng. J. Med., 294, 405-410.
3. Bonadonna, G., Valagussa, P., Rossi, A., Zucali, R., Veronesi, U. (1978). Im-
    provement of disease free and overall survival by adjuvant CMF in operable
    breast cancer. Presented at 69th Annual Meeting of American Association for
    Cancer Research.
4. Crile, G. Jr., Esselstyn, C.B.,Jr., Herman, R.E., Hoerr, S. (1973). Partial
    mastectomy for carcinoma of the breast. S.G.& O.,136, 929.
5. Crile, G., Jr. (1973). How much surgery for breast cancer. Modern Medicine, 41,
    32.
6. Cronin,T.D., Gerow, F.G. (1964). Augmentation mammoplasty:a new "natural feel"
    prosthesis. Transections of 3rd International Congress on Plastic surgery.
    Excerpta Medica Foundation, 41.
7. Euster, S. (1978). A system to meet the psycho-social needs of the chronically
    ill. Presented at National Conference on social welfare, 105th annual forum.
8. Gallager, H.S., Martin, J.E. (1969). The study of mammary carcinoma by mammo-
    graphy and whole organ sectioning. Cancer, 23, 855.
9. Gallager, H.S., Martin, J.E. (1969). Early phases of the development of breast
    cancer. Cancer, 24, 1170-1178.

10. Haagensen, C.D. (1973). A great leap backward in the treatment of carcinoma of
    the breast. Editorial, JAMA, 224 #8, 1181.
11. Handley, R.S., Thackray, A.C. (1969). Conservative radical mastectomy - Patey's
    operation. Annals of Surg. 170, 880.
12. Huvos, A.G., Hutter, R.V.P., Berg, J.W. (1971). Significance of axillary micro-
    metastases and macrometastases in mammary cancer. Annals of Surg., 173,44-46.
13. Mackenzie,I. (1965). Breast cancer following multiple fluoroscopies. Brit. J.
    Cancer, 19, 1-8.
14. Maguire, P. (1976). Psychological and social sequelae of mastectomy. Modern per-
    spectives in the psychiatric aspects of surgery. Brunner-Marzel, 19, 390-421.
15. Myrden, J.A., Haltz, J.E. (1969). Breast cancer following multiple fluoroscopies
    during artificial pneumothorax for treatment of pulmonary tuberculosis. Can-
    adian Med. J., 100, 1032-1034.
16. Phillips, C.M. (In Press). Reconstructive surgery following classical radical
    mastectomy using omental pedical grafts and fascialata. Breast - Diseases of
    the Breast. CPC Communications.
17. Rissanen, P. (1969). Comparison of conservative and radical surgery combined
    with radiotherapy in the treatment of early stage 1 carcinoma of the breast.
    Brit. J. Rad., 42, 423-426.
18. Rissanen, P., Holsti, P., Vergleich. (1974). Zwischen konservativer und radikal-
    er chirurgie, kombiniert mit, strahlentherapie, bei der behandlung des brust
    krebs im stadim 1. Strahlentherapie, 147, 370-374.
19. Schain, W.F. (1978). Facts every woman should know about breast reconstruction.
20. Shah,J.P., Rosen, P.P., Robbins, G.F. (1973). Pitfalls of local excision in the
    treatment of carcinoma of the breast. S.G. & O., 136, 721-725.
21. Torrie. (1971). Like a bird with broken wings. World Medicine.
22. Urban, J.A., Marjani, M.A. (1971). Significance of internal mammary lymph node
    metastases in breast cancer. Am. J. Roentg. 1, 130-136.
23. Urban, J.A., Castro, E.B. (1971). Selecting variations in extent of surgical
    procedures for breast cancer. Cancer, 28 #6, 1615-1623.
24. Urban, J.A. (1973). Partial mastectomy - unproven treatment for patients with
    potentially curable breast cancer. Clinical Bulletin, Memorial Sloan Kett-
    ering Cancer Center. 3 #4, 123-126.
25. Urban, J.A. (1976). Changing patterns of breast cancer. Cancer, 37 #1, 111-117.
26. Urban, J.A.(1977). Is there a rational for an extended radical procedure. Int. J.
    Rad. Onc., Biol. Phys. 2, 985-988.
27. Wanebo, H.J., Huvos, A.G., Urban, J.A. (1974). Treatment of minimal breast cancer.
    Cancer. 33 #2, 349-357.

Doctor-Patient Relationship in Oncology

Isaac L. Luchina*

*Doctor in Medicine, Member of the Argentine Society of Cardiology
Member of the Argentine Psychoanalytic Association
Founder of G.E.P.E.M. (Group for the study of new medical perspectives)
Gelly y Obes 2219, 1st Floor, Buenos Aires, Argentina

ABSTRACT

A new psychosocial model for medicine, amplifying and questioning the perspectives that the biomedical model offers is confronted and revalued. This delimits the medical field as a more technological field every time bounding the illness not to the 'person's' suffering but to externalizing biophysical or biochemical alterations as a measurable alteration of variables. The medical action is circumscribed to the domain of what Technology could detect or correct of that altered biological profile. With this perspective operating the 'person's' human factor that underlies the patient becomes increasingly blurred within the panorama of the 'illness' which means a withdrawal from the medicine of the patient's ailment or suffering in order to become transformed in a corrector of the altered variables trying to eliminate the causal psysical factors. This peculiar concept of healing involves more and more an special profile of the 'illness' which withdraws from its historical–anthropological meanings. The doctor embarked in this conception loses worth as a person in order to be of more consequence as a technician. Therefore all interpersonal relation between doctor and patient loses worth and the medical object becomes blurred and dehumanized.

The criticism of this model of such gravitation and importance in contemporary medicine comports a re-dimensioning of the 'illness'. It involves a revaluation of the patient, the doctor and their bond. The medical action transcends its technological possibilities and the medical 'person' reacquires value. This revaluation is not a humanistic appeal but an evidence extracted from a critical analysis of the perspectives offered by a technological medicine that would not only state the use of technical resources for the person's service but that it transforms itself in a perspective in itself.

The theme of the 'Doctor-patient relationship in oncology' appears somewhat abridged and perhaps strange in this Congress and it is unquestionably so, if we subscribe to the biomedical model in medicine.

Opposite the importance of the 'technical' resources, the human resources appear somewhat blurred. The field seems to circumscribe itself between scientific-technology and illness.

The doctor appears each time more like a simple administrator of technics and in certain cases he only has to mediate between the aforementioned resources and the patient.

In this scientific-technical display, man is losing relevance, not only in his role of doctor. This perspective, nevertheless, has enlarged the horizons of the fight against 'illness', at the same time that it conferred a peculiar imprint to the field. This technological seal not only stamps itself upon medicine but also upon all the contemporary civilization.

In this biomedical approach we understand the 'illness' as a biophysical or bio-chemical alteration made evident by the deviations from the rule of the measurable biological variables. This approach considers that the complex phenomena of the illness derive from a unique physical primary principle that excludes the mind-body problematic. The biomedical model requires the illness to be faced as an entity in-dependent from social behaviours and its congruent application requires that the alterations of the behaviour be explained on the basis of altered somatic processes (biochemical or nerophysiological). This biomedical model is now dominant in contem-porary medicine.

In a recent seminary on health of the Rockefeller Foundation, 1976 (1) a member ga-ve a detailed account of what we believe can be the paradigm of this position, me-dicine was asked to concentrate upon the 'real' illness and not to lose itself among psychological thickets. The conclusion was that the doctor should not be burdened with problems that have arisen from the claudication of the theologian or the philo-sopher.

George Engel (2),an eminent American psychosomatist says that psychiatrists have acknowledge the crisis by adopting two ostensibly opposed positions. Some of them lead by Szasz (3) want to exclude psychiatry from the field of medicine. Mental illness would be a 'myth' for them, inasmuch as it does not conform itself to the accepted concept of illness. A new discipline unfolds itself based on the 'behaviour-al sciences' that should take care of the re-education of people with 'problems of living'. Psychiatry disappears from medicine. Those disorders directly related with mental disturbances would be treated by neurologist and Psychiatry together with Medical Psychology would disappear as medical disciplines. This exclusionist point of view allows for the independent development of this new field that separated form medicine would not find apparently inconveniences for its development. In the second position the psychiatrist reduced to the biomedical model has a field of development limited to his conceptual model that considers that mental illness arises from 'natural' causes and not from metapsychological interpersonal or social ones.

Illness, emphasizes Fabrega (4), is a linguistic term that is employed in its gene-rical sense in order to refer to a certain class of phenomena towards which all the members of all the social groups from all the ages of the history of mankind have been exposed. He expresses a deviation or discontinuity centered in 'the person' that he finds injurious and undesirable and that is associated with impairment or malaise.

The terms of this definition acquire with the present biomedical approach a restric-tive sense that excludes 'the person' in order to refer to something impersonal centered in the biological alterations of this constituting parts.

We are facting a significant omission. Either we condense the definition of illness and change its linguistic sense in the history of culture or we change the word and invent another one that fits better in the technological culture of our age.

If 'the person' is included in the definition of illness, a series of variables are
they should necessarily be considered. The coherent exclusion of the word 'person'
in the definition of illness would be justified, if the illness was automatically
detected through technological means withouth passing through the total person. It
would be transformed then in a mere deviation of the variables registered by the
machine, this which could be, perhaps, a desideratum would scientifically imply talking about robots and not about persons. The biomedical model, which is after all an
explainable model, is insufficient for centering the problem of the illness and it
is referring itself to something more limited than is the biological alteration.
The criticism of the biomedical model in Cancerology does not turn out to be a here-
sy. The registers with which the human being detects or qualifies illness do not
have a precise relationship with the modified biological variables. It happens then
that situations are codified at different levels, with two different languages,
whilst the doctor tries to register the biological modifications that indicate to
him the illness and tries to eliminate them, supposing that that is his function,
the patient detects and codifies his illness with the peculiar code of his suffering and registers his recovery also in those terms. That can lead to different distortions, there can be gross biological alterations with no detection on part of
the bearer (negation of symtoms) (5) or on the contrary, brilliant biological cures
with a deep residual suffering. This make us ask if the healing should be codified
by the doctor with his biological-technical register or by the patient with a register bound to the personal meaning of his illness. To cure is it to satisfy technical
results or to cure is to relieve and to improve human suffering? To cure is it a
satisfaction for the doctor or the system that heals, or is it a satisfaction for
the patient? (6).

It is possible at present to try a new series of explanatory hypothesis that articulate themselves in a new model that includes the variable of the 'sick person'. A
qualitative leap is made and then a new biopsychosocial model is stated at a new
level. The doctor-patient relationship acquires a particular relevance for a medicine that is set in a biopsychosocial model. For this model the 'sick person' is opposed to the 'medical person'. The doctor acquires again a meaning per-se, clinical
medicine is revived, the clinical history and the word acquire a new meaning. A new
way for the de-alienation of man is attempted and the disease acquires sense as a
vital crisis (7). The doctor's dialogue with his patient is revitalized and the therapeutics stops being only a medicinal action in order to transform itself in a
'therapeutical process'. The 'therapeutical process' sets de doctor's biopsychosocial reality with the patient's biopsychosocial reality and tries by using all
the technical resources amplified by the discerning inclusion of sociological and
psychological facts to produce a modification of the total alternatives of that
being in the 'situation of being sick' whom the clinic calls patient, by associat-
ing him to the word ailment. What is important then is to assist the 'other one',
to make him recover himself, to understand him in his total significance and to
help him transit through the crisis of the disease. Death and life acquire peculiar
and unique meanings. Their sense is de-massified and there exists then an only life
and an only death. Life and death desalienated are supreme aspirations of this model.
All the postulates that I have stated are not a humanistic apellation that would
not have a strict sense in this Congress but a scientific statement, which acknow-
ledges a more ample truth and which sets into categories and interrelations variables that the biomedical model excludes. Man, the 'human person' scientifically
trascends his biological essence and creates due to his peculiar functioning an
area of variables that cannot be isolated from the disease unless their isolation
be due to a conjointed tactical reason and would not signify a totalizing and reducing perspective of the field. The technification towards which the biomedical model
leads, not only alienates and depersonalizes the patient but it produces similar effects upon the doctor. The man underlying the cancerologist suffers the same as his
patient, maybe in a different degree or zones. This is a constant that arises
through the dialogue with the cancerologist (8).

The exclusion from the field of the illness of the rational and discriminative dimension with the use of thought as a resource in the fight against the disease im-
poverishes the field, rigidifies it and ails him with a new disease that produces
a new suffering: alienation. The dealienation in this area produces the consciousness of a discriminate suffering, but this is the inherent reality of the human
condition and of the medical situations in Cancerology. It is impossible to eliminate it, one can only try to displace it. Its approach in the medical field avoids
that the suffering appear in non-medical zones and which maybe less controllable
within the total situation of the sick being, which can confer a different hue to
the suffering but cannot eliminate it.

For the medical 'person' to think is the only hygiene of his work and for a work
so exposed as the cancerological one it is seriously questioned if in order to
avoid situations that may produce suffering, it would be convenient to eliminate
thinking and with it, sometimes, criticism or common sense, or would it be more
suitable to face the situations, to learn how to handle them and to acquire new
resources for them (9).

Noting this perspective says Gerry P. Cream (10) director of the Investigation Center for Diagnostical Methodology of Glasgow: "The computer, a technical brain, must
be useful for helping the doctor classify the patient's symptom and signs and to
render possible a better diagnosis, but this method serves only as a support for
the clinical doctor because it cannot replace him, nor could it ever do that because the machine does not think.

The inclusion of the biopsychosocial model enlarges the register of therapeutical
possibilities, because by including the medical person within the therapeutical
process, the pharmacological and technical resources are set and may be potential-
ized. The doctor stops being only an informed technician, his criterion, his personality, his ability to organize the psychological and social resources in the
fight against illness are dramatically placed in the scale for the resources for
the illness since he does not exclude himself as the protagonist of the medical
situation that has the patient as the other protagonist of the medical situation
that has the patient as the other protagonist of this singular and unique situation
set in the social milieu where he situates himself and which also conditions the
interaction of both characters (11). This vision allows to bestow on the scientific
study of the placaebo effect a dimension of operability, and it jointly renders effective the scientific possibility of studying how do hope, confidence and a whole
series of mobilized maginal beliefs, operate in the patient and his family, within
the therapeutical resources of other cultures, and resources esteemed in a small
degree within a scientific-technical medicine that does not set into categories
the 'doctor as medicine' (12)(13).

This point of view renews the importance of the field upon the factors breaking
loose the illness. It sets it's eye primordially upon the correlation of the field
with the person's total ecology and in this way it includes a dynamical psychosocial ecology (14)(15). The dynamical inclusion of the total ecological point of
view of clinical epidemiology in the production of many diseases in such a way that
the etiological factors are enriched with this optic that articulates the sickening
factors with man's vital counterbalancing factors.

Cancer is the paradigm of a generally long diseases, that always has a reserved prognosis, that is frequently ominous, with an uncertain evolution that generates intense sufferings of every type and which means a vital crisis to the patient which
compromises him and his social micromilieu in a massive way. To sum up at present
we believe that in the same manner as the patient with cancer can be taken as the
best field of application of the biomedical model seeing that all the technical
diagnosis and therapeutical resources, the pharmacological and chirurgical ones

find an exceptional field of application due to the same causes, they also turn out to be the best field for the application of a biopsychosocial model.

Both models imply different perspectives and different resolutions that can in no manner be dissociated from the total perspective of the culture where they are inserted. It is necessary to know what is searched for in order to know what resources must be mobilized.

Lastly two quotations one belonging to von Krehl (16) quoted by Lain Entralgo (17) in his "Universal History of Medicine". This great master of pharmacology says: "Contrary to what I have wished and waited for during half of my life therapeutics is not a consequence but a complement of physiopathology, at the present time a doctor cannot say taht since such is the real cause of what I see by means of such a medicine I shall be able to attain with a scientific certainty the healing of the patient". Lain Entralgo then asks himself, "Why cannot the degree of action of a medicine be foreseen with the perfect exactitude that an astronomer can foretell the apparition of an eclipse?"

A journalistic news that appeared in "La Nación" on the 6th February 1978 answer this question in part: "The World Health Organization called attention to the fact of the increase in the so called diseases of civilization". The importance that regains the family doctor and the mother is emphasized in its conclusions.

The biopsychosocial model is coherently articulated with his field of application through the doctor. The medical figure transcends its technical and artisanal implications in order to transform itself in a vital part of the 'therapeutical process'. The adequate training of the doctor within this perspective is transformed together with the curricular change in a sine-qua-non goal. It aims to bestow on medical training the importance that arises from the imperative of creating a new doctor, heir to his retrieved dimensions. The doctor-patient relatioship is for this medical profile, the field of operation of all his technical effects and not a mere complication that as such he must try to avoid.

BIBLIOGRAPHY

(1) (1976). R.F. Illustrated, 3.5 .
(2) (1977). ENGEL, George: A new medical model necessity: a challenge to biomedicine Medical Orientation, 27, 1184. January, 1978.
(3) (1961). SZASZ, Thomas. The myth of the Mental Health. Harper and Row, New York, 1961.
(4) (1972). FABREGA, H. Arch. of Gen. Psychiatry 32. 1501.
(5) (1968). LUCHINA, I. The knowledge of the disease in Cancer, a psychological approach. In: "Cancer: contributions to its problematic" by Shavelzon, J. and collab. Ed. Paidós, Buenos Aires, 1968.
(6) (1978). LUCHINA I. Reports at the IVth International Congress of Balint Groups. London, 1978.(To be published in the Proceedings of the Congress).
(7) (1971). FERRARI, H., LUCHINA, I., LUCHINA, N.: "The medical-psychological inter consultation". Chapter 2. Ed. Nueva Visión, Buenos Aires, 1971.
(8) (1968). LANGER, M., LUCHINA, I.: The doctor before cancer. Chapter IV in "Cancer: contributions to its problematic", by José Shavelzon and collab. Ed. Paidós, Buenos Aires, 1968.
(9) (1973). LUCHINA, I., MEREA, C. Groups for the therapy of the medical practise. Latin Amer. Psychiat. Psychol. Acta, 19, 462.
(10)(1978). The computation as a support for prognosis. "La Nación", Buenos Aires, 21-4-78.
(11)(1973). SAPIR, M. Medicine d'accompagnement. Schw. Rundschau fur Medizin, 48, 1472-1476.

(12)(1975). SAPIR, M. Le corps dans la relation medicin-malade. Encycl.Med.chir.,
           Paris S-1975. Psychiatrie 37402 E-10.
(13)(1975). BALINT, M. The doctor, the patient and the illness. Int.Univ.Press,
           1975.
(14)(1975). RAHE R. Epidemiological studies of life changes and illness. Int.Journ.
           Psycho-Anal., 6, 1/2, 1975.
(15)(1975). EASTWOOD, M.R. Epidemiological studies of Psycho.Medicine. Int.Journ.
           Psycho-Anal., 6, 1/2, 1975.
(16)(1933). VON KREHL, R. Entstelung Erkennung und Behandlung. Innerer Krakheiten.
(17)(1974). LAIN ENTRALGO, P. Universal History of Medicine. Chap.: Towards a gene-
           ral anthropological therapeutics. Tome VII, Ed. Salvat, 1974.

The Emotional Impact of Breast Cancer and the Question of Premorbid Personality

Jimmie C. Holland

Chief, Psychiatry Service, Memorial Sloan-Kettering Cancer Center,
1275 York Avenue, New York, N.Y. 10021
Professor, Department of Psychiatry, Cornell University Medical College,
York Avenue & 68th Street, New York, N.Y.

ABSTRACT

The emotional impact of mastectomy is diminishing as less radical surgery is used, reconstruction becomes more available and feelings are discussed more freely. More attention is needed to those women who have a mastectomy followed by adjuvant therapy. 25 women were studied immediately after mastectomy and during adjuvant radiotherapy by use of an analysis of verbal content. They were studied at three points: prior to radiotherapy, during the second week and near the end of treatment (4-6 weeks). Mean scores showed a significant ($p < .05$) decrease in anxiety about body damage, and an increase in levels of anger and depression. Mean scores also showed increased anxiety related to separation at the end of treatment, a less hopeful outlook and, a decrease in overall anxiety. Women showed considerable emotional distress, particularly near the end of radiotherapy treatment, suggesting a need for more attention to the emotional stress of adjuvant therapy.

Longitudinal psychoendocrine studies of a group of women prior to breast biopsy and 10 years later revealed that reactivity to emotional distress and cortisol production rates were stable over time. The women with breast cancer had significantly higher sustained cortisol production rates than the women with benign lesions. Among those women who survived 10 years, there was a trend toward greater emotional expression of distress and higher cortisol production rates at the time of biopsy and 10 years later. Lower weight was also found with longer survival. A central hypothalamic mechanism is suggested which produces the pattern of greater emotional reactivity to stress, higher cortisol production rates and lower weight associated with longer survival.

The psychologic study of breast cancer provides a model from which the interaction of psychologic and biologic parameters of disease can be studied.

INTRODUCTION

The emotional impact of breast cancer, and particularly mastectomy, has recently become the subject of numerous autobiographical books, stories and psychologic studies in medical and nursing journals. A disease that was kept a shameful, guarded secret by women 25 years ago has now become a "fashionable" subject for open and frank discussion. While mastectomy will always represent a significant emotional stress by its threat to life, self-esteen and femininity, the exceedingly rapid change in society's attitude toward breast cancer has already altered

251

the psychosocial impact. Women now freely"compare notes"about feelings, ask for
the full facts of their medical situation and participate in decisions about their
care. If the woman is emotionally healthy, acute feelings of loss, emotional la-
bility and depressed mood usually diminish by four to six weeks. In a study of
40 women who had a mastectomy at Montefiore Hospital, Bronx, New York for breast
cancer, most women had returned to work and normal social life by four weeks.
Those women who had more trouble adjusting could be identified early in the post-
operative period by having poorer personal psychologic resources or fewer social
supports. A study of psychosocial intervention given by a nurse, social worker
and patient advocate (who had had a mastectomy) revealed that the women who had
an uncomplicated mastectomy needed the least help and for the shortest period.
The group next most in need of psychosocial support were those who had a mastectomy
followed by adjuvant chemotherapy and radiotherapy. The patients most in need of
continuing help were those with advanced disease, particularly the older woman who
lived alone (Wieder, Schwartzfeld, Fromewick, Holland, 1978).

Women now routinely inquire and are told about the presence and number of positive
axillary nodes found at mastectomy. When positive nodes are present, the importance of beginning adjuvant therapy is accepted. The stress of mastectomy must be
laid aside to deal with the stress of adjuvant therapy. While mastectomy is a
discrete loss that can be mourned, the new threat to life and body integrity im-
posed by adjuvant radiotherapy or chemotherapy requires an adaptation to treatment
and its side effects continuing over weeks to months. The possibility of breast
reconstruction is much less likely. Mastectomy followed by adjuvant therapy poses
a dual psychologic threat that has not received adeqate attention. A study of
the emotional stress during adjuvant radiotherapy following mastectomy is reported
here (Holland and co-workers, 1978).

EMOTIONAL IMPACT OF MASTECTOMY FOLLOWED BY ADJUVANT RADIOTHERAPY

25 women, 21 with breast cancer and 4 with gynecologic cancer, were studied in
the Radiotherapy Department of Montefiore Hospital, Bronx, New York. The mean age
was 61, with a range of 31-83. Slightly fewer than half (40%) were married. Most
of the women (80%) were white; 2 were black and 3, Hispanic. After the initial
visit with the radiotherapist, each woman was seen by one of two psychiatrists who
asked her to participate in a study of "how women react to radiotherapy treatments."
Patients were studied at three points in time: 1) prior to the first radiotherapy
treatment (Test Period 1); 2) during the second week of treatment (Test Period 2);
and , 3) near the end of treatment at approximately 4-6 weeks (Test Period 3). The
patient was interviewed briefly and was asked to speak (with a standardized instruction), into a tape recorder for 5 minutes to obtain a sample of speech for
analysis by the Gottschalk-Gleser Content Analysis of Verbal Behavior. This verbal technique yields useful projective information somewhat like that provided by
visual projective tests. Psychological mood states were measured by the Gottschalk-Gleser technique on each of the 5-minute transcribed samples of speech. The
Gottschalk-Gleser techinque is highly sensitive to affective states, and is not
distressing to patients. It also has the marked advantage of having no test-retest
habituation and may be used repeatedly with the same patient. It has been widely
used to study medically ill patients. The content scales have been carefully constructed and subjected to intensive validity and reliability testing (Gottschalk,
Gleser, 1969).

Five areas of emotional distress were assessed in this study: anxiety, hostility
(anger), depression and hope. The Overall Anxiety Scale, designed to measure total
manifest anxiety, yielded a sum of the six types of quantitated anxiety:
death, mutilation, separation, guilt, shame and diffuse. Hostility was reported
by two scales: hostility-outward (anger), and hostility-inward (depression). The

construct of hostility toward self, recording self-critical, self-destructive or
self-punishing feelings has been shown to correlate with depression. Hostility-
outward (anger) documented destructive, injurious or critical thoughts or actions
towards others. The Hope scale measured thoughts and expectations (positive or
hopeful) or (negative, pessimistic or hopeless) for the future.

Figure 1 is a graph of the mean scores for the 25 women at the three points in
time. The following changes were significant (p < .05): 1) an increase in hos-
tility-in (depression) over time; 2) an increase in hostility-out (anger), apparent by the second week and; 3) decrease in anxiety reflecting fears of body injury
(mutilation). Changes in mean scores which showed trends but did not reach significance were: 1) increase in anxiety related to separation, 2) decrease in
overall anxiety over time, and a decrease in hopefulness.

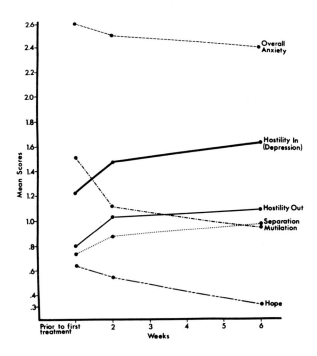

Fig. 1. Mean scores on six scales of emotional distress
         for women undergoing radiotherapy following mas-
         tectomy at three points in time: prior to first
         treatment, during the second week and near termin-
         ation of treatment (4-6 weeks).

Comparison of these data with other studies utilizing the Gottschalk-Gleser Scales,
revealed that women undergoing a regimen of postmastectomy radiotherapy exhibited
higher levels of Overall Anxiety and Hostility-Inward (depression) than several
other groups of medically ill patients, including men in a coronary care unit.

Based upon the common assumption that emotional distress is highest at the beginning of treatment, our hypothesis was that this would dminish over time. Data confirms that the women were most fearful as they began treatment with large strange machines and which, to many, was associated with palliation for cancer. Adequate explanation and information at this critical juncture, with reassurance by the radiotherapist and interaction with radiotherapy technicians alleviated some anxiety. The general leveling off of overall anxiety, although not statistically significant, would be expected as the patients became familiar with the environment, with the staff, and with the routine over the period of treatment. Also consistent with this hypothesis was the fact that as treatment progressed, anxiety about bodily harm or disfigurement, expressed by levels of mutilation anxiety, decreased significantly, being the highest prior to the first treatment, with a sharp drop at the second week, and a gentle lowering of level by the sixth week. However, the other two significant changes, an increase in both hostility-inward (depression) and hostility-outward (anger) represented a seeming contradiction to our hypothesis and required further interpretation.

It was of some surprise to find that the patients were more - not less - depressed as the end of treatment approached and they spoke with significantly more frequent expression of overt anger. One possible explanation is that patients often felt less well than they did prior to radiotherapy because of unpleasant side effects which include anorexia, fatigue, and general lack of well being. While transient, the new symptoms caused by the treatment might very well make patients feel both depressed and angry that they are worse instead of better as a consequence of their therapy. Such an explanation may also account for the less hopeful outlook which was noted.

Of considerable interest were the feelings of increased anxiety related to separation expressed at the end of treatment. Anxiety was expressed also with concern of being more vulnerable to recurrence of cancer when treatment stopped. In addition, the close, almost daily, monitoring of their medical condition would stop. The women appeared fearful of the future without the promise of continuing close medical surveillance and care, though they intellectually recognized it was not necessary. The anticipated end of close daily contact with the Radiotherapy Clinic staff threatened the feeling of being "protected", both medically and emotionally, which was present as long as treatment continued. This observation has also been made by oncologists who have noted that patients become more fearful about discontinuing long chemotherapy regimens, despite the discomfort of side effects and regular disruption of their lives. A similar phenomenon has been seen in patients leaving a coronary care unit, respirators and protected environments. Psychologic dependency requires "weaning" from the treatment situation and an accomodation to the feeling of diminished protection from disease.

Far more attention should be paid to the patient's psychologic state beginning and particularly, on reaching the end of radiotherapy treatment. We often assume that patients must feel relief upon reaching the end of a lengthy, arduous treatment regimen. Quite the contrary appears to be the case from our data: women felt less hopeful, were more depressed and angry than at the beginning of treatment and were anxious about loss of the frequent contact with staff and close medical surveillance. We speculate that these findings are generalizable to any therapeutic modality for cancer which requires major commitment and cooperation over a period of time. Several salient points emerge for psychological management: 1) There is a psychological need for the patient to be able to anticipate the end of treatment in advance, allowing ample time to control anxiety about termination. 2) Scheduling of an early re-visit for shortly after the end of treatment is indicated with reassurance of the physician's availability by telephone. 3)Awareness of the psychological dependence which patients develop upon the clinic staff is helpful in understanding emotional reactions. Identifying a single staff person, in addition to the radiotherapist to relate most closely to each patient, and who may continue to be available to them after active treatment ends, would contribute to a feeling of continuity of care and increase emotional security. The added psychologic support needed by many patients could (and often is) provided for by the radiotherapy nurse, social worker and/or radiotherapy technician.

PREMORBID PERSONALITY AND BREAST CANCER

Epidemiologic studies of breast cancer have defined several risk factors: late age of first live birth; late marriage; late menopause; early menarche; obesity; history of cystic mastitis; family history of breast cancer; multiple primary with contralateral breast, colon, uterus, ovary; ionizing radiation; higher social class, and exogenous hormones (Hoover, 1977; MacMahon, Cole, Brown, 1973). It is readily apparent that many of these factors are intertwined with psychologic and social phenomena. The identification of a particular personality or constellation of emotional conflicts as a separate and unique risk factor becomes more difficult in light of known risk factors which must be controlled to separate out any personality variables. Most psychologic studies to the present have not been controlled, have often been methodologically flawed and have usually been retrospective (Fox, 1978). Animal data (Riley, 1975; Henry, Stephens, Watson, 1975) however do suggest that in strains of mice which develop spontaneous mammary gland carcinoma, the incidence of tumor development can be enhanced by stress.

The work of Monjan and Collector (1977) has also provided animal data supporting a stress-induced modulation of immune function. The recent link of stress with hypothalamic-pituitary-adrenal axis stimulation and immunosuppression, has sparked renewed interest in patterns of emotional response to stress in development of hormone-dependent tumors, particularly breast. Some workers have suggested that a particular pattern of expression of anger is associated with breast cancer (Greer & Morris, 1975), and others related longer survival in women who expressed anger and had more emotional expressivity (Derogatis & Abeloff, 1978).

Katz and co-workers (1970) showed that women awaiting breast biopsy whose psychologic defenses were inadequate to cope with the stress, and who expressed more emotional distress, had greater activation of the hypothalamic-pituitary-adrenal axis as evidenced by higher cortisol production rates. Gorzynski and co-workers (1978) undertook to find the 30 women studied by Katz for a 10-year follow-up to determine their survival, psychologic state and cortisol production rates when not under the acute stress of impending breast biopsy. Of the 30 women (8 benign, and 22 with malignant lesions), at 10-year follow-up, thirteen had died (12 with malignant lesions and 1 with benign). Seven women were lost to follow-up. Eleven women were found; one woman refused to cooperate, leaving 10 of the original 30 women available for study; 7 who had malignant and 3 who had benign lesions. The women had no evidence of disease, were not on medication and were post-menopausal with a mean age of 64. None had experienced a recent significant trauma or acute stress at the time they were seen.

Women were studied for endocrine and psychologic function in the same way as 10 years earlier. A semi-structured interview was done with each woman in her home or at the hospital. Independent ratings of the patient on the Katz Defensive Adequacy Scale, (without knowledge of her rating in the initial study) were made by two psychiatrists yielding scores on affective distress, degree of impaired psychologic function and defensive adequacy. Cortisol production rates were obtained by 72 hour urine collection at home for determination of hydrocortisone metabolites, tetrahydrocortisone(THE), tetrahydrocortisol (THF), and allotetrahydrocortisol (ATHF). This technique provided production rates calculated from endogenous metabolites, a technique comparable to the C_{14} tracer method used 10 years ago.

No significant difference was found in the excretion rates of hydrocortisone meta-

bolites (THE, THF, ATHF) in individual women nor were mean values changed for the
entire group. The women with breast cancer, however, had higher mean values than
women with benign disease, both 10 years earlier and at follow-up (benign, 3.7 mg/g
creatinine to 4.3 mg/g; malignant, 5.9 mg/g. (Fig. 2).

MEAN EXCRETION OF HYDROCORTISONE METABOLITES
(THF·THE·ATHF) PRIOR TO BIOPSY AND 10 YEARS LATER

	Benign N=3	Breast Cancer N=7	Total N=10
Prior To Biopsy	3.7	5.9	5.2
10 Year Follow-up	4.3	5.5	5.1

Fig. 2

Thus, individual rates showed stability over time in all women, while those with
breast cancer had significantly higher rates than the women with benign disease.

On psychologic assessment, socres on Katz Defensive Adequacy Scale taken 10 years
earlier and at follow-up showed no statistical difference in scores despite the
contrast of anticipated surgery 10 years earlier and lack of acute stress at the
second evaluation. The women with breast cancer scored higher with a greater
emotional reactivity and affective stress than women with benign disease.

The primary patterns of psychologic defenses also were unchanged in individual patients. Major defensive patterns observed fell into five categories: denial/ra-
tionalization (3); mixed defensive pattern (3); stoicism/fatalism (2); prayer/faith
(1); and projection (1).

DISCUSSION

Adrenocortical stimulation, emotional distress and psychologic patterns of coping,
determined immediately prior to the acutely distressing situation of breast biopsy and/or mastectomy, were found to be insignificantly changed 10 years later in
the absence of acute stress in any of the women. These data suggest that the hy-
pothalamic-pituitay-adrenal axis stimulation response may be more stable and biologically patterned than previously assumed. They suggest further that adrenocortical reactivity may be a constant characteristic for an individual and a function of biological "programming". Psychologic reactivity and response to stress
appeared also to be patterned for each woman. These findings support the hypothesis
proposed earlier by Hamburg.

It is of considerable interest that the women with breast cancer had higher rates
of cortisol production than did women with benign lesions. A trend toward higher
cortisol production and greater emotional expression of distress was also seen in
the 10-year survivors as compared to those who died earlier. Gorzynski and co-
workers (1978) have confirmed both higher cortisol production and greater emotional
expressiveness of distress in a second group of 15 women who have survived 10 or
more years following mastectomy. These data do not support the hypothesis of Bul-

brook (Bulbrook, Greenwood, Hayward, 1960) that a low ratio of cortisol production in relation to androgen is a correlate of longer survival. They do support, however, need for further study of expression of anger in women with breast cancer as suggested by Greer & Morris (1975) and Abeloff and Derogatis (1977). In light of animal data that immune function can be modulated by stress (Monjan & Collector, 1977), and the finding of altered IgA related to overt expression of anger (lower IgA) or suppression (higher IgA) of anger in women prior to biopsy (Pettingale, Greer & Tee, 1977), further studies are indicated related to these findings.

Donegan, Harts & Rimm (1978) report that, after negative nodal status at mastectomy, lower weight is the most significant correlate of longer survival with breast cancer. We are exploring the hypothesis that the constellation of greater emotional reactivity and expressivity of distress, higher cortisol production rates and lower body weight associated with longer survival may reflect a central hypothalamic mechanism which can alter survival.

These data attempt to explore the possible rational links between psychologic and biologic parameters of breast cancer.

REFERENCES

1. Bulbrook, R., F. Greenwood, J. Hayward (1960). Selection of Breast Cancer Patients for Adrenalectomy or Hypophysectomy by Determination of Urinary 17-Hydroxycorticosteriods and Actrocholanolone. Lancet 1, 1154.

2. Derogatis, L., M. Abeloff (1978). Psychological Coping Mechanisms and Length of Survival in Advanced Breast Cancer (abstract). Proceedings of American Society of Clinical Oncology.

3. Donegan, W., A. Harts, and A. Rimm (1978). The Association of Body Weight with Recurrent Cancer of the Breast. Cancer 41, 1590-1594.

4. Fox, B. (1978). Premorbid Psychological Factors as Related to Cancer Incidence. Journal of Behavioral Medicine 1, 45-133.

5. Gorzynski, G., J. Holland, B. Zumoff, D. Fukushima, and J. Levine (1976). Ten Year Psychoendocrine Follow-up of Women Studied Before Breast Biopsy. American Psychosomatic Society Proceedings, March.

6. Gorzynski, G., M. Massie, B. Zumoff, J. Holland (1978). Unpublished data.

7. Gottschalk, L., G. Gleser (1969). The Measurement of Psychological States Through the Content Analysis of Verbal Behavior. University of California Press, Berkeley.

8. Greer, H.S., T. Morris (1975). Psychological Attributes of Women Who Develop Breast Cancer: A Controlled Study. J. Psychosomatic Res. 19, 142-153.

9. Henry, J., P. Stephens, and F. Watson (1975). Force Breeding, Social Disorder, and Mammary Tumor Formation in CBD/USC Mouse Colonies: A Pilot Study. Psychosomatic Medicine, 277-283.

10. Holland, J., A. Lebovitz, R. Rusalem, J. Rowland, F. Mincer, J. Davis (1978). Levels of Anxiety During Radiotherapy in Women with Breast Cancer. Abstract Proc. ASCO, March.

11. Hoover, R. (1977). Breast Cancer: Epidemiologic Considerations. Reserpine and Breast Cancer Task Force. HEW.

12. Katz, J., P. Ackerman, Y. Rothwax, E. Sachar, E. Weiner, L. Hellman, and T. Gallagher (1970). Psychoendocrine Aspects of Cancer of the Breast. Psychosomatic Medicine 32, 1.

13. MacMahon, B., P. Cole, and J. Brown (1973). Etiology of Human Breast Cancer: A Review. Journal of National Cancer Institute. 50, 21-42.

14. Monjan, A., M. Collector (1977). Stress-Induced Modulation of Immune Function. Science 196, 307-308.

15. Pettingale, K.W., S. Greer, D.H. Tee (1977). Serum IgA and Emotional Expression in Breast Cancer Patients. J. Psychosomatic Research 21, 395-399.

16. Riley, V. (1975). Mouse Mammary Tumors: Alteration of Incidence as Apparent Function of Stress. Science 189, 465-467.

17. Wieder, S., J. Schwartzfeld, J. Fromewick, J. Holland (1978). Psychosocial Support Program for Patients with Breast Cancer at Montefiore Hospital: Team Effort. Quality Review Bulletin 4, 10-13.

Antecedents of Important Psychical Traumas in Neoplasic Patients

Angel O. Masotta* and Jorge Caldera

**Director of the National Bank of Antineoplasic Drugs,
Paseo Colon 568, Buenos Aires, Argentina*

ABSTRACT

The authors state that they have found a relation between the appearance of neoplasic lesions and psychical traumas. Said traumas must necessarily have three fundamental characteristics:
1) Duration, 2) Intensity, 3) Obsessive character.
There is also a latency time between grief and the appearance of neo plasia, which is closely relately with the age of the patient.
Finally, the authors affirm that subjects who had psychical traunas with the mentioned characteristics, will not necessarily develop can cer; but every individual who has cancer, has had a psychical trauma with said characteristics.

KEYWORDS

PSYCHICAL TRAUMA – INTENSE – LASTING – OBSESSIVE – CANCER – LATENCY TIME

The relation between important psychical traumas and neoplasic disease is not certainly new, and has already been mentioned.

LeShan revised the literature and demonstrated that in 1902, there were papers that related psychological factors to the appearance of different types of cancer.

Thomas and Greenstreet followed up 1076 graduates of the John Hopkins Medical School, and found a higher grade of depression, anxiety and anger in subjects that later developed cancer.

We have carried out a retrospective survey which is less exact that a prospective work, however, we consider that the result are significant.

We surveyed 1830 patients from 3 to 85 years old, or their direct relatives.

METHODOLOGY:

We considered, as reference, the appearance of the first symptom. Our questionnaires started from this point and turned back to the past life of the patient.

At the beginning we carried out a kind of survey in which the patient was asked if he had lived determined situations, and when it had happened.

Once we received many answers, we realized, that a few similar situations were always repeated; then we made a list of these situations for the surveyed to read and find his own situation.

When we presented the list to the patients, we told them that it was not pretended that they had lived similar situations, but "that tipe" of situations.

Through this technique we tried that the questionnaire was not influenced by the personality of the interviewer.

In the first part of this study, only adults were surveyed, afterwards adolescents and children were included.

These two groups cover less number of patients, due to its later inclusion.

Obviously, in the case of little children we surveyed the mother or the closest relative.

LIST OF PSYCHICAL TRAUMAS MORE COMMONLY REPORTED

1) Death of relatives or very dear close friends.
2) Serious illness (of a certain duration) of relatives or very dear close friends.
3) Abandonmet of relatives or very dear close friends.
4) Not wanted lasting or definite separations.
5) Serious accidents with long lasting consequences (with depression and anxiety related to the future).
6) Major surgery with complicated and long post operatory process, that caused lasting depression and anxiety in the patient (no less than 15 days).
7) Great fears, with or without reasons, that remained obsesively more than 15 days.
8) Felonies conmited in the presence of the patient, who suffered later obsesive fears during more than 15 days.
9) Serious and lasting economic problems which become and obsesive problem.

10) Intense and enduring physical efforts without adequate rest, (often ocurring as a result of taking care
of a seriously ill close relative) with depression,
anxiety and fear for the health of said relative.

11) Serious labour injustices that are not overcome by
the patient (specially after 40 years of age. Denial
of improvements waited for a long time).

CHILDREN AND ADOLESCENTS

1) Death of relatives.
2) Not wanted separations.
3) School problems.
4) Great obsesive fears.

We detected a precocious maturity and hypersensitivity in children.

When whe have talked about these problems withs a colleague or with
any person, we heard them say: Who has not sometime been grieved ?

The comment has certainly sense, but according to our results, any
grief can not be related to cancer.

The psychical trauma must have three fundamental conditions.

1) INTENSITY: It must be an intense sorrow. The subject
feel fear, anguish, uncertainty, sorrow, moral affliction, sadness.
There is a deep disturbance of the personality.

2) DURATION: The psychical trauma that could be related to
cancer must be lasting. We have verified that in general, the
conflicting situation lasts no less than 15 days, being possible to
last several months.

We have verified that there are not among the frequent antecedents
of these patients, very intense buy short griefs, after which the
personality gains rapidly its equilibrium (that is to say, a serious
surgical operation of a dear relative who rapidly recovers himself).

3) OBSESSION: The psychical trauma must have an obsessive
form in the life of the patient, who broods over his problem the
whole day, and even awakes several times at night thinking of his
problem.

We want to state that our view is that subjects who undergo situations as those before mentioned, will not necessarily develop a
malignant tumor, but we believe that every patient who has a tumor,
has had some antecedent of this type.

LATENCY TIME: Some researchers have stated that the latency time, that is to say, the time passed between the grief and the appearance of the disease, can vary from 1 to 15 years.

We do not agree with this statement; we have proved that the latency time is related to the age of the subject. The latency time according to age is as follows:

> Children and adolescents: 1 to 12 months
> adults of 21 to 40 years of age: 12 to 20 months
> adults of 41 to 50 years of age: 20 to 30 months
> In adults older than 50 years of age, the latency time is
> of more than 30 months, but never less than five years.

These times may vary in more or less 6 months.

We believe that in tumors of slow development, these latency times are not exact only in appearance.

In little children who had cancer o who were born with cancer, (there is no bibliography enough available), we could verify that the mother had had very important emotional problems during pregnancy.

We think that the fetus acted possibly as the receiving organ.

Through this method we have proved that in 89 % of the cancer patients, it was possible to detect a psychical trauma with the before mentioned characteristics and within the mentioned latency times.Of the remaining 11 %, only 40 % denied firmly the existence of any important circumstance. It was impossible to obtain sound valid answers from the remaining 60 %, due to old age, bad general condition,etc.)

We do not intend to state that psychical trauma plays an etiological role, but we think that it can be a "facilitating" agent by way of immunological depression or other factors.

We have not verified any relation between psychical trauma and a determined type of tumor.

REFERENCES

Greene, W.A.(1966)The psychosocial setting of the development of leukemia and lymphoma. Ann. NY Acad. Sci. 125:794-801

Hagnell, O.(1966.)The premorbid personality of persons who develop cancer in a total population investigated in 1947 and 1957. Ann. NY Acad. Sci. 125:846-55

Kissen, D.M.(1966.)The significance of personality in lung cancer in men. Ann. NY Acad. Sci. 125:820-26

Kissen, D.M., Brown, R.I., Kissen, M.(1969.)A further report on personality and psychosocial factors in lung cancer. Ann. NY Acad. Sci. 164:535-45

LeShan, L.(1959.)Psychological states as factors in the development of malignant disease a critical review. J. Natl. Cancer Inst. 22:1-18

LeShan, L., Worthington, R.E.(1955.)Some psychologic correlates of neoplastic disease. J. Clin. Exp. Psychopathy. 16:281-88

LeShan, L., Worthington, R.E.(1956.)Some recent life history patterns observed in patients with malignant disease. J. Nerv.Ment. Dis. 124:460-65

LeShan, L., Worthington, R.E.(1956.)Loss of cathexes as a common psychodynamic characteristic of cancer patients. Psychol. Rep. 2:183-93

Psychodynamics of the Cancer Patient

Fernando Rísquez*

Apartado 60.143, Caracas 106, Venezuela

ABSTRACT

To a psychiatrist with many years of research into the psychotherapy of cancer patients, it appears that malignant disease is probably related to the patient's personality, particularly the psychological effects of personal suffering due to loss or to a serious disease. It is hoped that the investigation of such relationships will help in the prevention and treatment of cancer in a positive manner.

Key words: Aggression; desolation; psychotherapy; psychological impact

Being a doctor, I share with other doctors a terrible dread of death. As a psychiatrist, more than once I believed that I was getting far from it into the archipelago of mental illness, but, in one way or another, suicides kept reminding me that it is useless for a doctor to try escaping from omnipresent death and that he should face with courage its unlucky presence.

In 1956, I was induced to go on thinking about this subject when I visited, at the Experimental Medicine Institute (1), Doctor López Herrera, a specialist in endocrinology and oncology, who was experimenting with rats which he submitted to the sound of sirens. These sounds originated different changes in the rats and a systematic study was made of the effects of chronic aggression in experimental animals. (2) I wish to say that the ideas I am trying to express are based on concepts thought out day by day and week by week while keeping in constant touch with doctor López Herrera at first and, a few years afterwards, with many oncologists from the "Luis Razetti" Institute, also of Caracas.

The field of cancer is an extremely large one, also an extraordinarly profound one. (3)

(1) Instituto de Medicina Experimental. Universidad Central de Venezuela.
(2) López Herrera,L. (1956) Factores endocrinos de Agresión crónica y de Irritación local que condicionan el Aspecto de los Frotis mucosos. Asociación Venezolana Pro-Avance las Ciencias.
(3)
Bahnson, C.B. (1969). Psychological Complementarity in Malignancies. Pastwork and future Vistas. Ann.N.Y.Acad.Sci.164: 119
* Central University of Venezuela. "Andrés Bello" Catholic University in Caracas. (full Professor)

I won't speak specifically about cancer and only in a tangential manner, will I speak about its sociological consequences, to keep myself
within the limits of phenomenalistic observation and evade the ghost
always lying in ambush of the psychiatrical investigator: speculation.

I intend, with this paper, to give my personal impressions on cancer
patients and to be able to give a clear and understandable message.

Many times, in Psychiatry Courses, and when invited by oncologists or
surgeons, have I said that the first impression of a psychiatrist,
when he visits a cancer hospital is one of great uneasiness and bewilderment. Psychiatrists are professionally distorted; this we can cor-
roborate based on psychiatrical literature. We find in almost everything some pathological trait. And, when invited to visit cancer hospitals and observe its patients, we take for granted that the psycho-
pathology to be found there, will be as gloomy and frightful as cancer itself. We are therefore greatly surprised at finding out that
these patients, instead of voicing complaints and frustrations, are
extremely sensible and quiet people.

During 1956 and 1957, when surgery was still in a radical stage in
this field, and our cancer surgeons removed (meaning well), entire
parts of the body, I saw people who had no face, who were missing
half of their neck, who had no legs...real catastrophes from the anatomical point of view. These persons, instead of complaining, of showing their pain and heart-breaking sadness, asked me about horse-ra-
ces, talked to me about the most unimportant, brief and light things
of life. Years afterwards, reading some papers on this matter, I realized that other psychiatrists, who had also entered this field, had
felt the same uneasiness and surprise.

Definitely, cancer patients are not mental patients.

This is the first conclusion reached after a few days with these patients. Nevertheless, I went on looking for literature on this subject; I was surprised but still stubborn, in the manner of all good
psychiatrists; I said to myself: "there must be something; I must
use the instrumental method."

I took over the projective tests work myself, but after thinking that
my prejudices could modify the course of the investigation, trying also to follow scientific rules, I got help from several psychologists.
Finally, during the years 1967 and 1968, a Psychology professor and a
very gifted pupil collaborated in this investigation: it was impossible for me to have any kind of influence on them as they did'nt communicate directly with me. These psychologists, used the Rorchach, the
Bender, the Minnessota Tests, and many others, all well-known. We
then observed two things: in the first place that the psychologists
had felt as I had: confused and perplexed at not making any finds. After a short time, bored, and also depressed, they all were inclined
to leave the matter as it was. Their reports were all exactly the same: there was nothing, in this cancerous suffering mass of people,
that indicated more neurosis and, even less so, more psychosis than
in the general population. Nor when we compared statistics, in other

hospitalized patients, and kept observing them.

Subsequently, as the years passed, I meditated upon the fact that many patients died but many others did survive;; this made me think of a connection between personality and the desease's progress. I remember a Margariteño (4); he was a quiet man, not like his island'sinhabitants, lively and talkative. He used to tell me "about this thing, doctor, it's not so bad, I don't even feel like scratching it..." This was in 1956. The last time I saw him was in 1966 and "that thing" had 'nt changed much...The diagnosis had been one of a particularly serious type of cancer. On the contrary, I have seen many times people die in an alarmingly short time (even in a month); these people were notoriously spiritual and had great taste for many things in life.

I wish to make now a little observation, both anecdotal and psychiatrical: how I see a man, or a woman, getting old in a few days time. One can stop seeing a person during a week and upon meeting her, a forty years-old person, she suddenly looks sixty-five, a week later, seventy five and still a week after, dead... I am not referring only to the physical aspect, but about everything, and this can be felt in the patients conversations. I learned this with several surgeons, when studying Medicine; we used to make surgical prognosis based on what the patients told me. A patient, who is always talking about his wound, is not well; if he starts talking about his bed, for instance, he is getting better, if he complains about his nurse, he is much better and if he says something like "there is a lovely sun outside", he is truly convalescent.

With cancer patients in the terminal stage, the contrary happens: they reduce a lot the field of their attention; they start speaking, and do so more and more, of things that interest elderly people. This demostrates that there is a double command: physical and psychological.

Marlzberg, (5) in his papers, which I think are very reliable, gives numbers that confirm the fact that there is little cancer in mental hospitals to the point that a cancerologist is not required to be in attendance. I had observed this both at the Psychiatrical Hospital of Caracas, first as a student, then as a practicing psychiatrist, and at the Verdun Hospital in Montreal, where I stayed three years.

I will quote now myself from a chapter I wrote for the book "Cancer on Day" (6). In this chapter, I speak about cancer and schizophrenia (a real psychiatrist must be interested in schizophrenia)

"The world of the psychiatrist is the world of schizophrenia, with its violent twists, strange symptoms and permanent changes alternating with a heavy immovability. All this is the way to express loneliness and fear which are destroying the patient's ego and rendering his psyche useless, in a withered and clumsy body. The psychiatrist is well aware of the tragic death of suicides, which contrast with the final

(4) The Island of Margarita belongs to the State of Nueva Esparta, in the oriental cost of Venezuela. Natives are most of them, sailors, and generally happy and extravert people.
(5) Marlzberg, B. (1934). Mortality among Patients with mental deseases. State Hospital Press, Utica, New York.
(6) Rísquez, F. (1975). Aspectos psiquiátricos en Cancerología. en Vera y Palacios,(Ed) "Cancer al Día", Vol.1, Cromotip, Caracas.

death of schizophrenia, caused by lung deseases, but statistics show
that cancer´s death rate or brain´s hemorrhage deaths, are significantly lower than the general population´s rates. Analysing with care
this we find that:

a1) Between twenty five and thirty four years-old, the proportion in
mortality rate by cancer in schizophrenics is of 2,5 to 1 in general
population.
a2) This proportion slowly changes and after fifty five years-old, the
general population increases its mortality rate over the schizophre-
nicsrate. This phenomenon is at its highest point between sixty five and seventy four years-old, when the proportion is of one for schizophrenics and 1,4 for the general population.
a3) There is a marked difference between men and women, as to cancer
mortality. Between twenty five and thirty four years-old, schizophrenic men exceed general population 2,8 to one. The rate decreases
from forty five to fifty four years-old, to one and two. Between twenty five and thirty four years-old, the mortality rate in schizophrenic women exceeds general population 2,4 to 1. The rate of women´s
death by cancer, in the general population, exceeds the schizophenic
women´s one, excepting between forty five and fifty four years-old;
during these years, death in schizophrenic patients exceeded rate in
general population 1,3 to 1.
a4) After forty five years-old the rate of cancer mortality in schizo
phrenic women is always higher than the men´s rate. There is also a-
higher mortality in feminine patients (51%) in general population,
where women exceed men´s mortality rate (made even) in 15%.
a5) Mortality rate for cancer in general population, exceeds mental
patients death rate from the same cause. As if madness, was an immu-
nity factor as mysterious as unquestionable. (7) (8)

There are two poles in emotions expression. (9) Emotion is the hinge
of physiology and is equally claimed by Claude Bernard and Sigmund
Freud, although this has been discussed all through the last hundred
years. It expresses itself in two ways: the mind is moved and one
is able to communicate it, or one gets depressed, hides it in the cellular biochemical mecanisms and somatizes.

A person is ill with cancer: I call this being desolated; the person
keeps her desolation inside, the cells become insane and a tumor makes it appearance; or a person hides carefully her devastating despair, which is something very different in schizophrenia, the ego becomes insane, and scatters.

These are the two ends of medical dialectic: insanity or death through suffering. Medical pathology is made up of expressing both.

In world literature, I have found four different points of view in relation to psychological factors, detectable or not in cancer patients.

(7) Marlzberg, Benjamin. (1934). Mortality among Patients with mental
Deseases. State Hospital Press, Utica, New York.
(8) Rassidakis, N.C., Kelepouris, M.and Fox, S. (1961). Malignant Neoplasms as a Cause of Death among psychiatric Patients. Internal Medical Health Research. Newsletter Vol.XIII, Nº2.
(9) Bahnson, C.B. and Bahnson, M.B. Cancer as an Alternative to Psychosis: a theoritical Model of somatic and psychological Regression.
D.M. Kissen & L.L. Le Shan. (Eds.) Pitman, London (1964).

We can read about the first one in northamerican, german and russian
papers alike. It points out a capacity for directing one's emotions,
what the British call "self-control" and we could call channelled aggressive feelings, or polarized emotions, using a psychiatrical expression. These people can be classified in the following manner:
persons who direct their emotions towards theie environment, trying
to, or being able to modify it. Persons who have a neurotic conduct,
with reiterative stereotyped behaviour. Freud referred this to unconscious transferences in early childhood. And persons who keep their
emotions well inside and keep silent about them. It is in this last
group that cancer causes havoc. (10)

The cancer patient keeps to himself his negative emotions.

I used the word silent because all investigators coincide about this
characteristic and I believe, definitely, that all manifestations of
suffering, which precede cancer, tend to be unspoken, contrarily to
what happens with other deseases, like asthma. It is very difficult
to think that an asthmatic may fall ill with cancer, but if, by any
chance, he gets cured, and his psychodynamic situation has'nt changed
I should worry a lot because this could mean that he is modifying his
own system of expressing suffering. From a psychiatrical point of
view, we oppose with histerical temperament, that is of dramatic and
emotional expression, this kind of temperament.

Leshan, has been working actively, for more than nine years, in cancer
patients psychotherapy and has reached several conclusions: he emphasizes aggression and passivity variables as modifiers of cancer evolution, that should always keep us very alert because of the desease's
seriousness and its prognosis. (11)

The second point of view is based on the study of the patient's biopa-
thographical antecedents,(or simply biographical)(Leshan and collabo-
rators). Studying a longitudinal section view of cancer patients lives, allows us to say, within a rather safe limit, statiscally significant, that there have been early family losses, specially in certain
types of early cancer, and that when the desease comes later in life,
certain losses have also happened later, reactivating former ones in
the family constelation. The third manner to approach the problem is
taking into account life relationships. Here, we have made a contribution that resembles a little the findings of some northamerican investigators. Socially, what we find in the life of a person who has cancer, is a wish to be of service asking for nothing in exchange. These people are ready to serve others, gratuitously.

Lastly, López Herrera and I, have contributed with a new approach to
the problem; we realized rapidly, that the actions of a human being,
in his life relationships, in his intrapersonal life, can be measured
with two parameters. The first one is related to the sensation of
being protected, of being stable, of belonging to a group, with others; at first we called this safety but afterwards included it in the
concept of socialization. To make it shorter, I could use a metaphor,

(10) Freud, S. (1953). The Standard Edition of the Complete psychological Works. J. Strachey (ed) Hogarth Press, London.
(11) Leshan,L.L.An emotional Life History Pattern associated with neoplastic Deseases (1966). Ann.New York Academy of Sciences. Vol.125:
780.

it would be the <u>niche</u> that everyone makes, or wishes for, in the society where they belong. It is the place where a person feels safe. The
second parameter of human conduct would be connected with "movement to
reach an aim", with dynamism, with ego reaffirmation, with artistic
creativity,or the scientist, the investigator's solitary search. All
this we called, at first, <u>freedom</u> and then gave it a more jungian name,
continent and related, on the bipolar plane to the former: <u>individua-
tion.</u> (12) (13)

Human conduct shows two big tendencies: a tendency to socialization,
that drifts to safety, conservation and cautiousness, and, on the other side, a whole series of relationships that imply individuation,
<u>search, creativity</u> and <u>risk.</u>

Following my own personality and upbringing, I am a psychiatrist who
believes in <u>the dynamyc unconscious</u> discovered by Freud, and who also
believes in some jungian observations about <u>archetypal complexes,</u> unconscious complexes that can be present as <u>images.</u> The initial complex of socialization is referred, in infancy, to <u>the mother archety
pe.</u> The complex of individuation is referred to <u>the father archety-
pe.</u> The mother is safety and protection; the fathers spurs on the
wish to be adventurous, to take risks, to look for renewal.

In all cancer patients, observed by us, there has been a sudden loss,
and they have been unable, because of their particular personality, to
find some kind of substitute right at that moment. These losses are
not necessarily deaths, althouth death of the life-partner and, more
so, of a child (of any age), is often closely related to these cases.
This has been studied not only by psychiatrists but by oncologists.
We remember the case of a doctor's mother, medically checked up by her
son every three months; she loses in a terrible accident several members of her family and falls ill with a breast carcinoma. Inmediate-
ly, cancer spreads in metastasis and the woman dies in a few days time. It is very difficult not to correlate a sudden loss that made impossible for that woman to repair the niche of her socialization, with
the appearance of a malignant growth.

In another investigation (14), based on the study of twenty sick children, the psychiatrist knew practically nothing about them, and his only parameter was that all children had leucemia, which he thought of
as "liquid cancer". We found out that all of them had lost <u>the mother
figure.</u> Some of the mothers were dead, others had left the child, but
almost all of them, were incompetent. I witnessed in this group, real
secret tragedies. Two of the mothers were openly homosexual and for
them the birth of a child had been a monstrous event in their lives.
Two of the fathers were sadists, psychopaths who kept torturing their
wifes,who, in turn, had only one thought in mind: taking revenge and
cared nothing about their child. All children observed were"old", spoke like adults and had a special characteristic in common: they wanted
to protect their mothers, in what we afterwards called: "inversion of
the mother and child roles".

(12) Jung, C.G. (1957). <u>Collected Works.</u> Bollingen Series, Pantheon
Books, New York.
(13) Jung, C.G. (1970). <u>Arquetipos e Inconsciente Colectivo.</u> Biblio-
teca de Psicología Profunda. Editorial Paidos, Buenos Aires.
(14) Complete Results of this investigation, carried on at the Caracas University Hospital, several years ago, have'nt been published.

During this investigation, I happened to talk with a little boy who
had an osteosarcoma of the knee and, because of this, had not been included in the group, as his cancer was "solid"; he was a "little old
man", like the others, but after I had talked several times with him,
I started doubting whether our theory was correct because this child,
had a mother apparently, who took care of him, visited him and brought
him chocolates. All this the child kept telling me. I was extremely
surprised when, having asked about him the head-nurse, she told me that
the little boy's mother had only gone once to the hospital, the day she
had brought him; the nurse herself had bought the chocolates and he had
made up the rest of the story.

At once, we have here two characteristics made evident. First, there
is <u>a theatrical play,</u> but a serious play, not a histerical one, of the
phantasy of a good mother, a loving mother, and, on top of this, <u>the
child is protecting her good name</u> with his inventions.

In adult patients, we also find an early loss, seemingly, successfully
compensated, but at the expence of the patient who kept "selling himself for affection", sacrificing himself for others and losing his in
dividuality. Later on, any incident makes this plain. Twenty, thirty years afterwards, this person suffers a new loss, isolates himself,
is not "approved of" by his own people: a malignant desease makes its
appearance. We can see how this is true in the case of great workers,
of people well-known because of their social activities, who, five or
six months after a situation of death or separation, fall ill with cancer. Relating the type of cancer to the type of loss, we see that <u>the
violence of the desease is in direct proportion with the amount of lost
affection.</u> A few years ago, an excellent poet saw his best friend,
the head of the State, die; a month after, the poet died too. At least
we can put forward a question-mark connecting Allende and Neruda's
deaths.

There are also the people who, little by little, lose their security,
not getting love or satisfactions of any kind, in exchange of their
personal achievements. These people have what we call a <u>"slow-waste
cancer"</u>,which is the most frequent one. I had a widower as a patient;
his wife had died of cancer: she had been a mother to him and a mother
for everyone at home. He was not a well-educated man but had made a
lot of money. He had been born with a lesion that had never given him
any trouble. After a few years, this man fell in love with a youngish
woman and everything was getting settled for the better when his daughters started opposing this relationship, in the most violent manner,
and he left the young woman: "I have to choose between her and my daughters, who have no mother...". Six months passed. The lesion with
which he had been born, started bothering him, he had it examined, and
a particularly malignant cancer was discovered. An oncologist put me
in touch with the patient to whom I said, after having learned all this
"you are making a choice between life and death"-"Doctor, you don't
know...have a talk with my daughters". I did speak with them and was
appalled at their hostile and aggressive feelings and attitude and, also, at the passivity and stoicism of their father. Six months afterwards, he was dead and buried.

<u>I am not saying</u> and it is not my theory nor my experience, <u>that cancer
is caused by</u> this or that, I don't believe in causalism or in mechanism. I say that the factors of desolation and despair are <u>connected
with</u> the appearance of malignant tumors and their getting worse and,

that the increase of hope and freedom feelings and creative capacity,
diminishes the seriousness of the desease and may often prevent it.

These psychological observations allow us to find, not so much a personal, individualized formula for cancer patients, as a series of dynamyc characteristics that could be summed up as follows: the cancer
patient is sensible, serious, active and responsible; he slowly lets
all the activity of his family group, or/and his community and social
group, gather around him and in this way becomes what I have often called, "the garbage can", the silent and heroic continent of the whole
family's suffering. This patient, when first showing some kind of
symptomatology, worries more about his work and his family than about
his illness. At a later stage, he worries more about those he will
soon be leaving, than about what is happening to him. He tranfers to
others a great wish to be accepted and to be recognized. It is the
type of man, or woman, who absorbs in kleinian bipolarity of envy and
gratefulness, envy, and uses only the pole of gratitude. (15) In one
word, he is the image of what a good socializing person should be, giving a lot and getting very little, and also being able to hold a certain amount of fatalistic desolation.

The doctor may try dividing the problem the patient puts out to him
with his illness and he may use three different methods in his diagnosis, his therapy, and his prognosis.

If the doctor starts with this question: " where is the problem? where can I look for it and find it?", his therapy will be ablative or
reconstructive and his prognosis will depend upon the space gained o-
ver by the desease. This medical attitude implies the use of fire or
metal, a surgical or physical action into what is relatively inmedia-
te but, intentionally, into what is to be definitely changed. In the
second attitude, the doctor will ask himself: " when did this problem
start? what is to be done to change its rhythm and direction?" The
therapy will be substitutive or cathartic and the prognosis will depend upon how long the desease has been present, that is, it will depend upon time. All this implies the therapeutical use of medicines
and food and the careful observation of their effects during a prudent
but armed watch trying to educe rather slow changes. In the third attitude, the doctor will start thinking: " who is this person? who is
the patient?" or " in what way has the desease modified him as a person and in his vital relationships?" The therapeutical action will
be very subtle and rather passive, to be able to make good use of the
crucial moments in vital dynamics. This prognosis will be more in accordance with the idea of the greek Asclepiades about the "kairos",
the need to follow closely any symptom indicating a change towards
the preservation of life or towards its waste and death.

During the last twenty years, we have been actors and observers of the
medical struggle against cancer; we have seen how these three positions
have followed each other in almost imperceptible manner, to render more visible the great complexity of Cancerology and its place within
a full medical program.

The doctor bears the anxiety, the guilt and despair of the patient;
this is why it is so difficult to take care of people ill with cancer.
The only way to meet this difficulty is to increase the medical team

(15) Klein, M. (1960) Envidia y Gratitud. Nova, Buenos Aires.

taking care of these patients; this has been slowly happening. Twenty
years ago, we had, more or less, a surgeon pathologist and a nurse;
now we have a surgeon, a pathologist, an internist, nurses, specialists
and technicians in radiology, radiotherapy, bioanalysis, biophysics,
immunology, social communication, social work and, finally, psychiatrists and psychologists. But somebody must"own"the case. There is
nothing that annoys more these patients than to be taken care of by
an impersonal group of people, without names. This is to lack "mother" by antonomasia.   We think that the members of this much enlarged team must keep exchanging their different points of view, to reach
a top efficiency.   It would also be of benefit if they exchanged their
own ideas on the myth of cancer as a desease that the person gets or
that happens to him in an unexpected manner.

We believe that the cancer patient is a result of a process of"canceration" which includes, very specially, a "manner to be in the world"
which, in turn, is the result of a series of factors. One of these,
would be the attitude of the person towards life and its vital values.

We believe that nobody "gets" a cancer but that people find their own
cancer because this desease is the result of the individual's suffering in his struggle for life and to live his way.

In the case of children's cancer, we have to realize the enormous influence of the mother's negative attitude or behaviour. (16)

But to be able to realize these things, it is necessary to be acquainted with the secrets of the dynamic unconscious. If the tumor is at
the furthest end of a reactive "continuum", we can make three essential
reflections. First, it is absolutely necessary to study in a very detailed manner, the biopathography of the cancer patient, observing
with care his own way of being affected by the problems of life. Second, one is able to suspect more often the possibility of"canceration" and take more efficient therapeutical measures. Lastly, one
could even prevent "canceration".

The organization of this medical program, is a real challenge that only a complete team can accept, knowing that experimenting and dialo-
guing are not opposed methods. on the contrary: they complement each
other as psychiatrical and anatomo-clínical languages can get to complement each other.

The cancer patient is an individual manifestation of a process of social interacting begun by his family, parents and brothers and sisters
that goes on with his particular relationship with his life-companion
and children, and reflects itself in the ecological environment, society, time and culture interrelations.

All alive organisms have a structure apparently opposed to entropy,
(17) and this phenomenon is permanently present in homeostasis, which
depends upon cellular functions but is subordinated to the organization of the nervous central system, which in turn depends on his re-

(16) Bahnson, C.B. and Bahnson, M.B. (1964). Denial and Repression
of primitive Impulses and of disturbing Emotions in Patients with a
malignant Neoplasm. D.M. Kissen & L.L. Leshan. Pitman (Eds) London.
(17) López Herrera, L. (1960). Entropía y Cáncer. Boletín del Ins.
de Oncología "Luis Razetti". Vol.III. Nº3, Caracas.

lations with the other nervous systems in a constant interchange involving two very complex parameters that, for practical operational reasons, we have summarized into these words: safety and socialization,
freedom and individuation.

Future experiments will have to be designed to understand all the variables and respect their hierarchy. It is no longer possible to go on
experimenting only on a microscopical or even a molecular level without trying to interpret finds or discoveries from an anthropological
point of view. Both concepts, far from opposing each other, can integrate themselves within their own hierarchy. So much complexity is
discouraging but the difficulty of the task, can't keep us from carrying it on, in a lucid and harmonic manner.

As we believe that cancer is directly connected to a loss of safety,
in a repetitive and very afflictive way, we think that it is useless
and dangerous to make psychological experiments with cancer patients
unless we include in them a therapeutical medical action with all the
delicate net of intimacy that this implies. It is not conducive at
all, to try to discover mental aberrations in their behaviour as, precisely, they have somatized their suffering to keep their minds clear
and obedient to their companion's, family or social group's will. It
is absurd to try opening "canceration"'s intimacy kept so well closed
by the patient with the key of his hidden or unconscious feelings and
thoughts, with the keys of cold reason in an impersonal, constrained,
technological and distant communication.

We believe that Cancerology teaches us, in surgery, to cut up each day
less, to inject drugs more cautiosly each time, and to irradiate in a
much more accurate manner than before; to keep company to our patients
with humility but firmness, and to talk with moderation but precision,
to encourage at all times, whatever our medical method, a change in
the patient's vision of life and in his family's idea of death, so
that we can accomplish our therapeutical mission with these patients:
to fight desolation.

In this manner we can carry out Medicine's sacred purpose which is understanding suffering in sickness, and to increase vital hope in human
creativity. Decision and harmony against desolation, desintegration
and death. (18)

Before concluding, I would like to point out one or two more things.
There has been a lot of talk about a resistance to the desease; this
could be explained through Lewin's relation (19)(20) It is simply a spec-
tre through which resistance to desease has a direct connection with
the person's attitude in facing it. If the patient starts to bother
and annoy people, if he is not cured, at least he is getting better.
The prognosis can be made listening to the comments of the people who
are taking care of him: "he never used to ask for anything...now he
is always wanting something special..."

I want to insist on the importance of dialogue in all these things be-

(18) Lewin, K. (1935). A dynamic Theory of Personality. McGraw Hill,
New York.
(19 Lewin, K. (1938). The conceptual Representation and Measurement
of psychological Forces. Contr.Psychol.Theor.: I.
(20) Rísquez, F. (1975). Aspectos psiquiátricos en Cancerología en
Vera y Palacios,(Ed) Cancer al Día. Vol.1, Cromotip, Caracas.

because while the doctor is waiting for a therapeutical chance, he has to keep. his patients in a hopeful mood and has only one tool to do it and have them trusting him: dialogue. (21) The doctor-patient relationship has to be adapted to the changes in the cancer patient's personality which goes through three stages, exactly correspondent to antomo-clini cal discoveries: First the stage of cancer that has just been diagnosticated; second, the stage of advanced cancer and third, cancer in its terminal stage. (22)

It is possible that we doctors are sober and prudent in excess in the use of clinical records to the point of not presenting interesting cases that could be easily identified, because of their dramatic characteristics, avoiding in this manner the betrayal of professional secret. All the same, I wish to bring up for discussion, a testimony that confirms what I have been saying, in a non-medical manner, one of hurt innocence. It is given by journalists, and taken from a Caracas paper dated January 1976.

"X...had been a wonderful comrade, he had the will to be of service; you could say that his, complemented the reporters work. When papers became more graphic in expression, he was ready: although not a young man, he was quick on the job and could take spectacular photographs, whenever ir was required. He used to be a sportsman and had enjoyed excellent health; even more, hardly a month ago, he still looked healthy and well. He did'nt know it but in his insides, his cells were growing in a disorderly manner; the process....was unpainful, silent and traitorous, it attacked his stomach and his liver, then the metastasis set in. When we went to visit him at the clinic, he did'nt even have the will to talk; his wife admitted that he had collapsed: "he has'nt been able to touch any food...", she said, waiting for the doctor..."We went out with him several times during our work: he never showed any bad will when he had to put up with some extra work because he really loved his profession. Once, during his holidays, he decided to travel by car from Caracas to Buenos Aires and many years afterwards, he would tell us with pride, again and again, about his experience, maybe the most important one in his life., Not everybody could undertake it..."we just had will and courage and left by the Pacific Road, along the Andes..." He saw the inmense jungles, compared the Pampa with our Llanos, the sun looking different at midday...the "Cumparsita" was still popular; he went to the parisian show of the "Bal Tabarin", not far from Corrientes street, the cobblestone boulevards, Carlos Gardel's grave at the "Chacarita" and Palermo's Park and racetracks...He would tell us about the automobile in which, twenty years before he had set forth in this trip: "it was a simple but noble motor...we only stopped because of a few flat tyres" and predicted: "one day, there will be wonderful roads and they will bring people to know better each other".

"He was fifty-three years-old and had been awarded the National Prize of Journalism. Lately, he was working for the sports column; his comrades in that section will miss him: he was an excellent collaborator and could describe as well a by the head arrival in a race as any other event. He had been as efficient in other departments...We are grieving for the loss of an excellent worker, an honest man, an uncommon one. He always did all he could, as a human being and as a professional and asked nothing in exchange of his wish to be of service..."

(21) (22) Rísquez, F. (1975). Aspectos psiquiátricos en Cancerología en Vera y Palacios (Ed) Cancer al Dia. Vol.1, Cromotip, Caracas.

The desease that took him away from us was traitorous; he had only o-
ne symptom: a loss of weight; he felt no pain but kept getting thin-
ner and just said he wanted to lose weight..." "We did'nt know what
to think, said somebody else; some said he had an ulcer, others, an
esophageal hernia, some hinted of a mental illness but then we learned
the sad truth when the surgeon operated on him and declared that there
was nothing to be done: a carcinoma had destroyed him. The burial ce-
remony is today".

In all the papers, we find "the will to serve", "the wish to be of service" and that he was devoted to his home and family "after work, he
always went home to his loving wife and children who fulfilled all he
needed and all he hoped for" "he was austere, a model husband and a
model father; he was a good man, biologically..."

In the last twenty years, I have been interested in all these problems.
Basing my opinion on my personal observations, on the observations of
the oncologists who have been good enough to acompany and direct my
work, on the opinion of other psychiatrists who have interested themselves in this, I feel I can state, without fearing to be mistaken,
that the characteristics of the cancer patient are: an exagerated wish
to be of service in a gratuitous manner, an ability to take on, alone,
the whole family's personality and good sense, a dignity in accepting
suffering, a capacity to hide it and a need to feel affection at all
times.

It is possible that in the investigation we are now undertaking on
sub-clinical cancer, and in others we are preparing (I hope that many
other people will join us in this task), to look in the difficulties
of life, taken in a lengthwise section, for connections between socialization and suffering, individuation and suffering. we may be able
to discover the source that will help us as much in the prevention of
cancer as in its treatment.

But the last point I wish to emphasize is that we can warn people that
they are not playing in the right manner the game of life. We can
warn them if we see they are too responsible, too sensible, too bent
on sacrificing themselves, specially if they don't demand anything
from others and if they don't show any symptom of mental illness, that
they are potential cancer patients.

Sigmund Freud, Pope John XXIII (23) (24) are good examples of what I
am saying. We really have to open our eyes and say to this kind of
people: "do not give all the time, demand sometimes, do not feel responsible for everybody, leave them alone, and you will survive".

Lastly, I would like to say again a sentence I have often repeated;
in the memory of all cancer patients I have met and who have died, I
wish we could write on their tombstones the following words: "dead
in the fulfillment of duty".

(23) Stone, I. Pasiones del Espíritu. (1971) Emecé, Argentina.
(24) Roncalli, A.J. (Papa Juan XXIII). (1964) Diario del Alma. Edi-
ciones Cristiandad, Madrid.

Data Processing in Cancer

Methods of Monitoring Cancer Rates

J. A. H. Waterhouse

*Birmingham Regional Cancer Registry, Queen Elizabeth Medical Center,
Birmingham B15 2TH, England*

ABSTRACT

There are many purposes today which call for the regular monitoring of cancer rates
in specific population groups. They may refer to a limited group of sites only, or
to the total rate of malignant disease.

Common uses of such figures are to estimate health care requirements, and for the
provision of cancer treatment facilities; and for the detection of changes in the
rates of cancer, usually by individual sites, which may betoken new cancer hazards,
possibly ascribable to environmental factors such as new industrial processes or
products. An important consideration in all applications is the long latent period
between first exposure to a carcinogen and the development of the disease.

A valuable source of cancer morbidity data for monitoring purposes is a cancer
registry, population based and with good registration efficiency. A number of
additional factors which can affect the interpretation of such data in monitoring
are discussed, with illustrations drawn from data from the Birmingham Cancer
Registry over a fifteen year period.

Many influences have combined to focus attention upon the contemporary impact of
malignant disease on the community. The degree of control of infectious disease
which is now attainable has thrown into greater prominence other diseases, of which
the cancers form a significant group. Their relative intractability of treatment
places particular emphasis on all aspects of prevention - and thence on aetiological
studies, and on early warning systems to pick up possibly significant changes as
soon as may be possible.

We are all familiar with current estimates of the proportion of cancers which can
be related to environmental influences - a figure of 80% or more[1] - and we are also
well aware that the assessment of such a figure does not at the same time clearly
indicate each of the aetiological factors responsible. Where we do possess reasonably good evidence of causative factors - such as cigarette smoking, or various
dietary constituents - they are often so closely related to culture patterns in a
population, or to habitual life-styles, as to be very resistant to change. For
this reason, aetiological factors traceable to the environment - taking this term
in its widest connotation - tend to receive most attention. Such factors may be

man-made, or naturally-occurring: they may be climatic (such as the influence of
the sun on unpigmented skin), or they may be due to industry (such as asbestos,
mineral oil, and various chemicals).

It is this last group, essentially man-made, resulting from the highly sophisticated patterns of life in the developed countries of the world today - and extend-
ing very rapidly to the less developed countries - which excites particular
attention. New products and new processes are being developed and exploited on a
scale, and at a rate, which leaves inadequate time or facilities for the evaluation of their potential hazards to health and to safety, whether at work or in the
home. Thus, as a back-up, it is essential to be able to monitor the rates of
cancer - since we are here concerned primarily with the malignant disease risks -
lest other screening tests (or indeed the complete omission of testing) fail to
detect those products or processes which may be carcinogenic to man. Essentially,
of course, man himself is the ultimate test, and epidemiology provides the method
of evaluation. For no other screening procedure at present known can infallibly
substitute - whatever may be the dictates of prudence or of ethics. Nonetheless,
the long latent period required for the induction of most human tumours makes it a
slow and tedious process, and again stresses the importance of early detection of
changes of rate, or of secular trends.

But it is not only as a means of detecting new environmental hazards that it is
important to monitor cancer rates. They are a necessary input feature in the calculation of health care provision in the population. In planning for the provision
of cancer treatment facilities, they are of especial importance because of the very
high costs they involve. In addition to the basic requirements of hospital beds
and services, the treatment of cancer today forms usually the most costly constit-
uent of the drugs account, and calls also for very expensive equipment for radiation therapy as well as sophisticated radiographic methods of diagnosis and surveillance. Thus a knowledge of trends in cancer rates - often by sites of disease,
too - is an indispensable component of planning for health care and services.

For a long time, the chief source of information on cancer rates has been
mortality statistics. As indices of trend, or indeed as an early warning device,
statistics of cancer mortality show wide variations of usefulness, according
largely to the site of the disease and its survival rate. For sites which
commonly have a very short survival - such as cancers of the liver, lung, or
stomach - mortality rates form a useful guide to the behaviour of the disease at
those sites, and can well illustrate trends. For others, where survival is better,
their value progressively diminishes as survival improves, until for instance with
basal-cell cancers of the skin, where mortality is exceptionally low, it is
non-existent.

The increasing availability of morbidity rates of cancer by site has greatly
improved the usefulness of cancer rates, especially for the purposes outlined
earlier, where they can perform a monitoring role.[2] Figures of cancer morbidity
usually have their origin in a cancer registry, and their usefulness therefore
very much depends on the situation and efficiency of that registry. If it serves
a reasonably large population (anything from two to eight million preferably, with
some extensions at each end of the scale, perhaps); and if furthermore it is of a
high order of efficiency of registration (usually 90% or above), then it is likely
to be able to fulfil most of the functions enumerated above; and if it has been in
operation for some time, it can provide also a good basis for the calculation of
trends.

Example

To examine the subject more precisely and to discover what methods may be usefully
employed in this field I have taken a practical example. I have used the data of
the Birmingham Cancer Registry, over a period of fifteen years, during which time
its efficiency of registration has been 95% or greater. The Registry is situated
in the midlands of England, covering an area of 13,014 square kilometres and a
population of just over five million. It includes industrialised areas as well as
agricultural areas, and in fact is very similar in its make-up to the population
of England and Wales as a whole.

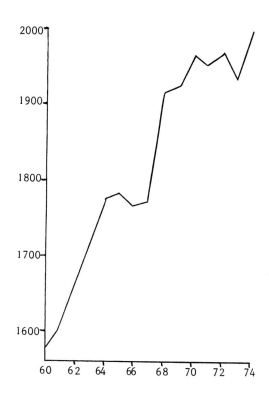

Fig. 1. Numbers of cases of Breast Cancer by calendar year: all ages

The site I have selected is the female breast - the commonest site in the female,
forming a quarter of all new registrations in the Birmingham region. The actual
numbers of cases range from 1,577 in 1960 to 2,003 in 1974, at the end of the
fifteen year period. Figure 1 shows the pattern of numbers of cases by calendar
year. Clearly there has been an increase, of the order of 30% in the whole period.
The actual number of cases observed is however the product of two more fundamental
quantities - the incidence rate of cancer of the breast, and the size of the population to which the register refers. Clearly, an increase in population would
increase the observed number of cases, although the rate might remain unaltered.
Is there evidence that the population has increased? The answer is - yes, it has

282   J. A. H. Waterhouse

increased, according to the two censuses included in the period under examination
(1961 and 1971), by an amount just exceeding 7%.

These figures refer only to the gross size of the population, and not to its
composition by age. The age structure of a population depends on many factors –
its history, in terms especially of its patterns of birth and death rates, and on
the extent of migration. In a disease which shows an exponential relationship to
age, as cancer does, the age structure of the population plays a central role in
determining the numbers of cases. For this reason I next examined the numbers of
cases in each five-year age group for every one of the fifteen calendar years. I
am only showing here a selection of typical graphs to indicate the pattern of
change in numbers of cases by age group.

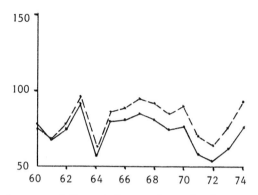

Fig. 2. Numbers of cases of Breast Cancer by calendar year in the age group 35-39

Figure 2 shows, in the full line, the actual numbers of cases by year for the age
group 35-39. It appears to show a slight decline as a very general trend over the
period. If allowance is made for the change in size of that age group however, for
each calendar year, we obtain the curve shown in a broken line. The pattern now no
longer shows evidence of decline, but is more stable.

The next graph (Fig. 3) refers to the age group 50-54, and again the two lines
correspond to the actual numbers (full line) and to the population-adjusted numbers
(broken line). In this age group the difference between the two lines is rather
less than previously: the "swing" from year to year is greater (though not propor-
tionally so), and there is possible, but not strong, evidence of a slight increase.

Figure 4 shows the age group 65-69, with again an oscillation of numbers in both
lines, but whereas the numbers actually observed show a clearcut rising trend, the
population adjustment makes the trend unmistakably horizontal, at least after an
initial small rise. Much the same pattern is shown by the next age group (70-74)
in Fig. 5, although there is a discernible slight upward trend in the adjusted
numbers – much less, however than in the actual numbers.

The last age group I have chosen to illustrate – 80-84 – in Fig. 6, is rather less
clearcut: the adjusted line shows a decreasing trend, while the actual numbers
show first a rise, and then some stability, or a possible decline. The numbers in
this age group are not large, so random fluctuations may obscure the delineation of
trends. For this reason I have not included in these illustrations age groups
either above this, or below 35, although I have examined each one.

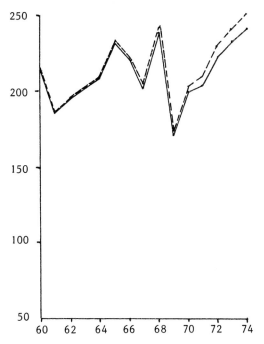

Fig. 3.   Numbers of cases of Breast
           Cancer by calendar year in
           the age group 50-54

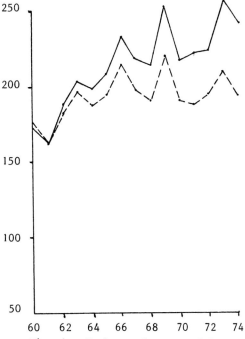

Fig. 4.   Numbers of cases of Breast
           Cancer by calendar year in
           the age group 65-69

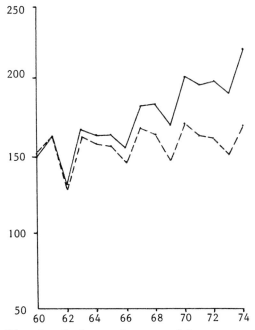

Fig. 5.   Numbers of cases of Breast
           Cancer by calendar year in
           the age group 70-74

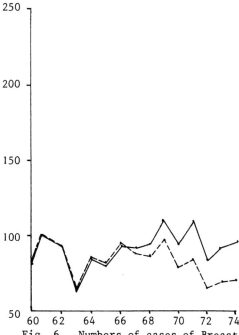

Fig. 6.   Numbers of cases of Breast
           Cancer by calendar year in
           the age group 80-84

Having shown the effect of allowing for population size changes in individual
quinquennial age groups, which invariably has reduced the apparent increase over
the period, and often has shown a stable resultant pattern, it is perhaps of value
to apply the same technique to the gross total of cases. Figure 7 shows this line
for the grand total of cases, and its comparison with the original line of Fig. 1
for comparison. These two lines are comparable in a general way with the pairs of
lines - actual and adjusted numbers - of the preceding sequence of graphs. The
large increase of Fig. 1 has now been reduced to about half its size (15%), but an
increase is very clearly discernible.

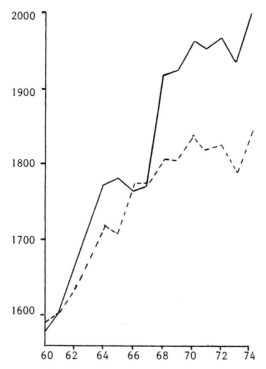

Fig. 7.   Numbers of cases of Breast Cancer by calendar year: all ages: actual and
                           population-adjusted

The application of this adjustment to the gross total of numbers takes no account
of possible changes in the age composition of the population. It makes the
implicit assumption in fact that the proportionate composition by age is unaltered.
In most actual circumstances this assumption is not justified, because age structure alters in a more irregular way. If we take the two census years, for which
the population is most reliably available by age group, the ratio of the proportionate structure by age of 1971 relative to 1961 for the Birmingham Region is
shown in Fig. 8. Clearly there has been a consistent and escalating increase in
all age groups above 50. As a result, the totals by year require an additional
adjustment to allow also for age composition, as well as overall population
changes. Fig. 9 shows what effect this adjustment has, in relation also to the
previous graphs of Fig. 1 and Fig. 7. Although smaller than the effect shown in
Fig. 7, there is also a further reduction of the numbers, suggesting perhaps a
plateau or levelling-off from about 1966 onwards.

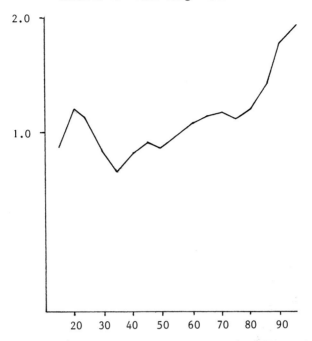

Fig. 8.   Ratio of proportionate age structure of female population: 1971 to 1961

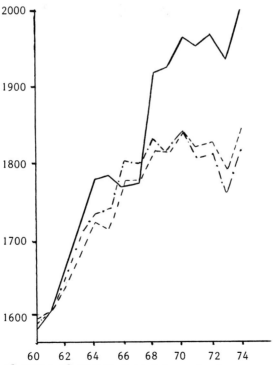

Fig. 9.   Numbers of cases of Breast Cancer by calendar years: all ages: actual;
          population adjusted; age and population adjusted

If we are looking for changes in the impact of the disease itself over the specific
period of fifteen years, then a better indication of secular effects is afforded
by a cohort analysis. Figure 10 shows a succession of cohort segments, formed
each from three points, and relating to central birth-years ranging from 1879 to
1939. For birth years from about the turn of the century onwards there is evidence
of some increase in each successive cohort, except perhaps for 1934 which shows a
slight reduction from 1929 - but 1939 returns to the pattern of increasing rates.

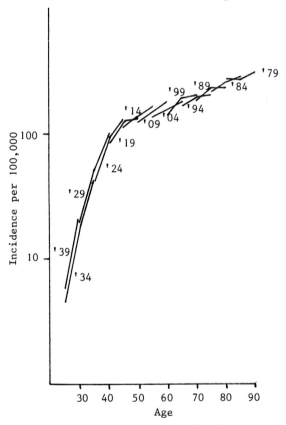

Fig. 10.   Cohort segments for breast cancer age incidence rates, from central
                   birth years 1879 to 1939

CONCLUSIONS

Although a result of this kind might form the starting-point for study to investigate possible reasons for these increases, it is not our place here to pursue such
considerations any further. If we are concerned with the planning of health care
provision, perhaps with special reference to breast cancer, then we are likely to
be more interested in the overall numbers of cases occurring each year (Fig. 1).
Whatever the direction of our interest in figures of this kind however, my chief
concern has been to demonstrate that a number of distinct components contribute to
the ultimate computation, and that they may need to be assembled into different
groupings for different purposes. Furthermore, the extent of sporadic variation -
primarily random fluctuations - is large, and can very easily mislead the investigator into too ready acceptance of an apparent trend which turns out to be only

transient and of no significance. In my example the total size of the population was five million, and the annual number of cases of the order of 2,000. They are large numbers, and yet they still exhibit considerable fluctuation. With smaller numbers, the effects of stochastic variation become more evident, and only sizable trends will be discernible.

REFERENCES

1. Higginson, J. (1976). Importance of environmental factors in cancer. In Rosenfeld, C. and Davis, W. (Ed.), *Environmental Pollution and Carcinogenic Risks*. International Agency for Research on Cancer, Lyon. (*IARC Scientific Publications No. 13*). 15-24

2. Doll, R., Payne, P., and Waterhouse, J. (1966) *Cancer Incidence in Five Continents*. Springer-Verlag, Berlin.

    Doll, R., Muir, C., and Waterhouse, J. (1970). *Cancer Incidence in Five Continents, Vol. II*. Springer-Verlag, Berlin.

    Waterhouse, J., Muir, C., Correa, P., and Powell, J. (1976). *Cancer Incidence in Five Continents, Vol. III*. International Agency for Research on Cancer (*IARC Scientific Publications No. 15*), Lyons.

The Pathogram of the Cancer Patient
EDP-controlled Clinical Cancer Registry and Documented Cancer Follow-up

G. Ott, R. Schunck and Ch. Baunach

Abstract

Presented is a program of recording all facts in the fate of a
cancer patient relevant for therapy and prognosis in a maner suitable
for EDP. Beside optimal medical treatment it is the substance of the
documentation system to produce the complete pathogram of all
registered cancer patients. From the day of establishment of the
diagnosis and the begin of clinical treatment in the Evgl. Krankenhaus up to the following 5 years the cancer patient runs through a
strongly termed and tumor specific follow-up.
All informations and facts are registered in a codable medical
record, a basic documentation for tumor patients, a follow-up and a
final questionaire. In the so coded pathogram of the cancer patient
we only use international binding classifications and coding systems.
The pathogram is the result of a longer development and testing time
in the surgical department of a smaller hospital. The presented
prinziples of documentation include all basis necessary for the
establishment of a clinical cancer registery and documentation
follow-up.

Keywords

Pathogram, Organisation, Cancer Patient, Clinical Cancer Registry,
EDP, Follow-up, Documentation.

The fight against cancer is a chain of functions: it extends, apart from cancer prevention, from early detection via therapy, reconcalescence, follow-up to rehabilitation which includes coping with these diseases psychologically. Whosoever aims at improving this fight against cancer, must not improve early detection alone, not cancer therapy alone, not follow-up alone; he must consider this chain of functions as an entity.

In each case, many experts and many institutions are involved. Starting from the family doctor or general practitioner via the practising specialist up to the diagnostic centers and hospital physicians, all medical experts and institutions may be found at the wayside of the cancer patient, this will necessitate a control center starting from the diagnosis up to the definite cure or the death of the patient. This central function can best be taken over by an EDP-supported clinical registry.

Among other things it is the task of cancer-follow up to safeguard therapeutic success and to prevent, eliminate or mitigate secondary diseases or injuries as a consequence of cancer therapy. Here it is the task of the clinical cancer registry to collect and pass on the most imprtant data of all concerned, to coordinate dates, to cecure economically permissible monitoring programs and to control the timed and standardized sequence of treatments (Tab. 1).

TAB.1:   Tasks of the Clinical Cancer Registry

TASKS OF THE CLINICAL CANCER REGISTRIES

1. INTERDISCIPLINARY PATIENT MANAGEMENT
2. ORGANIZATION OF THE FOLLOW-UP
3. COMPLETE DOCUMENTATION OF THE FACTORS WHICH ARE RELEVANT FOR THE PROGNOSIS (SETTING UP THE „PATHOGRAMS")
4. STATISTICAL EVALUATIONS
5. PROGRAM DEVELOPMENT (RATIONALIZATION, ECONOM, ETC.)
6. SUPRA-REGIONAL COLLABORATION (COMPOUND STUDIES)
7. EPIDEMIOLOGICAL COOPERATION

The findings must be classified according to internationally accepted
guidelines and coding systems in order to safeguard a comparable
evaluation for supra-regional compound studies. Only complete
coverage of the entire fate of many cancer patients with all
prognostically important treatments will permit evaluations and
analyses of methods of treatment, even if, as usual, we measure our
successes by survival times only.

An example: There was a dispute between urologists and radiologists
about the question as to who was in a better position to treat the
penis carcinoma. There were 52% five-year cures by amputating
urologists as opposed to 52% five-year cures by radiologists (who were
able to proudly present the "unshortened male member"). Only a joint
comparative study showed, upon clarification of the late fate of the
patients, that most of those who had been radiologically treated had
to be amputated in addition during the first few years.

So far, we have been accustomed to measuring the success of a method
by defining survival rates after 3, 5 and 1o years. The survival
curves are somewhat more accurate. The UICC has established obligatory
methods of calculation for this purpose. All this was sufficiently
reliable when, ten or twenty years ago, cancer patients were mostly
subjected to only one method of treatment, when recurrences could not
be cured and questionable additional therapies or long-time therapies
could be left out of consideration. However, this won`t do any longer.
Our analyses of success must take into account the varying complexity
of measures relevant for prognosis in our patients. Today we must
make comparable "pathogram of a cancer patients" the basis of our
judgments of success. By "pathogram of a cancer patient" we mean the
reco ding of all factors in the fate of a cancer patient which are
relevant for therapy and prognosis, in a manner suitable for EDP.

PATHOGRAM OF A CANCER PATIENT

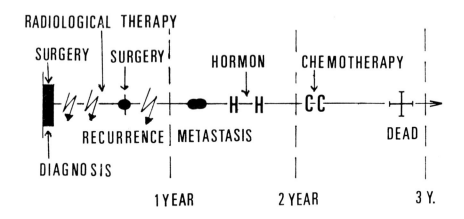

FIG.1: Pathogram of a Cancer Patient

Only by comparative analysis of a considerable numer of comparable
pathograms will be able to judge the value of new chemotherapeutica,
of various methods of surgical treatment of new radiation techniques
and to find the best possible therapy for every individual cancer
patient. In order to anable us to arrive at a scientitic analysis of
the methods of treatment in clinical oncology from the collected data,
the following conditions must be fulfilled.

1 QUESTIONNAIRES SUITABLE FOR DOCUMENTATION
2 BINDING CODE SYSTEMS
3 STANDARDIZED FOLLOW - UP
4 SUFFICIENT NUMBER OF PATIENTS
5 AGREED METHODS OF CALCULATION

TAB.2: Conditions for Clinical Cancer Statistics

1. A centralized, evenly timed cancer follow-up with comparable diagnostic level;
2. data acquisition suitable for EDP;
3. Internationally binding classification and coding systems;
4. agreed methods of calculation;
5. the complete recording of the entire pathogram for a sufficient number of patients.

FOLLOW-UP OF A COLON-CA PATIENT

```
AFTER 3 MONTH     LOCAL,LABOR,RÖ:THORACIC,ENDOSCOPY
      6           LOCAL,LABOR,RÖ:COLON
      9           LOCAL,LABOR,RÖ:THORACIC,ENDOSCOPY
AFTER 1 YEAR      LOCAL,LABOR,RÖ:COLON
      1 1/2       LOCAL,LABOR,RÖ:THORACIC,ENDOSCOPY
      2           LOCAL,LABOR,RÖ:THORACIC AND COLON
      3           LOCAL,LABOR,RÖ:THORACIC AND COLON
                  ISOTOPE:LIVER
      4           LOCAL,LABOR,RÖ:THORACIC AND COLON
                  ISOTOPE:LIVER
      5           LOCAL,LABOR,RÖ:THORACIC AND COLON
                  ENDOSCOPY,ISOTOPE:LIVER
*******************************************************
AFTER 10 YEARS    LOCAL,LABOR,RÖ:THORACIC AND COLON
                  ENDOSCOPY,ISOTOPE:LIVER
```

TAB.3: Follow-up-Program for a Cancer Patient

Our own organization of an EDP-assisted clinical registry has been developed and tested during the last 15 years together with Prof. Wagner and Dr. Köhler of the German Cancer Research Center, during the last eight years in the Surgical Department of the Evangelisches Krankenhaus in Bonn-Bad Godesberg ("Bad Godesberger Modell")

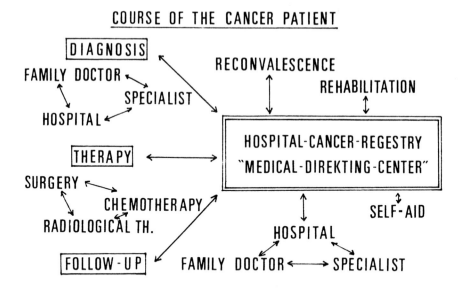

FIG.2: Bad Godesberger Modell

An important prerequisite has been that we should be able to operate
a small size EDP installation independent of a large central computer.
The programs developed by us are conceived in such a manner that
they can be run without the assistance of an EDP specialist. In most
cases, it has not been possible to comply with the justified request
of physicians to be assisted by such installations in their daily
work for the benefit of their patients. This has been due to the fact
that so far only large centralized installations have been tested in
the hospitals which, not being directed towards daily clinical
activities, were to fulfil a wide range of different tasks
simultaneously for many institutions. These large installations do
but burden the physician with additional work. He hardly sees any
benefit for his routine work. He feels that he is forced to complete
crossword puzzle-like forms with which non-physicians feed their
EDP installations without daily benefit to him and his patients.

In order to obtain a "pathogram" of the cancer patient it is
essential to limit the data collection to an extent that makes it

reasonable to expect the physician's cooperation. For this purpose, we developed a basic program for surgery.

DOCUMENTATION - PROGRAM

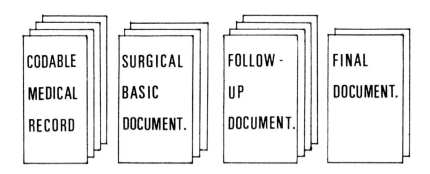

FIG.3:   Documentation Program

1. The basis is formend by a <u>codable medical record</u> including the standardized medical record face sheet. Here the personal data, the most important diagnoses and therapeutical measures are recorded.

2. At the time of discharge from the hospital a "<u>basic documentation for tumour patients</u>" is established in the clinical cancer registry. In addition to the medical record, all cancer-relevant factors are recorded here, for instance risk groups, secondary tumours, recurrences and follow-up findings of the patient. Here, too, the TNM-classification (pre-operative, intra-operative and post-operative) is recorded. Moreover, the varying diagnostic certainty is to be coded.

3. At each re-examination a follow-up questionnaire is filled out.
   This covers
   a) any factors that have come up in the corresponding interval
      since the last examination and documents,
   b) the results of the clinical examination including diagnostic
      measures on the day of examination.

4. Whenever a patient is discharged from the follow-up, a final
   questionnaire is made up. It forms the end of the pathogram and
   gives an unequivocal statement about the reason fo r the finali-
   zation of the follow-up.

We only use internationally agreed coding systems. The data fixed by
the UICC for the basic documentation of tumour centers are used. A
small computer with 24 K storage capacity, two floppy disks and two
cassette drives meets the requirements. It is capable of taking in
the data obtained, of storing and listing them and of carrying out
simple calculations. Apart from that, it comprises a use-oriented
text processing system and copes with the automated appointments for
our tumour patients. We are also able to link up any extended program
for organ-oriented studies with our basic documentation are urgently
required for other medical disciplines, too, in particular for
internal medicine, radiotherapy, paediat rics and pathology, but they
have not been developed up to this date. Our tumour follow-up system
makes it possible to detect local recurrences and metastases early
enough and to cure a high percentage of them. While in earlier times
80% of local breast cancer recurrences reached the surgeon in a non-
operable state, wo today succed in re-operating about four out of
five patients, half of whom will be cured. In the case of colon
cancer about 1o to 15% of those that have undergone surgery will
suffer local recurrences. In the case of erarly detection including
the use of modern endoscopic possibilities, these patients can be
subjected to surgery once again.

Furthermore, it is possible to prevent secondary injuries as a
consequence of therapy or at least to subject them to timely
treatment or achieve mitigation. This, for instance, goes for oedema
of the arm subsequent to breast cancer surgery, to scar hernio,

stitch fistulae, the problems of anus praeter carriers and the
manifold psychological problems and rehabilitation difficulties of
our cancer patients.

SURGERY OF RECURRENCES

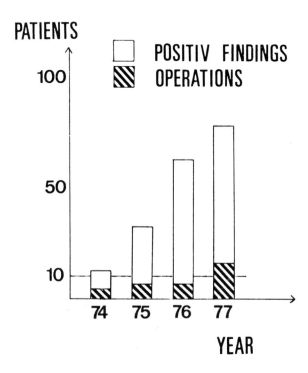

FIG.4:   Positiv Findings and Operations of Recurrences

Since curable recurrences and regional metastases are mainly observed during the forst two years, the routine follow-up examinations are carried out quarterly in the first year and twice in the
second year after operation. In the following three years we carry
out the routine re-examinations once or twice yearly. With the aid
of the EDP installation the clinical registry guarantees the regular
appointment scheduling and the monitoring of our cancer patients.

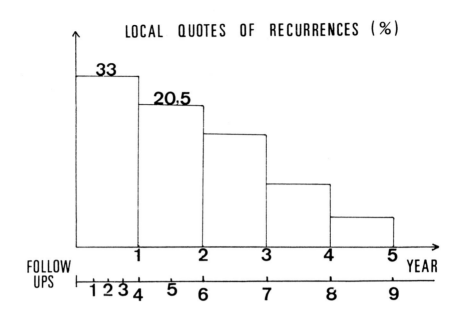

FIG.5:   Local Quotes of Recurrences

It was our idea to try out a practicable EDP-controlled cancer
follow-up in smaller hospitals, too.

In order to safeguard a really patient-oriented medical care, the
cancer follow-up should be realized as a joint task of practising
physicians and hospital physicians. Therefore, the clinical cancer
registry invites the mutual patient to visit his family doctor in the
first instance. Thus, it is warranted that the family doctor receives all the information concerning his patient. Nothing happens
without his knowledge. The family doctor carries out any examinations
of which he is capable. He communicates his results to the clinical
cancer registry in order the guarantee the complete recording of all
findings. Documentation is secured in the hospital by the hospital
physicians. Moreover, they carry through the necessary complementary
examinations, such as endoscopy, scintigraphy, ultrasound or computer
tomography, and the control of the local findings.

In order to improve hospital treatment and to permit interdisciplinary consultation for the patient, we first established an

"Oncological Working Group" in 1963 within the framework of a large
clinical complex of the University of Heidelberg. Standardized
therapy recommendations were worked out which serve as a basis for
consultation (Ott, Kuttig and Drings, 1974). An internal oncological
working group is to be recommended for every medium-sized hospital
so that therapeutic guidelines in the different departments may be
matched and secured.

To begin with, we gained our experience retrospectively with roughly
2o,ooo cance ɪ patients of the years 1943 to 1963 at the Surgical
University Hospital in Heidelberg. With the support of Prof. Linder,
director of the hospital, we covered the survivors, tried out organ-
oriented afer-care centers and began to care for these cancer patients
medically for years. Since 197o we have set up this model in Bonn-
Bad Godesberg, characterized by the collaboration with the family
doctors, as of 1974 supported by an EDP-controlled clinical cancer
registry. Up to now, more than 1,ooo cancer patients have been registered (prospectively) and the first appreciable number of pathograms can be evaluated.

We are convinced that the organized cancer follow-up of this type has
improved the survival chances of our patients. We attein a five-year
survival rate of more than 6o% for all stages of breast cancer taken
together. If we add the results of the last two years to our
calculations, then it is 68%. Taking all cancerous diseases together
every second cancer patient will survive the five-year limit
following his cancer operation. The effect of such an EDP-controlled
clinical cancer registry, however, cannot be measured by the improved rate of cures alone. Of much greater importance are the improvements in the quality of life for our patients which are
realized daily. However, we have not so far developed a method for
measuring these effects in cancerology.

Moreever, our organized standardized cancer follow-up has also
proved its worth in monitoring cancer risk patients. As regards
breast cancer, this concerns proliferating mastopathy, carcinoma
lobulare in situ and papillomatosis of the milk duct, with regard
to the digestive tract proliferating polyps, villous tumours, poly-
posis intestini and colitis ulcerosa. Here we blend in organ-

oriented examinations at time intervals of six or twelve months, for
instance mammography with breast cancer risk patients, coloscopy
with colon cancer risk patients and gastroscopy with stomach cancer
risk patients. Only histologically secured facultative pre-neo-
plasias are considered by us to be risk patients. Such an expensive
organ-oriented follow-up of histologically secured cancer risk
patients has so far been rare in medical care. It can easily be
carried through and is most effective.

CANCER RISK PATIENTS (1975-76)

	NR.	MALIGNISATION	DEATH
BREAST	170	12	-
STOMACH-INTESTINES	74	4	1
TOTAL	244	16	1

TAB.4:   Number of Cancer Risk Patients 1975 - 76

Should we be successful in coordinating this model of clinical cancer
follow-up in a compound system among numerous hospitals, we will then
have the chance of adapting our medical measures according to
scientifically valid optimal chances of cure from an appreciable
number of comparable pathograms and to extablish a standardized
cancer therapy with starting situations that can be clinically
determined.

Let me summarize: an improved comprehensive cancer control requires
a follow-up in smaller interdisciplinary centers. Here cancer follow-
up will have to be centrally organized, documented and adequately
timed with the aid of a reasonably economic program for routine
examinations. The management of the tumour patients calls for a
clinical cancer registry. A small to medium-sized EDP installation
is recommended for its support. Independent minicomputers should
definitely have precedence over terminal stations of large installations. We may state that such a well-documented and organized
interdisciplinary cancer therapy and cancer follow-up (including
cancer risk patients) will permit improved cancer control and
already today guarantees very much better chances of cure for our
cancer patients.

Large-scale Patient Information Systems— Design Considerations

Vincent F. Guinee and Gerald D. Everett

Department of Epidemiology, University of Texas System Cancer Center,
M. D. Anderson Hospital and Tumor Institute, Texas Medical Center,
Houston, Texas 77030, U.S.A.

ABSTRACT

To an ever increasing degree, research and treatment efforts in cancer are relying on large-scale patient information systems.

In considering alternative systems, investigators and administrators must choose the most advantageous approach from a variety of information processing strategies.

Of prime importance is consideration of the inescapable compromise between efficiency of maintenance and ease of retrieval.

Maintenance (updating) of a large system affects a signficant portion of stored data. Whereas, even complex data searches act on only small segments of a data base.

Thus in these decisions, design of the maintenance component is proposed as the dominant factor to be considered.

KEYWORDS

Computer
Cancer Patient Data
Data Base Maintenance

To an ever increasing degree, research and treatment efforts in cancer are relying
on large-scale patient information systems.

Maintenance (updating) of these large systems interacts with a significant portion
of stored data. Whereas, even complex data searches act on only small segments of
a data base.

Thus in these systems, design of the maintenance component is proposed as the
dominant factor to be considered.

This presentation will discuss alternative computer systems that can assist a
cancer center in managing its cancer patient data. Our conclusions will be
specifically related to the management of data bases of ten thousand or more cases.

The devices available for computer data storage range from the simple computer data
storage of punch cards and magnetic tape to the more complex storage form of the
computer disk.

In this spectrum of data storage devices, there are a variety of data storage
structures that can be maintained by computer programs.

By sequential data storage we mean that individual records of information can
only be accessed by scanning the file in a simple set order or sequence, always
starting at the front of the file.

Direct access data storage refers to the capability of accessing any individual
record without regard to its sequential place on the file.

The essential element of direct access storage is an index or search key.

An index is an ordered list of values of a single data item maintained independently of the master file. This index can be used to identify all records
on the master file with the specific key value.

A commonly used index would be a list of patient identification numbers. When
only one index is used a storage structure is termed "indexed sequential." When
more than one is used the storage structure is termed "partially inverted."

When an index is maintained for every data item the constellation of indices
becomes the data file itself and the master file ceases to be functional. This
storage structure is called "fully inverted."

A simple index includes all values of a single data item. In a hierarchy system
values from different data items are tied together to be retrieved as a group.
For example, a simple index retrieval would ask for the results of a particular
type of x-ray. Whereas a hierarchical retrieval would ask for the results of all
tests performed on a patient during a particular visit.

The functions of updating, full record editing, and retrieval are affected by their
location on this spectrum of storage structures.

The updating process is an important function of a cancer patient data system.
We are interested in changes in the patient's status, treatment and ultimately his
survival.

In actuality, considering the day-to-day work of maintaining a large file of
information on cancer patients, the update is the major production activity. The
update function includes: changes, additions, and deletions of data item values.

This must take place at each location of a value and at each reference connection of that value. Therefore, the more complex the structure the more complicated the update.

Thus, when 90% of all records on a file must have an update the simple storage of a sequential file is most appropriate.

When less than 10% of records on file must have updates the structure expedites location of items to be changed. The complex storage of a fully inverted file is not amenable to numerous or frequent updates.

The full record edit takes place at the time a record is updated. New values to be entered are compared for consistency with values already on the file. This type of edit is necessary for the achievement of high quality data which must be processed in large volume.

To the extent that all values of a record are in a single location (sequential) or at least that all values remain in a master file, a full record edit is practical. Storage structures that distribute the values of a record over numerous files make a full edit increasingly difficult.

Retrieval functions of a system must follow the reference paths of the storage structure. The reference paths of a fully inverted system are efficient in seeking out isolated data values because each value has its own retrieval or reference path. However, to retrieve all the values of a record you are still obligated to use individual paths. A reference path to a record as a whole does not exist in these systems. In contrast, retrieval of values from a large percentage of records on a file is most efficient from a record oriented structure (sequential) which does not have and does not need the multiple retrieval path for each value within each record.

When one chooses a computer system these factors must be considered. It should be stressed that no one system currently available can support all functions at an optimal level.

In considering alternative systems, investigators and administrators must choose the most advantageous approach from a variety of information processing strategies. Of prime importance is consideration of the inescapable compromise between efficiency of maintenance and ease of retrieval.

V. F. Guinee and G. D. Everett

LARGE SCALE PATIENT INFORMATION SYSTEMS -- DESIGN CONSIDERATIONS*

STORAGE DEVICE	Punch Cards	Magnetic Tape	Disk				
STORAGE STRUCTURE	Sequential	Sequential	Sequential	Indexed Sequential	Partially Inverted	Fully Inverted	Fully Inverted Hierarchy
UPDATE	X	>90%	>90%	<10%	<10%	Archive	Archive
FULL RECORD EDIT	X	Yes	Yes	Yes	Yes	No	No
RETRIEVAL	X	>75%	>75%	>75%	<25%	<10%	<10%

*More than 10,000 patients

Department of Epidemiology
M. D. Anderson Hospital

Interactive EDP in a Cancer Research Institution

G. Wagner

Heidelberg

The German Cancer Research Center (DKFZ) employs at present more than 1,000 people (among them about 250 scientists) in 8 institutes. Each of these institutes is divided into 4 to 5 departments - the scientific units of the center. The research program of the DKFZ mainly covers basic research, but also applied research on cancer prevention, early detection, treatment and cancer control.

Several computers are at the disposal of the center for processing the large number of data coming up. The processing of data in radiology and nuclear medicine takes place in a separate computer system; the remaining computers in the different institutes are connected to the central computer IBM 370/158 of the Institute of Documentation, Information and Statistics. The institute built up a computer system, the philosophy of which is to take the computer to the user and not the user to the computer. The system enables all scientists - even those without any knowledge of EDP - to carry through simple tasks on the computer after a training period of but a few hours. In dialog with the system the user may even ask the computer in which manner he should proceed.

The paper gives some examples for the interactive mode of working with the system.

Key-Words: Interactive EDP, Computer Network, System AVAS, Cancer Research Center, DKFZ.

G. Wagner

Cancer Control is one of the most important tasks of our time in the
fields of natural sciences and medicine. The problems of cancer research
are multifacetted and complicated; a prerequisite for their solution is
the concentration of existing research capacities, last not least the use
of modern computer technology.

Recognizing the socio-political importance of the cancer problem, the
Government of the Land Baden-Württemberg, by order dated January 28, 1964,
founded the German Cancer Research Center (DKFZ) in Heidelberg as a
foundation of public law. In 1975 the Center was taken over financially
by the Federal Ministry for Research and Technology in Bonn and was
recognized as one of the twelve so-called "Big Science Institutions"
of the Federal Republic of Germany. As defined by the statutes, it is
the task of the DKFZ to investigate the etiology and pathogenesis, the
prevention and the control of cancerous diseases - a long-term research
commission of special public interest.

At the present time more than 1,000 people (among them about 250 scientists)
are employed at the eight institutes of the DKFZ (Fig. 1). Each of these

The Institutes of the DKFZ

1) **Institute of Experimental Pathology**
    (Director: Prof. Dr. med. K. Goerttler)

2) **Institute of Toxicology and Chemotherapy**
    (Director: Prof. Dr. med. D. Schmähl)

3) **Institute of Cell Research**
    (Provisional Director: Prof. Dr. rer. nat. D. Werner)

4) **Institute of Biochemistry**
    (Director: Prof. Dr. rer. nat. E. Hecker)

5) **Institute of Virus Research**
    (Director: Prof. Dr. med. K. Munk)

6) **Institute of Nuclear Medicine**
    (Director: Prof. Dr. med. K. E. Scheer)

7) **Institute of Documentation, Information and Statistics**
    (Director: Prof. Dr. med. G. Wagner)

8) **Institute of Immunology and Genetic**
    (Director: Prof. Dr. rer. nat. V. Schirrmacher)

Fig.1: The Institutes of the DKFZ

institutes is subdivided into four to five departments - the scientific
units of the Center. Although the research program of the DKFZ (Fig. 2)

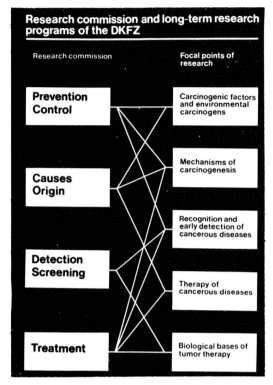

Fig.2:   The Research Program of the DKFZ

is mainly directed to basic research on the causes of cancer and carcinogenesis, applied research on cancer prevention, early detection, treatment
and cancer control is also covered. Clinical oncology remains in the
background in Heidelberg, since the Center has no beds for in-patients.
Thus, therapeutic research can only be carried through in collaboration
with the hospitals of Heidelberg University; nevertheless, the DKFZ is
engaged in intensive research work in the field of nuclear medical
diagnostics.

The research program of the DKFZ comprises the following focal points:
1.) Carcinogenic Factors and Environmental Carcinogenesis

Eventually, all measures of cancer control are based on the knowledge
about carcinogenic factors in our environment. Various working groups
of the Center are engaged in analysing the effect of individual carcinogens
or the joint effect of several carcinogenic factors in the human environment
and in working out measures to eliminate them as much as possible. This

topic also includes investigations about the effect of chemical carcinogens
on offspring of animals treated during pregnancy, questions of the viral
etiology of malignant tumours and leukemias as well as epidemiological
research.

2.) Mechanisms of Carcinogenesis

Research in the field of carcinogenesis on a molecular and cellular level
is of great importance to the understanding of the origin of cancer. Viral
research offers relatively favourable model systems to this purpose; but
molecular-biological, biochemical, histomorphological and mathematical
models and investigations, too, serve to widen our knowledge in this
important field.

3.) Recognition and Early Detection of Cancerous Diseases

Experimental pathology is endeavouring to work out refined methods for
the recognition and early detection of cancer. Radiophysics, biophysics,
radiopharmacology and electronic data processing offer promising attempts
at further development of tumour diagnostics.

4.) Therapy of Cancerous Diseases

Here in particular improvements of the chemotherapy of malignant tumours
are attempted - for example by a synthesis of new chemotherapeutics,
an improved combination of cytostatics and the synchronization of
cell division during chemotherapy -, but also new forms of radiotherapy with incorporated sources of radiation and fast neutrons.

5.) Biological Bases of Tumour Therapy

The projects of this focal point mainly cover molecular-biological,
biochemical, immunological and morphological investigations of the
cell kernel, of the mitotic apparatus and the cell membranes.

On account of its complexity and the high costs arising, modern
cancer research depends to a special extent on interdisciplinary
collaboration on a national and international level. Ever since
its foundation the DKFZ has endeavoured to foster such a collaboration;
today it maintains contacts with numerous German and foreign researchers
and scientific institutions and participates in a series of international
multicentric projects.

For the large number of data coming up in such a big research center,
various computers of different origin are available to the institutes
of the DKFZ. They are connected in a compound system with the central

computer IBM/370-158 of the Institute of Documentation, Information
and Statistics. Merely the evaluation of radiological and nuclear
medical measuring data takes place in a separate system consisting
of a central PDP 10 and several PDP 11 installations.

With about 40 employees the "Central Data Processing Department"
headed by Dr. C. O. Köhler is the largest department of the Institute
of Documentation, Information and Statistics. It considers as its
main task the development of an on-line computer network for all
institutes and working groups at the Center which is to permit an
optimal flow of information and make it possible for all scientists
to use the computer directly and to process their data independently.
The philosophy underlying this concept reads: "Do not take the user
to the computer, but the computer to the user". In a research center
directed toward medicine and natural sciences it cannot be expected
that all scientists have the time, the previous knowledge and the
will to acquire special knowledge about programming. If, therefore,
a compound computing system is to succeed and be applied on a broad
basis, all scientists, even those without any knowledge about data
processing, must be in a position to become familiar with the
functions of the system within a relatively short time and to carry
out themselves at least rather simple operations on the computer
(such as building up data bases from their own data, searching
these data bases, evaluating data in the form of tables, carry
through statistical analyses etc.). This aim has today been reached
to a large extent (3).

Since November 1974 the "Central Data Processing Department" of the
DKFZ has had at its disposal an IBM/370-158 with 2 mega bytes main
storage capacity, 1 drum IBM 2305 with 11 mega bytes storage capacity,
16 magnetic disk drives with 100 MB storage capacity each, magnetic
tape units with 320 bit per second transfer speed, 2 fast printers
and 1 punch card reader/puncher unit. At present 49 terminals and
15 typewriter terminals are connected to the central computer,
furthermore 1 graphic terminal TEKTRONIX 4015 as well as a CALCOMP
plotter. Also connected is an EVANS & SUTHERLAND picture system with
three-dimensional data display which is controlled via a PDP 11/40
with 64 KB main store.

As already mentioned above, several computers in other institutes of
the Center (e.g. PDP 11/40, Gier-Datapoint, Siemens 306, Plurimat

Multi 20/Multi 4) are linked with the central computer IBM/370-158

via the self-developed system ODIF (Ön-line Öata Interface) (Fig. 3).

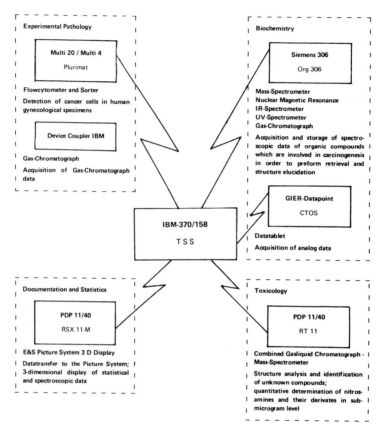

Fig.3:   Computers in Different Institutes Linked
         to the Central Computer IBM-370/158

Thus, for example, the data acquisition for the Laser flow cytophotometry of the Institute for Experimental Pathology takes place on a
Plurimat Multi 20/Multi 4, the further analysis of the collected data
in the central computer. The Biochemical Institute acquires its
spectrometric and gas chromatographic data on a Siemens installation;
the evaluation again takes place in the much more powerful central
computer. The same applies to the data of the Institute of Toxicology
and Chemotherapy as well as to other peripheral computer installations
at present in the stage of development.

The central computer runs on the operating system TSS which was
launched by the IBM in 1965 but withdrawn from the market after a
relatively short period of time. This system is still being used

today by 10 large scientific centers (8 of them in the USA and Canada
and 2 in Germany). TSS is a time-sharing operating system built up
in modules and very much user-oriented which makes the best possible
use of the virtual store and the paging concept of the IBM 360/67
and the IBM 370/158. The system is particularly well suited for
scientific centers with many users with varying tasks - such as
the DKFZ -, since it permits "simultaneous" operation from numerous
terminals installed in different places.

In the sense of the above mentioned philosophy to take the computer
to the user and not the user to the computer the employees of the
institute developed the software package AVAS (a universally applicable
data evaluation and retrieval system) which runs in batch as well as
in dialog (4). Among other things AVAS contains an error detection
and an error correction program, a program for setting up tables,
a retrieval system and a statistical program package for data analysis.

The system is built up in modules, parameter-controlled and easily
extendable. Its basic functions can be learnt in a few hours. It
is even possible for the user to have the further procedure explained
to him by the computer in dialog.

AVAS makes it possible to cope with about 75% of the tasks with which
the central data processing unit is at present approached. Among the
user applications at present running under the system AVAS are:

1.) ALIS, the Animal Laboratory Information System of our animal
        laboratory test department for about 70,000 animals constantly
        kept in experiments by 25 working groups of the DKFZ (mainly
        rats, mice, hamsters). The subsystem "evaluation of experiments"
        which is also part of ALIS is at present in a pilot phase (1).

2.) CANCERNET (formerly SABIR-C), the cancer literature information
        system developed jointly by the French Cancer Research Center
        at Villejuif and the DKFZ in Heidelberg which today, with
        more than 100,000 stored titles, constitutes the largest
        computer-controlled literature information system in the
        field of clinical and experimental oncology (5, 6). An
        essential part of the system is the internally stored three
        language thesaurus of more than 5,000 descriptors and more
        than 12,000 secondary terms in German, French and English,
        which allows the results of searches to be printed out in
        one of these three languages. CANCERNET comprises the

G. Wagner

acquisition, error checking, storage and retrieval as well
as the output of the references which have been fed in. The
latter can take place in the form of lists or index cards
(Fig. 4).

SABIR-LITERATURDIENST DKFZ HEIDELBERG

RECHERCHE NR.   1690   VOM 17.11.75 CARD NO.   2

069769
35/3/1/75
KULAKOWSKI A.,DZIUKOWA J.
  KLIN.CHIR.ONKOL.,WARSZAWIE,POLSKA
PIERWOTNE NOWOTWORY KOSCI ZUCHWY.
NOWOTWORY,24:23-29,1974
  MANDIBULA (T),KNOCHEN (T),AMELOBLASTOM,CHIRURGIE
  RADIKAL,ALTER,EPIDEMIOLOGIE,UEBERLEBENSZEIT (MEHR
  ALS FUENF JAHRE),

SABIR-LITERATURDIENST DKFZ HEIDELBERG

RECHERCHE NR.   1690   VOM 17.11.75 CARD NO.   3

069201
46/3/2/75
LINDER F.,PIEPER M.,OTT G.,BECKER W.,WILLERT H.G.
  CHIR.UNIV.KLIN.,HEIDELBERG,DEUTSCHLAND
ZUR THERAPIE DER KNOCHENGESCHWUELSTE.ERGEBNISSE EINER
GEMEINSCHAFTSSTUDIE AN 527 FAELLEN.
CHIRURG.,45:54-62,1974
  KNOCHEN (T),SARKOM,KLASSIFIKATION TNM,
  THERAPEUTISCHER VERSUCH KONTROLLIERT,THERAPIE
  KOMBINIERT,CHIRURGIE RADIKAL,RADIOTHERAPIE,VERGLEICH,
  DIAGNOSTIK*DIFFERENTIAL-,DIAGNOSTIK RADIOLOGISCH,
  HISTOPATHOLOGIE,BIOPSIE*KNOCHEN-,UEBERLEBENSZEIT (
  MEHR ALS FUENF JAHRE),ALTER,STATISTIK,

SABIR-LITERATURDIENST DKFZ HEIDELBERG

Fig.4:   Computer Outprint on Index Cards
         - Cancer Literature Information Service CANCERNET

3.) - 5.) Further systems for processing literature are ILIDOK,
     our internal literature documentation system with the aid
     of which the annual publication lists of the DKFZ are
     compiled, then BIKAT, a system for setting up index cards
     for the books and monographs taken into the Central Library
     of the DKFZ permitting the allocation of up to ten key-words
     per title characterizing the contents and the setting up of
     up to 25 cards per title with varying headlines for the
     different types of catalogs in the international library
     format. Finally there is IBIS, our interactive library

information system for covering and making available all
literature in the possession of the DKFZ in book form. This
system also deals with the administrative tasks of the
library.

6.) VADS (variable address system) permits updating user-owned
address files and printing self-adhesive address labels
for any mailing lists existing in the Center.

7.) VIS, the information system of the administration of the DKFZ,
handles a number of tasks of the administration and the
technical service, among others matters of personnel,
supervising the household, supervising orders, setting up
the inventory, storekeeping etc.

Individual scientific projects running under AVAS are, among others,
the various spectroscopy data banks of the Institute of Biochemistry
(UV-, IR-, NMR- and mass spectrometers), the central bone tumor
registry for the Federal Republic of Germany, the international
CIOMS project for the standardization of the nomenclature of
diseases as well as the Clearing-House for On-going Research in
Cancer Epidemiology built up and operated jointly by the International Agency for Research on Cancer in Lyon and the DKFZ
within the framework of the International Cancer Research Data
Bank (ICRDB). Its Directory 1978 comprising 550 pages with 1,025
project descriptions and 7 different indexes, produced automatically in computer-controlled phototype setting, appeared recently.

The interactive system STAPRO is available for statistical evaluations. Here the user has the possibility of calling up each of
26 statistical test procedures. The plotter program PLOTTEN serves
the optical output of curves and results.

Apart from the system AVAS there are a number of special programs,
for example the cancer simulation model of the department of
mathematical models as well as the programs for the evaluation of
experiments of the department for the design of experiments, both
written in APL.

The graphic sub-system with the CALCOMP plotter and the Evans &
Sutherland 3 D terminal deserve special mention. The Evans &
Sutherland picture system permits dynamic viewing and manipulation
of three-dimensional graphic information. The presentation is vector-
oriented, that is to say each picture is composed of a multitude of

lines, dark vectors, points and texts (as opposed to the television principle where the picture is composed of a multitude of picture points of varying brightness or colour). The system is used to display arrays of histological specimens, serial scans, frequencies in space, for the visualization and manipulation of secondary and tertiary structures of nucleic- and amino acids etc.

Finally, I want to mention our Accounting System which makes it possible to allocate the services rendered to every user and to account for these services according to a detailed code. While these services are not charged to the co-workers of the Center, the system is in a position to render the central EDP Department, an excellent general account as to who worked when and how much on the time-sharing installation (2).

The problems of data protection have to be taken very seriously even in an institution of basic research such as the DKFZ, since here, too, although only to a moderate extent (e.g. in nuclear medicine, epidemiology, administration of personnel) person-oriented data are being processed. The Center appointed a person who is in charge of data protection. It is his task to see to it that data protection is warranted by hardware, software and organizational measures. All employees who have to work with person-oriented data are, moreover, bound to professional secrecy.

References

(1) Berg, H., Graw, J., Köhler, C.O., Naumann, D., Petrovsky, R. (1978).
     ALIS - Ein Versuchstierinformationssystem.
     Z.Versuchstierk., 20, 145-157.

(2) Böhm, K. (1975). Kostenabrechnung für einen Computer mit Time-Sharing-
     Betriebssystemen. On-line. Z.Datenverarb., 13, 133-136.

(3) Köhler, C.O. (1976). Interaktive Datenverarbeitung im Bereich der
     medizinisch-biologischen Forschung. In G. Wagner und C.O. Köhler
     (Hrsg.): Interaktive Datenverarbeitung in der Medizin. Mensch-Maschine-
     Dialog. pp. 77-87. F.K. Schattauer-Verlag, Stuttgart - New York.

(4) Köhler, C.O., Schadewaldt, K. (1974). AVAS - General Variable
     Evaluation System. In J. Anderson and J.M. Forsythe (Eds): MEDINFO '74.
     pp. 407-410. North-Holland - Elsevier, Amsterdam.

(5) Wagner, G., Sandor, L. (1978). Das Krebsliteratur-Informationssystem
     CANCERNET. Med.uns.Zeit, 2, 40-47.

(6) Wagner, G., Wolff-Terroine, M. (1972). Das Krebsliteratur-Dokumentations-
     System SABIR. Z.Krebsforsch.,78, 4-11.

Index

The page numbers refer to the first page of the article in which the index term appears.